ROUTLEDGE LIBRARY EDITIONS:
SPECIAL EDUCATIONAL NEEDS

Volume 22

CHILDREN ON MEDICATION
VOLUME I

CHILDREN ON MEDICATION VOLUME I

Hyperactivity, Learning Disabilities, and Mental Retardation

KENNETH D. GADOW

Routledge
Taylor & Francis Group
LONDON AND NEW YORK

First published in 1986 by Taylor & Francis Ltd

This edition first published in 2019
by Routledge
2 Park Square, Milton Park, Abingdon, Oxon OX14 4RN

and by Routledge
711 Third Avenue, New York, NY 10017

Routledge is an imprint of the Taylor & Francis Group, an informa business

British Library Cataloguing in Publication Data
A catalogue record for this book is available from the British Library

ISBN: 978-1-138-58532-4 (Set)
ISBN: 978-0-429-46809-4 (Set) (ebk)
ISBN: 978-1-138-59368-8 (Volume 22) (hbk)
ISBN: 978-0-429-48929-7 (Volume 22) (ebk)

Publisher's Note
The publisher has gone to great lengths to ensure the quality of this reprint but points out that some imperfections in the original copies may be apparent.

Disclaimer
The publisher has made every effort to trace copyright holders and would welcome correspondence from those they have been unable to trace.

Additional publisher's Note

These are re-issues of books published some years ago which are inevitably a reflection of the time in which they were published. The language used is indicative of that time and as such no offence is intended by the re-issuing of the books.

Children on Medication
Volume I

Hyperactivity, Learning Disabilities, and Mental Retardation

Kenneth D. Gadow, Ph.D.

Taylor & Francis Ltd
London

Published by
Taylor & Francis Ltd, 4 John Street, London WC1N 2ET

First published by College-Hill Press, San Diego, California

British Library Cataloguing in Publication Data

Gadow, Kenneth D
Children on medication, Volume I: Hyperactivity, learning disabilities, and mental retardation.
1. Classroom management. 2. Chemotherapy
I. Title
371.1′02 LB3013
ISBN 0 85066 574 4

This edition not for sale in the American continent.
Printed in the United States of America

Dedicated to the teachers, parents, and children who, by their participation in medical and psychological research, have made this book possible. Their unselfish support of clinical research will allow subsequent generations to reap the benefits of scientific inquiry, just as we all benefit from the efforts of those who have preceded us.

CONTENTS

FOREWORD

One of the most notable aspects about the topic of this book is the vast gaps in some areas of knowledge. Often these vast gaps in knowledge are in extremely important areas. The author cites several examples to illustrate the point being made. For example, in the chapter entitled "Mental Retardation," he notes that the arbitrary exclusion criterion of eliminating potential subjects in psychotropic medication studies with IQs falling within the mental retardation range has led to "a glaring gap in our clinical knowledge" (p. 155) about treating mentally retarded children and adolescents. A similar gap exists in regard to available information for educators, including teachers, special education teachers, supervisors, and principals as well as parents. Fortunately, this situation is being greatly reduced by the publication of the second edition of *Children on Medication*.

Another example of a glaring gap in the clinical data base pertains to information about reducing and terminating psychotropic medication for hyperactive children and, for that matter, other handicapped children as well. To put this in perspective, consider that there are probably 750 articles in the medical literature describing how to use psychotropic medication (usually stimulants for hyperactive children), but probably fewer than 10 articles that address explicitly how to either reduce or terminate medication for a hyperactive child who no longer needs it (Reatig, 1984). Surely this is an unbalanced and one-sided approach to say the least. This book seeks to remedy such one-sided approaches.

Before leaving this topic, a few comments are in order about how this situation arose in the first place. There really is no evidence in medical literature that explains why there are glaring gaps in knowledge that have not been addressed by scholars or researchers, but it seems that the most likely explanation is the philosophical orientation of the medical scholars and researchers who write in this area. The primary orientation of these writers is the biomedical model which emphasizes biological etiology (causes) and medical interventions (treatments), in this case, psychotropic medication. Keep in mind that the biomedical model has been, fortunately for the welfare of mankind, quite successful in many acute biological disorders; the ancient scourge of mankind, smallpox, has now been eliminated from the world largely due to following techniques outlined by the biomedical model. In spite of such notable feats, the biomedical model is much less helpful in chronic disorders that are influenced by educational, behavioral, and sociological factors. Areas of high interest to parents and educators are often considered outside the purview of the biomedical model, thus such problems are all too often ignored by researchers.

This book fills an important need in the field of education and special education in particular. If one accepts the higher estimates of the number of hyperactive children in the United States on stimulant medication and assumes that these children were evenly distributed in the general population in the United States, on the average about one hyperactive child on medication would appear in each public school classroom. As Dr. Gadow's own unique surveys of the use of psychotropic medication in special education clearly show, the percentage of special education students who are on psychotropic medication is much higher than one per class, which means that it is the rule, not the exception, that the special education teacher has taught children who encounter problems with their psychotropic medication. Given this state of affairs, it seems very important that the special education teacher and associated colleagues have an accurate, readable source of information about psychotropic medication other than the current popular medical shows on television, *Reader's Digest*, or, worst of all, *The National Enquirer*.

Anyone with a chronic medical problem in the family quickly realizes how important it is to have readable, accurate, and nontechnical sources of information about the chronic disease of importance to them. At this point I am not writing about an abstract idea which seems valid on the basis of my reading and research, but I am describing a week-after-week situation in my own family involving kidney failure, a serious chronic medical disorder, in which pertinent, readable information is very important, sometimes involving life-or-death types of decisions. As many others have found to be the case, the printed material supplied by well-meaning staff members simply does not satisfy the information needs of a patient's family. In this context, it is with considerable pleasure that I write this preface and state that this edition fills a very important glaring gap in the psychopharmacological literature. In appropriately detailed fashion, with the introduction of technical terms and subsequent defintions only when needed, the edition covers a broad range of issues surrounding the often controversial question of administering psychotropic drugs to an exceptional child or adolescent.

Finally, as an instructor of a university course on psychotropic medication in children for the past 17 years, I certainly look forward to the appearance of this edition to use as a textbook for special education students who enroll and who are often bewildered by the mass of technical information that is available in the medical literature on the topic. So, for these prospective students and the families of the exceptional children receiving psychotropic medication, I endorse this volume for those seeking information about such medication use in children and adolescents.

REFERENCE

Reatig, N. (1984). Attention deficit disorder: A bibliography. *Psychopharmacology Bulletin, 20*, 693–730.

ROBERT L. SPRAGUE, Ph.D.

FOREWORD

In almost every school program that addresses the behavioral and educational needs of children, the topic of medication is at some time discussed. Be it from an anxious parent, teacher, administrator, or other caregiver, the topic remains a highly volatile one often open to many interpretations.

For years, teachers and other caregivers have been kept in the dark concerning the use of medications prescribed to their children. This situation has often led to a mystifying reliance on those who have prescribed the medications. In many ways this lack of information was used to excuse acceptable and valid reasons for inappropriate behavior or academic difficulties. By removing or at least clarifying the medication mystic, Gadow, in this book, attempts to provide for the first time critical information that is sorely lacking.

It is especially important to note that Gadow does not attempt to make everyone who reads this book into medical practitioners. He is quick to point out that his major goal is to provide much-needed pharmacological information that will help caregivers better understand medical decisions. This is especially important today in light of societies' growing obsession with drugs and their side effects.

Gadow clearly points out that important pharmacological work has been published in the past, but for *select* professional populations. This landmark attempt, however, puts all related and needed information together in a single resource to be read and referred to by diverse populations of professional and lay people.

Finally, Gadow, in what I have come to know as his typically thorough and persevering style, and in his effort to teach us as much as possible, has developed a suggested reading list and glossary that acts as an aid in clarifying fundamental medication concepts and terms.

In summary, this book is both a technically detailed resource and a reference guide. It is clearly written and succinctly outlines the path the reader is to take as he or she approaches different disability areas or child domains. In many ways this resource is unique in that it addresses the needs of a professional audience as well as those parents who for years have been left with unanswered pharmacological questions. Gadow's discussion of psychotropic drugs, how physicians prescribe drugs in everyday situations, and the timely discussion of trade versus generic names are but some examples that prove to be especially helpful.

Having been on the administrative and teaching side of working with handicapped children for almost two decades, and having had the opportunity to review Dr. Gadow's work, I can unequivocally say that those working with handicapped children now have a comprehensive resource to which they can turn much in the same way as the physician has had his or her desk reference (PDR).

As with most comprehensive resources, time will dictate how well this book is received. Personally, I have already found it to be invaluable.

Michael Bender, Ed.D.

ACKNOWLEDGMENTS

This book was made possible through the efforts of many people. The author would like to express appreciation to the following people for making prepublication materials, copyrighted figures and tables or lengthy quotations available to me: Ronald Brown, Magda Campbell, Susan Campbell, John Kalachnik, Richard Milich, K. Daniel O'Leary, William Pelham, Mark Rapport, Daniel Safer, Esther Sleator, Robert Sprague, Gabrielle Weiss, and Carol Whalen. I would like to thank Irv Bialer and Mark Rapport for providing valuable editorial assistence on individual chapters. I am also most grateful to Lucinda Lindgren and Gretchen Daly for their role in preparing the various drafts of manuscript.

I am very grateful to the literally hundreds of teachers and parents in Illinois who supplied the necessary information to describe therapeutic drug use patterns among children in special education programs and to the Directors of Special Education, school administrators, and school nurses who made these data collection efforts possible. A special thanks is extended to my interviewers, Jan Knecht, Tobey Fumento, and Norma Wilson.

I wish especially to express appreciation to my colleagues at the Institute for Child Behavior and Development (University of Illinois ar Urbana-Champaign), particularly Robert L. Sprague and Esther Sleator, for their encouragement and support over the years. They provided a most unique environment in which to learn about pediatric psychopharmacotherapy; one that emphasized both methodological rigor and clinical common sense.

Introduction

The primary purpose of this book is to provide information about the use of medication for several childhood disorders that require long-term treatment. It is the author's expectation that this information will allow caregivers to make better decisions about the use of medication. Unfortunately, knowing what to do is often not a simple matter of right versus wrong or correct versus incorrect, but rather the product of a complex set of evaluations pertaining to child characteristics and the family and school setting. Before addressing the text's role with regard to this process, it is important to explain exactly what kinds of drugs and disorders are discussed here.

Among the most commonly prescribed drugs for children that are administered on a long-term basis are the psychotropics, and they are generally prescribed to control mood, thought processes, and behavior. These drugs are familiar to most of us and include the following: stimulants, antidepressants, neuroleptics (major tranquilizers), antianxiety agents (minor tranquilizers), hypnotics, and sedatives. In children they are prescribed for a variety of disorders such as hyperactivity, aggression, nocturnal enuresis (bed wetting), anxiety, sleep problems, and so forth.

Early in my experiences with children in special education programs, it became evident that medication and the disorders for which they were prescribed affected the lives of many people, often in very important ways. Yet, there was little opportunity for caregivers to learn about drugs, their intended therapeutic effects, and their unwanted side effects. Moreover, the information that was available (e.g., in the child's school medical records) was often inaccurate or incomplete or too technical (e.g., medical reference books) for lay audiences. In recent years there have been numerous attempts to fill this void, a fact that can be readily confirmed by a casual perusal of the paperback books placed in the health care section of your local bookstore.

Although one might infer from this observation that the information problem has been addressed, it is my impression that many texts aimed at lay audiences are too superficial, incomplete with regard to treatment practices and controversies, and silent on the topic of the psychosocial aspects of pharmacotherapy. What is really needed is a technically detailed reference that is both readable and to the point. It should be thorough enough to be useful for medical personnel who have limited experience in this area (but who are nevertheless called upon to manage such cases after the specialist initiates treatment) and yet free of medical jargon so the lay person can appreciate the factual content. It should strive to focus on clinical management and refrain from speculating about the implications of laboratory findings that are loosely connected to real world situations. Moreover, it is probably fair to say that although much of our research efforts generate greater understanding of these children, their problems, and their reaction to medication, on a year to year basis, very few studies actually effect changes in treatment practices for a particular disorder. In fact, since the first edition of this book was published, very few "new" drugs (or new applications for existing drugs) have appeared on the scene (see, for example, Campbell et al., 1983, and Gualtieri et al., 1983).

The use of drug therapy in the management of childhood behavior, learning, and psychiatric disorders has received much attention in recent years. One can walk into almost any public school, special education facility, residential placement, sheltered workshop, or community-based program for the handicapped and, after engaging teachers and staff in a conversation about children and medication, discover that this is quite a controversial topic. Such discussions not only reveal a considerable interest in medication but also a variety of problems associated with drug therapy (see, for example, Gadow, 1982). Unfortunately, it is difficult for people outside the medical professions to learn about the therapeutic use of psychotropic drugs. It is not unusual, therefore, that many caregivers are poorly informed about medication. This lack of knowledge is often accompanied by uncertainties and misconceptions that are created, in part, by sensational articles in popular periodicals and newspapers. The fact that researchers and clinicians simply do not know all the answers to frequently asked questions about pharmacotherapy also complicates matters. Highly biased articles both for and against drug treatment have fueled a bitter controversy over the use of medication for certain childhood disorders. Because little is known about the etiology (causes) of most of these maladies, a number of prophets have surfaced who are willing to lead us to the truth. They have claimed that everything from bad lighting to tight underwear produces behavioral disturbance. In the center of this confusion, controversy, and uncertainty are the family, school, and health care providers trying to figure out what is the best thing to do for their children. And, they are not always in agreement.

WHY LEARN ABOUT DRUG TREATMENT?

The use of medication in the management of learning and behavior disorders is of interest to caregivers for several reasons:

1. The very behaviors that are altered by drugs are often interrelated with the educational, habilitative, and parenting process. For example, behavior disorders can interfere with the child's ability to benefit from instruction, as well as hinder the teacher's efforts to teach other children in the class. Physically aggressive acts can actually place the welfare of both caregiver and peers in jeopardy. Because chronic childhood disorders often precipitate serious emotional problems, caregivers can become involved in another aspect of child development—social adjustment. One way learning and behavior problems become a part of the teaching process is when they are identified as instructional objectives. This is particularly true in special education settings.

2. Medication is of interest to caregivers because the drugs used in the management of these disorders have a pronounced effect on behavior. In some children, medication suppresses behavior that is perceived as incompatible with accepted standards. For other children, drug therapy appears to make them more responsive to their environment by enhancing cognitive abilities. Parents may comment, for example, "The child is easier to manage," "You can get through to him now," or "He can sit still long enough to read to" (Gadow, 1977). Also of importance are the adverse effects of medication. Although many side effects are benign or eventually go away, others can be quite alarming if those responsible for the child's care are unprepared for what to expect. When side effects impair adaptive behavior (e.g., learning ability, social interaction) or create emo-

tional problems, they are not only distressing to caregivers but raise serious risk-to-benefit questions.

3. Studies have shown that relatively large numbers of school-aged children are on medication for hyperactivity, behavior problems, and aggressivity (Gadow, 1981; Safer & Krager, 1984). In fact, few child care providers have not had some experience with youngsters who were receiving medication for one of these problems. Exposure to pharmacotherapy is much greater for teachers in special education programs, particularly those for mentally retarded, emotionally disturbed (behavior disordered), and learning disabled children.

4. Studies have clearly demonstrated the importance of feedback from caregivers in making treatment-related decisions (Sprague & Gadow, 1976). Teachers, for example, can be helpful by providing the child's physician with behavioral evaluations during the diagnostic, dosage adjustment, and followup phases of drug treatment. Reports of side effects observed in the home, classroom, or community setting are also valuable. Because medication does not teach the child anything, many children with learning and behavior problems will require educational or habilitative programming as part of the total treatment plan. It has been my experience that caregivers are often very interested in therapeutic measures that impact upon their own efforts. Charles Bradley, one of the important historical figures in pediatric psychopharmacology, expressed his thoughts on the matter as follows:

> It is probably helpful for the teacher to have some understanding of the effect any medication may be having on the child's behavior. Teachers as well as parents can be more objective when they understand the true nature of a child's difficulty, and the physician may often wisely make the proper interpretation to them if the parents so desire. (Bradley, 1957, p. 1058)

OBJECTIVES OF THIS BOOK

After conducting three state-wide studies about how medication was being used with children in special education programs, I realized that teachers and parents were interested in drug treatment and were concerned about a number of treatment-related problems. Perhaps the greatest single problem is a lack of information about drug therapy. Caregivers have many questions about what medication is supposed to do to help children, what the side effects are, whether drugs can interfere with learning, what the dosage should be, what people should do in various treatment-related situations, what drug interactions may occur, and what kinds of drugs are used for specific disorders (Gadow, 1982).

Because there are few comprehensive references for parents, teachers, and health care providers about drug therapy, this book was developed to answer these and other questions about children on medication. It must be emphasized that making drug information available in this format does *not* imply that nonmedical caregivers should preempt a medical role! School personnel, for example, should not make medical diagnoses or recommend to parents that their child should be placed on medication. It is generally agreed, however, that teachers can be helpful to physicians by providing much-needed feedback about the response to treatment. The school is but a part of a team effort that involves the family, health professions, psychological services, and social welfare agencies. It is hoped that by making drug information available to parents and nonmedical professionals, they will be more effective in participating in an interdisciplinary treatment effort.

The primary focus of this book is a description of the behavioral effects of drugs and the primary side effects observable to caregivers. Although questions are frequently asked about how medication acts on the body to produce certain behavioral changes, this topic is not discussed here. A lack of understanding on the part of the reader about how a drug works should not interfere in any way with the expressed objectives of this text.

There is always a danger, of course, that a frank discussion of adverse drug reactions may deter parents from obtaining desirable and, quite possibly, necessary treatment. The reader must bear in mind that almost all forms of therapy are associated with some risk. These risks, moreover, may very well be *less* serious than the consequences of ignoring true therapeutic needs. It should also be emphasized that many psychotropic drugs are true miracles of modern pharmacological research. Their role in reducing human pain and suffering can be readily confirmed by simply reading about, or talking with someone who is familiar with, the situation that existed in our mental health facilities prior to the mid-1950s. Information about side effects is provided here not to alarm caregivers, but rather to prepare them for their possible occurrence and in so doing alleviate the intense anxiety associated with unexpected drug-related phenomena. Fortunately, the majority of commonly prescribed psychotropic drugs are associated with low levels of risk when used and monitored appropriately.

Of equal importance to discussing drug-related changes in behavior is describing how doctors use medication. This includes typical dosages, the time of day medication is taken, how long treatment will last, and under what circumstances medication is terminated. This is much more difficult than it sounds because few people study the behavior of physicians (or teachers or other professionals, for that matter). Although there are many statements of clinical experience in the literature, or "how to treat" articles, there is often a disparity between what experts say should be done and what really happens in everyday situations. In order to create a more realistic picture of actual practices, the available data on everyday medical procedures are included.

The effective use of medical technology is an art. Physicians, like most professionals, develop a variety of ways for handling similar problems based upon the responses of previous patients. The reader is cautioned, therefore, that the descriptions of medical practice presented in this text are not necessarily what one might encounter or what one should necessarily expect. Many people are uncomfortable with this underlying degree of uncertainty that characterizes psychotropic drug therapy for childhood and adolescent disorders. It is, nevertheless, a reality, and we should all recognize the limitations of medical science. Gualtieri et al. (1983) have described this situation as follows:

> Diagnosis and prediction of drug response are not exact sciences. The child, treated with a psychoactive agent, is in reality a research subject. The only real measure of good practice is an empirical approach to the individual child. Management of difficult behaviors by the administration of psychotropic drugs is justifiable only in the context of an individualized and comprehensive therapeutic program. (p. 202)

WHAT'S MISSING

There is a point after which detail becomes either impractical or counterproductive, and subsequently decisions about this book had to be made with regard to which topics were going to be briefly cited or omitted altogether. In this text, the following question aided in making this decision. Does an understanding of this topic provide insight into how a particular disorder should (or is) generally managed? Among the topics that have received more limited treatment are etiology (causes), diagnostic procedures, and neuropharmacology (how drugs affect the nervous system). The necessary focus on medical intervention has precluded any explanation of the social-emotional problems associated with chronic childhood disorders. It is hoped that this will not obscure the importance of *psychosocial* factors in the etiology, response to treatment, and long-term therapeutic outcome of behavior disorders. What may, to some, be a limitation is the secondary treatment of alternative therapeutic procedures. It would be truly unfortunate to infer from this decision that drug therapy is the sole treatment for learning and behavior disorders or even the best method for all or most children. Because many books and articles are available about nonmedical techniques, it seemed unnecessary to review them in any detail here. Instead, publications discussing alternative measures are cited as references.

TRADE NAMES VERSUS GENERIC NAMES

If for no other reason than financial ones, most people are aware of the fact that drugs possess both trade names and generic names. In general, if a particular medicine is available in both trade and generic forms, the latter is less expensive. A *trade name* is a registered trademark, and only the holder of the trademark or its legal representative can ever use the trade name to sell medicine. A *generic name* is a scientific name that is recognized throughout the world and is used by scientists and clinicians in scientific papers and textbooks.

To more fully understand the significance of the differences between these two terms, the reader should also know that a drug manufacturer typically patents a newly formulated agent and controls the right to manufacture it for 17 years. This time period is provided, in part, to allow the drug company an opportunity to recoup its financial investment into the product. In reality, however, it usually takes several years to obtain Food and Drug Administration approval to market a new drug in the United States, so the actual period of competition-free merchandising is actually much shorter. During this competition-free period, the drug company seeks to establish brand loyalty through the use of its trade name. In other words, after the patent has expired, many clinicians will continue to write prescriptions for the trade name. To help insure this response, drugs were often given complicated generic names that were difficult to spell and remember. For example, the generic name for Ritalin is methylphenidate hydrochloride. Obviously, it is much easier to write and remember the word Ritalin. This situation changed due in part to the passage of the 1962 Kefauver-Harris Amendments to the Food, Drug, and Cosmetic Act of 1938. Following the passage of this legislation, the United States Adopted Names Council, which is supervised by the federal government, was established to decide whether or not a generic name is suitable (Silverman & Lee, 1974, p. 37).

The importance of these facts is that when the period of patent protection expires, any drug company can then manufacture the drug and sell it either by its generic name or by a different trade name. The generic drug manufacturer profits by selling the drug in large volume at a lower price. There has been, and continues to be, a considerable debate concerning generic drugs. The primary issue has been the question of *bioavailability.* It has been alleged that certain generic drugs may not be identical to the trade name product because they do not reach and concentrate in the same body areas as the trade name product to a comparable degree. Some have even argued that generic products should undergo the same intense scrutiny by the FDA as new drugs.

This somewhat detailed discussion of generic and trade names is presented here for more than just educational purposes. It is also intended to help explain why trade names are used in this text and why this will be viewed as unacceptable by some. It could be said that, in view of the aforementioned discussion, the use of trade names in a textbook constitutes a form of advertising for a particular product. This having been said, the justification for using trade names here is threefold. One, most psychotropic drug prescriptions for children are still written for trade name products. Therefore, caregivers generally encounter trade names. Two, generic drug products are not necessarily available, even if the period of patent protection has expired. And three, a careful examination of the research on the topics addressed in this book will show that most studies acknowledge the fact that the drug(s) employed was supplied by the trade name manufacturer. In a certain sense, our scientific knowledge is based upon trade name products. Although this explanation will not satisfy everyone, the purpose of this text is to provide drug information to help people who are not medically trained in the use of a particular drug to make better treatment-related decisions. Suffice it to say, then, that the scientific literature generally uses generic names and that generic products, if available, will probably be less expensive than trade name products. For those who are more familiar with generic names, conversion from trade to generic name can be achieved quite easily by simply referring to Appendix D.

INTERNATIONAL AUDIENCE

This book has been prepared with the intent of reaching an international audience interested in the pharmacological management of child and adolescent disorders. Two steps have been taken in an attempt to achieve this goal. One has been the formulation of a special list of trade names and their associated generic names for *some* products marketed in Great Britain and Western Europe (see Appendix I). The formulation of an exhaustive list is an almost insurmountable task because there are no consistent rules for trade name use. The problem is compounded by the fact that there are hundreds of psychotropic drugs and an even greater number of countries. As was previously discussed, Appendix D can be used to resolve any confusion concerning a specific trade name.

The second step toward an international approach has been the inclusion of research and discussions of clinical practice from scientists and clinicians throughout the world. It is important to emphasize that there are often major differences of opinion from one country to the next on how medication should be used.

Reaching an international audience is made more difficult by the fact that (a) generic names are not always identical and (b) the rules for conducting research and obtaining governmental approval for the use of new agents vary greatly, so it is possible for a particular drug to be popularly used in one country and not yet available in another. The first problem, internationally inconsistent generic names, can be either minor or major depending upon the drug. For example, the drug known as phenobarbital in the United States has been referred to as phenobarbitone in Great Britain, a difference that would be of trivial consequence. However, the antiepileptic drug known as valproic acid (Depakene) in the United States is referred to as sodium valproate in Great Britain. This example is of course much more problematical. Interestingly, the actual chemical formulations of these two products differ slightly, hence the different generic names. The second problem, differential government regulation procedures, is more difficult to resolve. Basically, with few exceptions, the drugs discussed in this book are only those that are approved for use in the United States.

SUGGESTED READINGS

Given the varied background of the intended audience and its equally diverse information needs, each chapter closes with a list of suggested readings for those interested in pursuing a particular topic in greater detail. It has been my experience that it is very difficult to find a "good" article on a particular medical topic without knowing someone who is trained in that area. The suggested readings listed in this text are ones that may be particularly useful for more extensive study. These are not, however, exhaustive lists, and the failure to cite a particular reference should not be misconstrued as judgmental. The existing medical literature is so staggering (see Durack, 1978), that it was possible to cite only a few representative examples for each area. Each item in the list is coded for the audience for which it is most appropriate: P = parent, S = school personnel, and C = clinician. Many items in the last category are suitable for graduate students in the behavioral sciences. Because this book was designed to serve as an introduction to the medical literature, many of the sources cited as being appropriate for clinicians are also suitable for motivated parents and school personnel. Fortunately, the prudent course of action in many treatment-related situations is nothing more than common sense, providing one has access to all relevant information.

GLOSSARY

The demystification of scientific areas can often be achieved by simply adopting nontechnical terminology to explain fundamental concepts. This is successful in many instances, but in others it makes more sense to define and subsequently use the scientific term. This book employs both approaches. Although the decision to use a particular technical term may appear to be arbitrary, the author has attempted to select and use those which were deemed useful for interdisciplinary collaboration and further study. A glossary of terms appears at the back of the book to assist the reader in deciphering medically oriented discussions of drug therapy. Each term is defined in nontechnical language, and the reader is encouraged to refer to it whenever necessary. The glossary should help solve the problem of terms that are defined in earlier chapters of the text but are encountered for the first time by readers who select particular topics for reference purposes.

COMPANION VOLUMES

The first edition of *Children On Medication* attempted to present an overview of pediatric psychopharmacology in one volume. As the current revision progressed, however, with its expanded range of topics and increased depth of detail, it some became apparent that a single volume was no longer feasible, practical, or desirable. For example, one of the major impediments to acquiring medical information is an economic one. Most medical reference books are simply too expensive for the average reader. True, although some are available in public libraries, their treatment of medication for specific conditions is often greatly limited by their expressed need to discuss a variety of disorders. Rather than add another expensive text to the list of available medical reference books, we decided to divide *Children On Medication* into companion volumes. This not only allowed us to more closely approximate the goal of economic feasibility but also provides the reader with an opportunity to select topics of greatest interest. Fortunately, the content lent itself to such a division, and two separate books were formulated, one subtitled *Hyperactivity, Learning Disabilities, and Mental Retardation* and a second subtitled *Epilepsy, Emotional Disturbance, and Adolescent Disorders*. It was our goal to formulate two volumes that would be fairly equivalent in price to one large book.

In creating two volumes of *Children On Medication*, it was necessary to repeat some material such as the appendices and the glossary. An abridged version of the chapter "Fundamental Concepts of Pharmacotherapy" that appears in this book was prepared for *Epilepsy, Emotional Disturbance, and Adolescent Disorders* so that each volume could stand on its own as a complete text. It was also necessary to resist the temptation to make the discussion of each disorder even more comprehensive by adding peripheral but related topics because this obviously would have only resulted in the recurrence of the initial problem.

ORGANIZATION OF THE BOOKS

This book, *Hyperactivity, Learning Disabilities, and Mental Retardation*, focuses primarily on psychotropic drug use for hyperactivity and aggressiveness, two disorders that often co-occur. Because academic underachievement is often, but certainly not always, an associated problem, it seemed logical to include these three disorders in the same text. A separate chapter appears on mental retardation because hyperactive behavior and aggressiveness are often managed in very different ways for children and adolescents who are mentally retarded compared with their nonretarded peers. This is especially true for mentally retarded people who live in institutional settings, who are more severely retarded, or both.

The companion volume, *Epilepsy, Emotional Disturbance, and Adolescent Disorders*, describes antiepileptic drug therapy for epilepsy (seizure disorders), childhood psychoses such as infantile autism and schizophrenia, a variety of adolescent psychiatric disorders (e.g., schizophrenia and depression), and several miscellaneous conditions, such as enuresis and cerebral palsy, that are difficult to group under a particular heading. Many, but certainly not all, of these disorders share the characteristics of being (a) disabilities of relatively low prevalence (at least when compared with hyperactivity, learning disability, and mental retardation), (b) more commonly recognized as organically based, particularly seizure disorders and severe emotional disturbance, and (c) more readily accepted as medical conditions by the general public.

The general outline of each book is as follows: Chapter 1 explains some of the fundamental concepts and terms relating to drug therapy. Each of the following chapters covers the use of medication with regard to specific childhood disorders. However, their arrangement is somewhat different from that of most medical texts on medication. Instead of grouping the topics by psychiatric diagnoses, more functional categories were formulated from both the standpoint of drug therapy and the caregiver's frame of reference. Three categorical systems are used here: medical diagnosis, special education, and age. Two of the more common medical disorders for which drugs are prescribed (hyperactivity and seizure disorders) are discussed in some detail in a separate chapter for each. There are also separate chapters for three of the major (on the basis of prevalence) handicapping conditions recognized by special education professionals (learning disabilities, mental retardation, and emotional disturbance). This seemed prudent, given the relatively high rates of drug use among children and adolescents in these programs (e.g., Epstein et al., 1985; Gadow 1981; Safer & Krager, 1984). Moreover, parents and, of course, school personnel are more inclined to think of children in terms of special education categorical labels. The third categorical system is represented here with separate chapters about preschool-aged children and adolescents. Middle childhood is the primary focus of the other chapters. To facilitate pursuit of a particular disorder, careful attention has been given to the subject index, and many topics are cross-referenced within the text.

When available, prevalence figures are reported for each disorder and for the use of drug therapy in the general school population and in special education programs. Both therapeutic and side effects of the drugs employed are described, along with the pattern of treatment. The latter includes dosage, schedule of drug administration, duration of treatment, and drug combinations. Because drugs typically have many pharmacological properties, they are often used in the management of more than one disorder. To prevent the redundancy that would result from describing the same drug in different chapters, only the primary drugs associated with the treatment of each condition are discussed in any detail.

To repeat, by no means should the intent of these books be misconstrued as implying that school personnel, parents, or other nonmedical personnel should assume the role of a physician. However, if they enable caregivers to ask more intelligent questions during interdisciplinary interaction and to focus more clearly on educational and child development issues, then these texts will have fulfilled their purpose. It is hoped that one by-product of this increased awareness will be a more satisfactory life experience for the child, the true objective of our efforts as parents, educators, and clinicians.

Hyperactivity, Learning Disabilities, and Mental Retardation

Chapter 1: Fundamental Concepts of Pharmacotherapy. The first chapter is a brief introduction to the different kinds of drugs that are used to effect changes in mood, thought processes, and behavior. Central to an appreciation for the complexity of drug treatment is a basic understanding of the way drugs move through the body. Other topics include dosage adjustment, drug interactions, tolerance, and side effects. Using the treatment of hyperactivity as an example, an argument is made for the importance of caregiver participation in drug therapy.

Chapter 2: Hyperactivity. The most common childhood disorder for which psychotropic drugs are prescribed is hyperactivity. *Hyperactivity* is defined as a persistent developmental pattern characterized by excessive motor restlessness and inattentiveness. The latter *may* be the most important feature of the disorder. Other behavioral symptoms are frequently associated with hyperactivity, including poor school achievement, conduct problems, immaturity, impulsivity, and peer difficulties. In this chapter, research investigating the effects of stimulants (Ritalin, Dexedrine, and Cylert) on activity level, perceptual-motor skills, learning and cognitive performance, conduct problems, school achievement, and interpersonal relationships is summarized. The results of long-term followup studies on hyperactive children are also reviewed. Nonstimulant drugs occasionally used in the treatment of hyperactivity, and nondrug therapies are also described briefly.

Chapter 3: Learning Disabilities. On the basis of available prevalence data, more children are receiving special education services for learning disabilities in the United States than for any other handicapping condition. The disorder is defined as a significant discrepancy between ability and academic achievement. While no drugs are specifically approved for the treatment of learning disabilities as defined by federal law, much has been written about the effects of stimulant drugs on academic performance in hyperactive children. This chapter discusses the relevant literature on this topic and the limited research on medication for nonhyperactive learning disabled children.

Chapter 4: Mental Retardation. Drug treatment for behavior disorders is much more common among mentally retarded children and adolescents in comparison with their nonretarded peers. Surveys show that stimulants are the most commonly prescribed drugs for behavior disorders in mentally retarded children in public school programs, whereas neuroleptics are the preferred agents in residential facilities. Some of the commonly reported reasons for administering medication are the control of hyperactivity, aggressivity, self-injurious behavior, and stereotypies. This chapter describes the use of neuroleptics (e.g., Thorazine, Mellaril, and Haldol) and stimulants in the treatment of behavior disorders associated with mental retardation. Many of the issues concerning the use of psychotropic drugs with mentally retarded people are discussed, including recent litigation.

Chapter 5: Early Childhood. Prescribing psychotropic drugs for children under 6 years of age is associated with a greater degree of uncertainty because little formal research is conducted with this age group, for a number of obvious reasons. In spite of this situation, many preschool-aged children receive psychotropic medication, the two major categories being stimulants and neuroleptics. In this chapter the available literature on medication use with young children is reviewed to include existing treatment practices, clinical research, and the special issues that pertain to this population.

Epilepsy, Emotional Disturbance, and Adolescent Disorders

Chapter 1: Fundamental Concepts of Pharmacotherapy: An Overview. The first chapter presents a brief introduction to the different kinds of drugs that are used to effect changes in mood, thought processes, and behavior, and an overview of some basic concepts in drug therapy such as dosage adjustment, tolerance, and side effects.

Chapter 2: Seizure Disorders. There are a number of seizure disorders, and they differ from one another in terms of what the seizures look like, the age when attacks usually begin, and the type of drug most effective in controlling the seizures. The main focus of this chapter is a description of the various types of epilepsy and the drugs used to treat them. Other topics include febrile seizures, the management of seizures in the classroom, the circumstances under which drug treatment is terminated, and how antiepileptic drugs can affect classroom performance. Because many children who have a seizure disorder receive two or more drugs per day, drug interactions are also discussed.

Chapter 3: Seizure Disorders: Early Childhood and Mental Retardation. Antiepileptic drug therapy is particularly common among children in two special education categories, early childhood and mental retardation. This chapter addresses the special problems presented by seizure disorders for these two populations of children and their clinical implications.

Chapter 4: Emotional Disturbance. Unquestionably, two of the most disabling childhood disorders for which psychotropic drugs may be prescribed are infantile autism and childhood schizophrenia. At the present time, the neuroleptics appear to be the drugs of choice for children for whom this treatment is appropriate. Two additional childhood disorders for which the term *emotional disturbance* could be considered appropriate, at least as it is used by the special education community, are childhood depression and conduct disorder. This chapter discusses drug treatment for each of these disorders and presents a special overview of neuroleptic drug use for preschool-aged autistic children.

Chapter 5: Adolescent Psychiatric Disorders. This chapter addresses the use of psychotropic drugs for the treatment of adolescent psychiatric disorders. They are grouped here according to areas of functioning: mood (mania, depression), thinking (psychosis), conduct (aggression, hyperactivity), eating (anorexia nervosa, bulimia, obesity), and emotions (anxiety, phobias, and obsessional disorders). Although the most suitable drug for the management of these disorders varies depending upon the condition being treated, two broad groups of drugs, the neuroleptics and antidepressants, are the primary focus of this discussion. Special attention has been given to the behavioral characteristics of each disorder.

Chapter 6: Other Disorders. The final chapter briefly describes the use of psychotropic drugs for enuresis, school phobia (separation anxiety), cerebral palsy, and Tourette syndrome. The tricyclic antidepressants (e.g., Tofranil) have been used with some success in the treatment of enuresis (bedwetting) and school phobia. The two most commonly prescribed skeletal muscle relaxants for cerebral palsy are Valium and Dantrium. A variety of drugs have been used to treat Tourette syndrome, but the neuroleptics are generally considered the most effective agents at the present time.

REFERENCES

Bradley, C. (1957). Characteristics and management of children with behavior problems associated with organic brain damage. *Pediatric Clinics of North America, 4,* 1049–1060.

Campbell, M., Anderson, L. T., & Green, W. H. (1983). Behavior-disordered and aggressive children: New advances in pharmacotherapy. *Developmental and Behavioral Pediatrics, 4,* 265–271.

Durack, D. T. (1978). The weight of medical knowledge. *New England Journal of Medicine, 298,* 773–775.

Epstein, M. H., Cullinan, D., & Gadow, K. D. (1985). *Prevalence of psychotropic drug use with learning disabled, emotionally disturbed, and mentally retarded children.* Unpublished manuscript, University of Northern Illinois, Department of Learning, Development, & Special Education, De Kalb.

Gadow, K. D. (1977). *Psychotropic and antiepileptic drug treatment in early childhood special education.* Champaign, IL: University of Illinois, Institute for Child Behavior and Development. (ERIC Document Reproduction Service No. ED 162 494)

Gadow, K. D. (1981). Prevalence of drug treatment for hyperactivity and other childhood behavior disorders. In K. D. Gadow & J. Loney (Eds.), *Psychosocial aspects of drug treatment for hyperactivity* (pp. 13–76). Boulder, CO: Westview Press.

Gadow, K. D. (1982). Problems with students on medication. *Exceptional Children, 49,* 20–27.

Gaultieri, C. T., Golden, R. N., & Fahs, J. J. (1983). New developments in pediatric psychopharmacology. *Developmental and Behavioral Pediatrics, 4,* 202–209.

Silverman, M., & Lee, P. R. (1974). *Pills, profits, and politics.* Berkeley: University of California Press.

Safer, D. J., & Krager, J. M. (1984). Trends in medication therapy for hyperactivity: National and international perspectives. In K. D. Gadow (Ed.), *Advances in Learning and Behavioral Disabilities* (Vol. 3, pp. 125–149). Greenwich, CT: JAI Press.

Sprague, R. L., & Gadow, K. D. (1976). The role of the teacher in drug treatment. *School Review, 85,* 109–140.

Chapter 1

Fundamental Concepts of Pharmacotherapy

Pharmacology is the study of the chemical and physical properties of drugs; the effects of drugs on body chemistry, physiology and behavior; the mechanisms of action; the movement of drugs into, around, and out of the body; and their use in the treatment of medical disorders. One major subdivision of this science is *neuropharmacology*, which investigates the effects of drugs on the nervous system. As stated in the introduction, this topic is not covered here. There are, however, a number of fine sources that provide discussions of how drugs used to modify behavior alter the functioning of nerve cells, certain areas of the brain, and the autonomic nervous system (e.g., Abel, 1974; Gilman et al., 1980; Leavitt, 1982; Swonger, 1978). A second major division is *psychopharmacology*, the study of how drugs affect behavior. Broadly defined, behavior includes thinking, feelings, mood, perceptions, motor activities, and so forth. Because the bodies of children and the disorders for which they are treated differ in many ways from those of adults, there is a separate science concerning the behavioral effects of drugs in children. This is known as *pediatric psychopharmacology*.

There are approximately 10,000 prescription drugs available to American physicians, and an additional 100,000 products can be purchased without a prescription (Silverman & Lee, 1974). The latter are referred to as *over-the-counter* drugs, or, more simply, as OTCs. Of the prescription medicines, one category is of particular interest because these drugs have pronounced effects upon behavior and are used frequently in treating chronic childhood disorders. These are the *psychotropics.*

Drugs that are prescribed primarily for their effect on mood, thought processes, and behavior are collectively referred to as psychotropic drugs. A number of different classification schemes have been used to subdivide this category of drugs, and a variety of labels are used in the literature to describe given subcategories (Leavitt, 1982; Usdin, 1970). To minimize confusion, the psychotropic medications discussed in this text have been grouped according to six categories proposed by Usdin and Effron (1972). These are *stimulants, neuroleptics* (major tranquilizers), *antianxiety agents* (minor tranquilizers), *antidepressants, hypnotics,* and *sedatives.* An extensive listing of the drugs in each of these categories appears in Appendix A. A seventh category of psychotropic agents, the *hallucinogens,* have not proved to be effective in the treatment of childhood disorders. It would be inappropriate, however, to infer the reason for which a drug is prescribed from its assigned categorical label. For example, the antidepressant Tofranil (imipramine) is used not only in the management of depression but also to treat spontaneous panic attacks (Klein et al., 1980), enuresis (Blackwell & Currah, 1973), hyperactivity (Rapoport et al., 1974), separation anxiety (Gittelman-Klein, 1975), and even certain types of seizure disorders (Fromm et al., 1978).

To add to the confusion, drugs have both a *generic* name and a *trade* name. As was noted in the introduction, the generic name is typically used in the medical literature and is employed by the scientific community throughout the world. The trade name, however, is a registered trademark and is controlled by the manufacturer indefinitely. For reasons already discussed, drugs are referred to here by their United States trade names. In the case of drugs that are no longer protected by a patent, the original trade name is cited. After the first mention of a drug in each chapter, the generic name appears in parentheses.

Because generic products are often sold at a lower price than the original trade name product, compelling arguments have been made for more widespread use of generic drugs (Burack & Fox, 1975). In many states, the pharmacist can fill a doctor's prescription with a less expensive generic product unless the physician specifies no substitutions (Sonnenreich & Menger, 1977). (The actual guidelines for making substitutions vary from state to state.) The patient, of course, can always ask the doctor to write the prescription using the generic name if generic products are available. For this and other reasons, an extensive list of psychotropic drugs by trade name appears in Appendix D along with the corresponding generic name.

PSYCHOTROPIC DRUGS

Stimulants are among the most frequently prescribed psychotropic drugs for children and are used primarily for the management of hyperactivity. This group includes Ritalin (methylphenidate), Dexedrine (dextroamphetamine), and Cylert (pemoline). These drugs are occasionally used in the treatment of certain types of epilepsy and may be administered to control drowsiness, which is a side effect of some antiepileptic drugs. Stimulants are also used to treat *narcolepsy*, a disorder characterized by sudden attacks of sleep during normal waking hours. However, narcolepsy is an uncommon disorder and rarely develops in children under 12 years of age.

Neuroleptics are typically administered to control bizarre behavior in psychotic adults. These drugs are also referred to as *major tranquilizers* and *antipsychotic agents*. There are over a dozen neuroleptics that are used with some frequency, but the most common are Mellaril (thioridazine), Thorazine (chlorpromazine), and Haldol (haloperidol). In children, these drugs are administered to control hyperactivity, aggressivity, self-injurious behavior, and stereotypies and to facilitate general management. Compared with children in regular classrooms, surveys show that neuroleptics are used more frequently to control behavior disorders in mentally retarded and emotionally disturbed children in special education programs.

Antianxiety agents (also called *minor tranquilizers* or *sedative-antianxiety agents*) can be subdivided into three major groups of drugs that share similar properties. One category, the *benzodiazepines*, includes Valium (diazepam), Librium (chlordiazepoxide), Clonopin (clonazepam), Serax (oxazepam), and Tranxene (clorazepate). All have antiepileptic properties, but Valium (one of the most frequently used prescription drugs in the world) and Clonopin are more commonly used with epileptic children. Valium is also a frequently prescribed skeletal muscle relaxant for children with cerebral palsy. At relatively high doses, Valium has hypnotic properties and, therefore, may be administered to induce sleep. *Diphenylmethane derivatives*, a second category of antianxiety agents, include Atarax (hydroxyzine pamoate). They are infrequently used to control hyperactivity, and, in younger children, they may be administered to induce sleep. A third category, *propanediols*, includes Equanil (meprobamate) and related drugs. Although they are frequently prescribed for anxiety in adults, surveys show they are not used very often with children. The benzodiazepines are preferred over the propanediols for the treatment of anxiety because the latter are more apt to be fatal in suicide attempts and accidental poisonings.

Among the antidepressant drugs, there are two major categories, one of which, the *tricyclics*, is relevant to this discussion. As previously stated, the term *antidepressant* is somewhat misleading when one considers the variety of disorders for which these drugs are used. In children, Tofranil is the most frequently prescribed tricyclic drug. It is prescribed most often in the treatment of enuresis and occasionally for hyperactivity. Elavil (amitriptyline) is another tricyclic that may be used for hyperactivity but is more commonly prescribed for the treatment of depression in adolescents and adults. The other category of antidepressant drugs is the *monoamine oxidase inhibitors*, usually abbreviated MAOIs. They are used primarily with adults, typically for the treatment of depression.

Sedative drugs are used to calm anxious people, and hypnotics are prescribed to induce sleep. The separation of these two categories is somewhat artificial because higher doses of most sedative drugs (e.g., antianxiety agents) have hypnotic effects. One large group of hypnotic drugs, the barbiturates, has antiepileptic properties. In fact, phenobarbital and Mebaral (mephobarbital) are all used primarily to treat epilepsy in children. Examples of nonbarbiturate hypnotics are Noctec (chloral hydrate), Paral (paraldehyde), and Doriden (glutethimide).

HISTORICAL PERSPECTIVE

While it is true that people have been taking medication for thousands of years to either cure or alleviate the symptoms of illness, the modern drug therapy era did not begin until the 1930s with the discovery of the first sulfa drug (an antibacterial agent). The recency of this technological development can probably best be appreciated in terms of the number of effective drugs and the emergence of legislation to regulate the marketing of new medication (see Silverman and Lee, 1974, for an excellent discussion of the drug industry). Traditionally, most medicines were of questionable value, and when they did work it was due either to *spontaneous remission* (the malady improved simply with the passage of time) or to *placebo effects*. The latter refers to a variety of psychological processes associated with treatment that produce symptomatic relief (see Gadow et al., 1986, and White et al., 1985). To give some idea of what the premodern era was like, Bevan (1976) cited the following quote from an early paper by MacPhail (1933):

> For a perfect sight of the old medicine, let me conduct you to the bedside of Charles II: With a cry he fell. Dr. King, who, fortunately,

> happened to be present, bled him with a pocket knife. Fourteen physicians were quickly in attendance. They bled him more thoroughly; they scarified and cupped him; they shaved and blistered his head; they gave him an emetic, a clyster, and two pills. During the next eight days they "threw in" fifty-seven separate drugs; and towards the end, a cordial containing forty more. This availing nothing, they tried Goa stone, which was a calculus obtained from a species of Indian goat; and as a final remedy, the distillate of human skull.

In the 1700s, only a few of the literally thousands of drug products available and in use were actually effective, and by the end of the 19th century, the number had grown to only a dozen or so. In spite of the fact that thousands of different drugs were being sold commercially, it was not until 1938 that the United States government required drug companies to prove convincingly that their products were safe! Even more sobering is the fact that unbiased, scientific proof of efficacy was not required until 1962.

It follows from the aforementioned developments that pediatric pharmacotherapy for behavior disorders is also a recent development. It was not until the discovery of the clinical properties of stimulants (Bradley, 1937) and neuroleptics (Heuyer et al., 1953) that relatively safe and powerful therapeutic agents for children were available. Prior to this time, clinicians generally had to rely on sedatives, which often produced marked drowsiness and left the patient in a state of mental dullness or confusion.

Because pediatric psychopharmacology is a relatively new discipline, it is still experiencing "growing pains," as is evidenced by the storm of controversy generated over stimulant drug therapy for hyperactivity. It must be emphasized, however, that the major themes in this debate are applicable to *all* childhood disorders for which psychotropic drugs are prescribed. The essence of the controversy focuses on two broad issues: One, are the right children being treated? Two, is the treatment regimen being managed appropriately?

The first is a diagnostic problem that stems from the fact that caregiver opinions about the nature and severity of the child's symptoms are often the basis for deciding whether or not a trial of medication will be initiated. The controversy arises over whether or not the best interests of the child are the overriding concern. Critics argue that children are exploited by the treatment process, while proponents readily point to numerous examples of how the child's life experiences have become more rewarding.

The second issue (the questionable adequacy of treatment evaluation practices as they are currently employed) is equally and possibly more troubling than the diagnostic problem. There is some debate as to whether or not traditional medical treatment practices are adequate for evaluating and monitoring response to psychotropic medication. There are, of course, two sides to this controversy, but the fact remains that there are sufficient cases of mismanagement to warrant concern. Among the concerns that are subsumed under the rubric of treatment monitoring are risk-to-benefit ratio, behavioral toxicity, and the adjunctive status of pharmacotherapy. It is not the purpose of this text to resolve these issues, but it is, nevertheless, imperative to raise them when appropriate. Two excellent papers have been written on the clinician's perspective of these troubling aspects of psychotropic drug therapy; one is by Gabrielle Weiss (1981), some of which is presented in Chapter 2 of this volume, and the second is by Leon Eisenberg (1975), a brief segment of which is presented here:

> Benefit must still be weighed against risk, the risk of drug toxicity, the risk of the social consequences from an invidious label which, once attached, is not easily shed, the risk of the misapplication of drug treatment *as well as* the risk of *not* applying a treatment while symptoms flourish (Baldessarini and Lipinski, 1973). Society has learned, at great cost, how debilitating prolonged hospitalization can be by superimposing onto the patient's initial disorder a syndrome of social breakdown more pervasive than the dysfunction that brought him to medical attention (Gruenberg, 1967).
>
> With the range of treatments available, it is no longer tolerable to have "schools" of exclusive salvationism. . . . It has become unethical to deny relief to a patient with a profound depression because of an anachronistic bias that a drug cure is inferior to a talking cure, at a time when the former has been shown to be effective and the latter not. The argument is as strong for the failure to use appropriate medication for an acute schizophrenic. Yet both practices persist among duly certified psychiatrists. The use of drugs is not in contradiction to, nor a substitute for, respectful listening and judicious confrontation of psychic conflicts. The psychopharmacologist must be no less sensitive to personal and family dynamics than the psychotherapist . . . to be fully effective; [the] patient remains a person with problems in living, even if [the therapist] recognizes [the patient] as suffering from a neuropsychiatric syndrome with important biological roots (Eisenberg, 1973). (pp. 96–97)

PHARMACOKINETICS: MOVEMENT OF DRUGS IN THE BODY

In order for a drug to exert its characteristic effect, it must be absorbed into the body and transported to the tissues and organs in which it typically concentrates. For the effect to be terminated, the drug must be changed into an inactive substance or removed from the body. The movement of drugs into, through, and out of the body can be described in terms of four processes: *absorption* (movement into the blood), *distribution* (concentration in body compartments), *biotransformation* (breakdown of drugs into compounds that can be more readily removed), and *excretion* (movement out of the body).

Drugs can be administered either by mouth (*orally*) or by injection (*parenterally*). The latter method includes injecting the drug through various different routes such as *intravenous* (into the bloodstream), *subcutaneous* (under the surface of the skin), and *intramuscular* (into muscle tissue). Intravenous injections can produce relatively immediate effects because the process of absorption in the gastrointestinal tract is bypassed. When injected into a muscle, drugs are absorbed into the bloodstream via the capillaries in the muscle tissue. The rate of absorption can be increased by adding a substance that dilates blood vessels, or decreased with an agent that constricts blood vessels. Occasionally, neuroleptics are administered intramuscularly in a form that is not very soluble. This slows the rate of absroption, which in turn prolongs the effects of a single injection for several days. Subcutaneous injections are not used very often in the treatment of childhood medical disorders.

The relationships among four different routes of administration in terms of plasma concentration (amount of drug in the blood) are presented in Figure 1–1 for a hypothetical drug. As is clear from this figure, the speed with which a drug begins to act, the duration of its effect and changes over time (*time-course*), and the magnitude of the drug response are determined, in part, by the route of administration. While the general pattern of relationships presented in Figure 1–1 is characteristic of many drugs, time-course relationships for plasma concentrations vary greatly.

Absorption

Psychotropic drugs are usually taken orally. This is the oldest and easiest route of drug administration. To be absorbed, drugs in tablet or capsule form must dissolve in the fluids of the stomach and intestine. Drug molecules then pass through the cells that line the wall of the digestive tract and into the capillaries of the veins that lead from the stomach and gut to the liver.

A number of variables influence the rate of absorption, including the chemical characteristics of the drug, changes in the acidity of the stomach, other drugs present in the digestive tract, less than adequate supply of blood, and illnesses that result in a more rapid

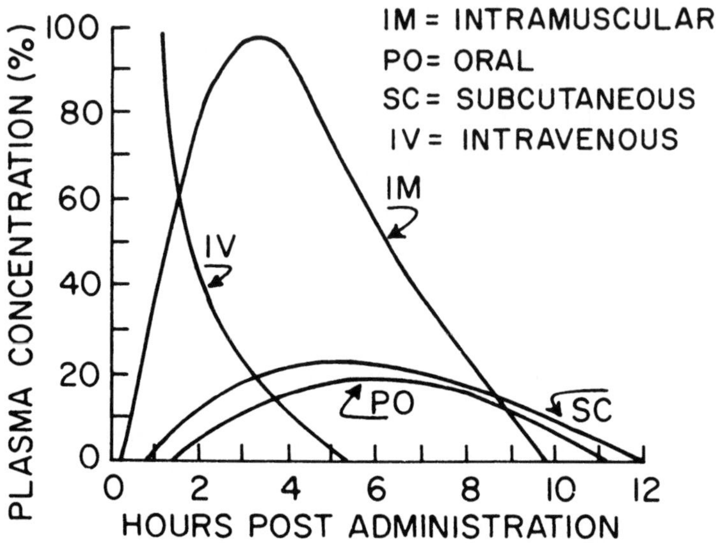

Figure 1–1. Plasma concentration of a hypothetical drug across time as a function of route of and time following drug administration. *Note:* From "Behavioral Pharmacology and Principles of Drug Action" by A. D. Poling and J. Henningfield, 1982, in *Drugs and Mental Retardation* (p. 93) by S. E. Breuning and A. D. Poling (eds.). Springfield, IL: Charles C Thomas. Copyright 1982 by Charles C Thomas. Reprinted by permission.

passage of food through the gut. Natural and added chemicals in the food we eat may also slow down or speed up this process. Because it is difficult to predict exactly how any change in the stomach or intestine may affect absorption, it is best to avoid, when possible, anything that might interfere with this process. For this reason, some drugs are administered at least 1 hour before or 2 hours after eating.

Distribution

Once in the bloodstream, drug molecules are distributed throughout the body, concentrating in various areas referred to as *compartments*. The characteristics of the drug determine the sites of distribution and the degree of concentration. Some agents are restricted primarily to the circulatory system. Others pass through the capillary membrane into the water that surrounds the tissues and cells (the extracellular fluid) or concentrate in the water inside the cells (intracellular fluid) of specific types of tissue.

The molecules of most drugs combine with large molecules in the blood (plasma protein). This process is referred to as *plasma protein binding*. Bound molecules, because of their size, are unable to pass out of the bloodstream, and, unlike unbound (free) drug molecules, do not have a pharmacological effect on the body. An equilibrium is established between bound and unbound molecules. As free molecules pass out of the blood, bound molecules are released so the ratio of bound to unbound molecules in the blood remains the same. Although the maximal effect of the drug is reduced by protein binding, it prolongs the effect of the drug by creating a reservoir of bound drug molecules that are released over time (Briant, 1978).

The movement of drug molecules from the bloodstream into the brain is made more difficult by the presence of a *blood-brain barrier*. This is not an anatomical structure per se but refers to the fact that the capillaries of the brain prevent certain classes of compounds from entering and affecting brain neurones. A closeknit layer of glial cells surrounds the brain capillaries, creating an additional barrier for compounds that are not lipid soluble. Without such a barrier, many chemicals in the foods we eat could directly alter the function of the central nervous system. Psychotropic drugs do, of course, pass through the blood-brain barrier.

Biotransformation

The liver is the primary organ responsible for the breakdown of drugs (biotransformation) into new compounds (metabolites). Substances (*microsomal enzymes*) within the cells of the liver bring about or increase the rate of the chemical reactions that transform drugs into metabolites. Generally, an active drug is metabolized into an inactive, more water soluble compound(s) that can be excreted through the kidney. If lipid soluble drugs (e.g., Valium) were not transformed into water soluble metabolites, they would be reabsorbed into the bloodstream by the kidney, and the effects of a single dose could, therefore, last indefinitely (Briant, 1978).

Not all drugs are metabolized into inactive substances within the body. Some are excreted unchanged, while others are transformed from inert substances into active metabolites.

The rate of drug metabolism in the liver can be greatly affected by the presence of another drug or chemical. This is one form of drug interaction. Genetic factors also play an important role in determining the speed at which compounds are transformed. When the same drug is administered to a number of different people, the rate of metabolism may vary greatly (Vessell & Page, 1968).

Excretion

The kidney is the primary organ responsible for the removal of drugs and their metabolites from the body in the form of water-soluble compounds. Other pathways of elimination are feces, perspiration, and the milk of nursing mothers.

The rate of excretion can be influenced by the pH of the urine. For example, basic drug molecules are excreted more rapidly when the urine is acidic, and vice versa. Therefore, the presence of another drug or chemical that changes the pH of the urine could alter the rate of excretion.

Many, but certainly not all, drugs have *linear kinetics*, which means that the body's drug elimination mechanisms excrete a constant amount or percent of the drug per unit of time. It is possible, therefore, to predict the relationship between drug dose and blood concentration. One of the most widely used expressions to describe drug elimination is *half-life*, which is the amount of time it takes the body to reduce the amount of drug in the blood by 50%. For drugs with linear kinetics, the half-life is *independent* of both dose and concentration. The average half-life is a useful guide for therapy because it takes five half-lives to reach a stable concentration (*steady state*) of drug in the blood after treatment has been initiated. A steady state is attained when the rate of drug intake is equal to the rate of output (removal from the body). Although blood concentrations do fluctuate between doses, during a steady state they are fairly stable. This is most important because a particular medication generally cannot be adequately evaluated until a stable drug concentration has been reached. Knowing the half-life is also useful when it comes to withdrawing medication because it takes approximately five half-lives for a drug to be completely eliminated from the body. It is also a helpful guide for dosing. When a drug is administered once per half-life, this will generally prevent fluctuations in drug blood concentrations.

Some drugs have *nonlinear kinetics*, which means that their elimination mechanisms can become saturated. In other words, as the dose or concentration of the drug increases, the body does eliminate more drug, but at a slower rate. Therefore, the apparent half-life increases. This complicates the picture because for any age group there is a wide range of half-lives, depending upon the dose and the initial concentration at which the apparent half-life is measured. For more discussion on how information about drug kinetics and blood concentration is used in making clinical decisions, see Dodson (1984) and Gualtieri et al. (1984).

DOSAGE

Before a drug is marketed, a considerable amount of information is collected about the effects of different amounts of the drug on laboratory animals and people. From reports of accidental poisonings and suicide attempts, it is even possible to determine fatal human dosage levels. In adjusting dosage, the physician starts with a small amount of the medication—usually below the therapeutic range. Over time, the dose is gradually increased until the desired response is achieved. This process is referred to as *titration*. Recommended dosage limits, both minimum and maximum, guide the physician in this procedure. If unwanted or intolerable side effects emerge, (a) the dose may have to be reduced, (b) the drug may be stopped completely and gradually reintroduced, (c) a different medication may be substituted for the offending agent, or (d) an additional drug may be prescribed to control the side effect.

Although we often do not consider this, people differ from one another internally as well as externally. Individual variability in the way we react to drugs may reflect differences in the biological systems that are responsible for absorption, distribution, biotransformation, and excretion or simply differences in body size. In order to limit some of this variability in drug response, researchers sometimes adjust dosage to physical size. A measured amount of medication is administered per unit of body weight in kilograms (kg). A kilogram equals approximately 2.2 pounds.

Medication is typically measured in milligrams (mg). One milligram is equivalent to approximately 1/28,000 of an ounce. The actual dosage in milligrams per kilogram of body weight (mg/kg) can be calculated as follows: $DW = M$, where D = desired mg/kg dose, W = weight in kilograms, M = actual amount of medication in milligrams. For example, let us assume the physician decides to administer drug A at a dose of 0.3 mg/kg. A child weighing 88 pounds (40 kg) would then receive 12 mg of drug A ($DW = M$; $0.3 \times 40 = 12$). For any given M, one can determine the mg/kg dose by a simple algebraic manipulation. Thus, for a child who weighs 44 pounds (20 kg) and is receiving 12 mg of drug A each morning, the dose would be 0.6 mg/kg $\frac{M}{W} = D$; $12/20 = 0.6$).

With some drugs, the amount of medication administered in milligrams has little relationship to the amount in the blood. Therefore, a more useful measure than mg/kg for dose would be one that indicated how much drug was in the blood. This is sometimes expressed as micrograms (mcg or μg) of drug per milliliter (ml) of blood. These are very small amounts. For example, there are 1,000 micrograms in 1 milligram. An even smaller unit of measurement is the *nanogram*. There are 1,000 micrograms in one nanogram. When expressed as an amount in the blood, it is often cited as nanograms per milliliter (ng/ml).

Psychotropic drug treatment for learning and behavior disorders is not typically monitored in this way (see Gualtieri et al., 1984). In fact, procedures for determining blood levels are not yet available for many of these agents. It is noteworthy that a reliable method for assessing blood levels of Ritalin in children is a fairly recent development.

SIDE EFFECTS

No drug is completely free of side effects. There are a number of terms used to denote side effects, including *untoward reactions*, *toxic effects*, and *adverse drug reactions*. There is also a newer term, *treatment emergent symptoms*, that is being popularized to some extent in the psychiatric literature. Some side effects are trivial, while others seriously impair health. The latter are sometimes referred to as *toxic effects*, but this term appears to be used somewhat inconsistently. Adverse effects may go away after a period of time (*self-limiting*) or they may persist. If the disorder being treated is severe, side effects that are not self-limiting may have to be endured. Side effects may appear shortly after the onset of treatment or may go unrecognized for months or even years. The pervasiveness of side effects often alarms people, but one must realize that the body is an extremely complicated chemical system whose functions are highly interrelated and that the alteration of one process affects others as well. It is noteworthy that what is an adverse drug reaction for one person may be the desired treatment response for another patient with a different disorder.

When drugs interfere with a person's ability to think, interact socially, and perform work-related behaviors (classroom activities in the case of children) or either induces or aggravates (*exacerbates*) a preexisting behavior disorder, this reaction is often referred to as *behavioral toxicity*. Unfortunately, such reactions often occur at dosages below or at therapeutic levels. In recent years, much deserved attention has been focused on behavioral toxicity with regard to *risk-to-benefit* decisions. In other words, do the benefits of drug therapy outweigh the risks? The latter consist of short-term side effects that are immediately evident as well as longer-term adverse reactions that are not apparent until long after the commitment to therapy has been made. Some long-term consequences of treatment are really the cumulative effects of chronic drug-induced impairment. Because the signs or symptoms of behavioral toxicity are often difficult to detect on the basis of behavior exhibited in the physician's office but may be clearly visible to care-providers, this topic has received special attention in this book.

While the current focus on behavioral toxicity suggests that this is a relatively recent development, the proposition that a standard battery of psychological tests should be developed (Hollingworth, 1912) and routinely employed in all drug evaluations (Gray & Trowbridge, 1942), including antiepileptic medication (Lennox, 1942), is certainly not new (see Wittenborn, 1980); nor is the idea that behavioral toxicity may outweight the benefits of treatment as is evident from a comment by Gray and Trowbridge (1942; cited by Wittenborn, 1980; see also Lennox, 1942): "When medication is followed by undesirable mental changes or personality disturbances, the results may be more undesirable than the symptoms which indicated the use of the drug" (p. 128).

Adverse drug reactions can be categorized into three groups (Zbinden, 1963). The first, and generally least serious, are *functional* side effects, which represent a change in the function of an organ. Examples of functional side effects of the nervous system are headache, slurred speech, incoordination, and dizziness. Most functional side effects are *reversible* (i.e., cease or gradually go away) when medication is stopped. Changes in the *biochemical* reactions associated with various organs are a second category of side effects. Two examples are alterations in the balance of hormones and changes in blood coagulation. Biochemical side effects are also usually reversed upon stopping treatment. A third group, *structural* side effects, involves an actual change in the structure of an organ. Examples of these are liver damage and cataracts. Obviously, functional and biochemical effects may also be associated with organ damage. The following chapters in this book discuss mostly functional side effects that are clearly visible to parents and teachers. Drugs that are known to cause biochemical and structural side effects must be carefully monitored.

Most side effects are predictable. They may take the form of (a) an excessive therapeutic response, which can typically be corrected by dosage reduction, or (b) physiological or behavioral reactions that are commonly associated with the pharmacological properties of the drug. For example, hyperactive children treated with stimulant drugs may become abnormally inactive (excessive therapeutic response) or may experience a temporary loss of appetite due to the drug's characteristic effect on the autonomic nervous system (pharmacologically predictable response). Other less common side effects are not predictable because they are due, in part, to the genetic or physiological peculiarities of the patient (*host factor*). One such side effect is an *allergic* reaction, also called *hypersensitivity*. Skin reactions are a common sign of drug allergy. Another unpredictable side effect is an *idiosyncratic* reaction, which is characterized by an excessive or abnormal unexplained response to a typical dose of medication.

DOSE-RESPONSE

As we all know from our experiences with either common substances such as coffee and alcoholic beverages or with prescription and nonprescription medication, the amount of drug intake is directly related to the experienced effect. Whereas one cup of coffee may make us more alert for our drive to work, several cups during a short period may leave us nervous and overly responsive to mild stress. This relationship between dose and drug effect is referred to as *dose-response* or *dose-effect*. While this may sound fairly straightforward, it is not. The complicating variable is the fact that drugs almost always produce multiple physiological and behavioral effects. Moreover, the dose-response *and* time-course relationships for these various treatment effects often differ.

This concept can be better appreciated by examining Figure 1–2, which is an adaptation of hypothetical dose-response relations for stimulant drugs in hyperactive children proposed by Sprague and Sleator (1975). They are presented here as more general response patterns to portray treatment issues associated with most psychotropic drugs. The target symptom curve represents any of the behavioral features for which these drugs are prescribed (e.g., activity level, aggressivity, academic underachievement). As the dosage increases, symptom control becomes greater and greater. There reaches a point, however, after which further dosage increments fail to improve the condition, at least to any appreciable degree. Equally important is the fact that there is an optimal range of dosages that produce a fairly similar degree of therapeutic improvement. For example, if the optimal range is 150 to 200 mg, the amount of improvement obtained with the larger dose is fairly similar to that for the lower dose. This idea of an optimal range has caused some people to argue that it makes more sense to use a *smaller* dose from the optimal range, particularly when side effects are an issue.

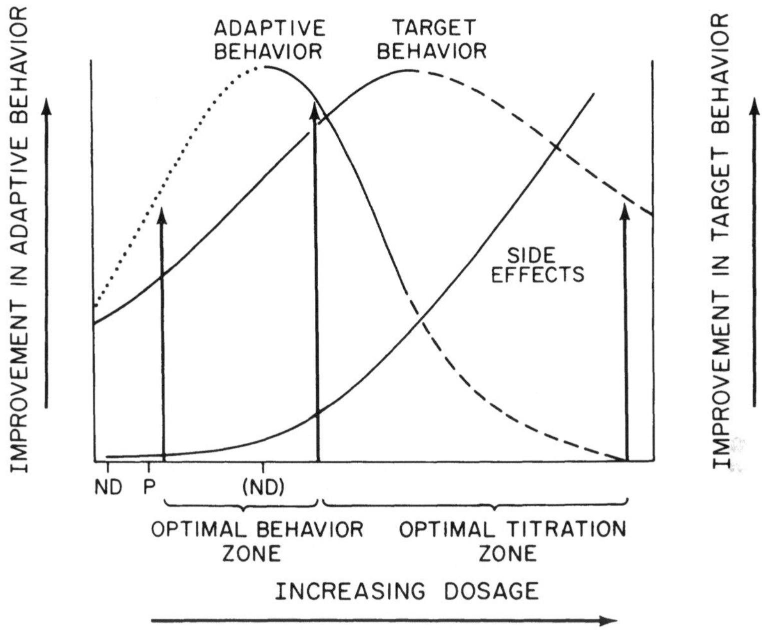

Figure 1–2. Dose-response relationships for target symptoms, adaptive behavior, and somatic side effects for a hypothetical drug. *Note:* From "What Is the Proper Dose of Stimulant Drugs in Children?" by R. L. Sprague and E. K. Sleator, 1975, *International Journal of Mental Health*, 4, p. 96. Copyright 1975 by International Arts & Sciences Press, Inc. Adapted by permission.

The descending part of the target symptom curve is shown as a dashed line because higher drug dosages may or may not exacerbate the target symptoms. For example, higher therapeutic dosages of Dilantin (phenytoin) may actually cause an *increase* in seizure frequency (Levy & Fenichel, 1965), which would be represented as a decrease in improvement, or a descending slope. For many other target symptoms, however, higher therapeutic dosages generally do not lead to a deterioration (e.g., increased frequency) in the symptoms for which the drug was prescribed. Unfortunately, the same cannot be said for adaptive behavior.

Because the ability to think clearly, solve problems, learn, and interact socially are so important to everyday life, drug-induced impairment of these behaviors is considered to be a serious treatment-related consideration. It goes without saying that this is particularly true for children in general and people with limited intellectual ability. The adaptive behavior curve in Figure 1–2 depicts two possible outcomes. One, the drug may actually enhance adaptive behavior, even though this may *not* be the primary target of intervention (dotted line). Such outcomes should be considered *serendipitous* (accidental but nevertheless beneficial), but they often have a way of becoming justifications for treatment. As is evident from the figure, medication enhances adaptive behavior, but, with increasing dosage, all the beneficial effects are nullified and performance even drops below baseline levels (dashed line) at higher dosages. While this type of reaction is rarely reported for psychotropic drugs other than the stimulants (e.g., Sprague & Sleator, 1977), it has been found with neuroleptic medication as well (e.g., Werry & Aman, 1975) and certainly depends, in part, on task characteristics. As with target symptoms, there is an optimum dosage range. Ideally, one would want to maximize therapeutic gain by selecting a dosage that benefited both adaptive and target behaviors.

Probably the more typical situation with adaptive behaviors is represented by the solid adaptive behavior line and the second baseline, which is designated here as (ND). In this case, the therapist does not anticipate improvement in adaptive behavior but is concerned about the extent to which adaptive behavior is *impaired* by medication (i.e., behavioral toxicity). In our example, only mild impairment is seen at the lower end of the therapeutic dosage range for treating target symptoms.

The side effects line in this figure represents somatic symptoms (e.g., heart rate, dizziness, gastrointestinal distress, and so forth). It is placed to the right of the behavioral toxicity curve because it has been hypothesized (e.g., Sprague & Werry, 1971, p. 191) that behavioral toxicity may be more commonly manifested at dosages lower than those associated with serious somatic complaints. It should be evident from this example that dosage titration on the basis of somatic side effects could lead to medication levels that severely impair adaptive behavior. While this may sound fairly simple, in real-world situations it is often very difficult to effectively evaluate behavioral toxicity, therapeutic response, and in some instances, even somatic toxicity.

TOLERANCE

When the same dose of medication no longer has a characteristic effect after repeated administrations, this is referred to as *tolerance*. The exact mechanisms underlying this alteration in response are not always well understood for each and every drug. Tolerance is reported in some children receiving Ritalin or Tofranil for hyperactivity who no longer react to medication in the same way as when treatment was first started. In the case of Ritalin, a modest increase in dose is usually sufficient to maintain the desired response (Sleator et al., 1974). Occasionally, some hyperactive children show a dramatic therapeutic improvement with stimulants but then develop a complete tolerance (Gross & Wilson, 1974). For such children, increasing the dose only helps for a short time, and medication must eventually be withdrawn. Tolerance for the therapeutic effects of medication that develops very rapidly, i.e., after the administration of a few doses, is referred to as *tachyphylaxis*. Fortunately, children also develop a tolerance for many side effects. For example, stimulant drugs often cause a loss of appetite when treatment first begins. However, after receiving medication for a couple of weeks, most children are not bothered by this reaction.

Because drugs often have many properties, children may develop a tolerance for only some of them. As noted in the previous example, although children typically develop a tolerance for the appetite-suppressing effects of stimulant medication, the behavior-controlling properties of the drug may not change. Adjustments are sometimes made in the dosage of medication as the child grows to accommodate for changes in body size, but this is not the same thing as tolerance.

When a person shows a decreased reactivity to one drug (B) after repeated exposure to another drug (A), the phenomenon is referred to as *cross-tolerance*. This generally occurs for drugs that are pharmacologically similar (i.e., related mechanisms of action and effects).

Tolerance to drug effects is achieved in three different ways. *Behavioral tolerance* develops when an individual learns how to counteract the behavioral effects of the drug. For example, the performance of two people under the influence of a drug may differ if one has practiced the task while taking the drug and the other person has not, given equal levels of drug exposure and task practice. This may explain, in part, the ability of some alcoholics to diminish the effect of alcohol, or "to hold their liquor."

Repeated drug administrations may also increase the rate at which drugs move through the body. This is referred to as *drug disposition* or *metabolic tolerance*. For example, the regular intake of some drugs actually stimulates the metabolic processes responsible for the breakdown of the drug. To achieve the same effect, the dose must be larger than the previous one. In one study of epileptic adults treated with Dilantin, 45% showed a drop in the blood level of the drug over several months of treatment (Reynolds et al., 1976). In some cases, the level dropped so low that seizures recurred in patients who were previously seizure free. The situation was remedied by increasing the dose. It should be noted that in the treatment of epilepsy, this does *not* end in a vicious cycle of dosage increments.

Pharmacodynamic or *cellular tolerance* develops when the cells of the nervous system actually adjust to the presence of the medication. In order to achieve the same reaction to the drug, the dosage must be increased to overcome the body's compensatory mechanisms. If a neurological adjustment is made to the larger dose, even more medication will be required, and so on. This type of tolerance is encountered with the euphoric effect of opium and related drugs.

Tolerance is an important clinical concern because repeated dosage increments may lead to drug levels that produce serious or troublesome side effects. In the treatment of hyperactivity, for example, clinicians have described individual cases that showed a highly favorable response to one stimulant (e.g., Ritalin) but later had to be switched to another (e.g., Dexedrine) because tolerance developed to both lower and higher doses of the initial drug during the course of treatment. Of course, if cross-tolerance is a problem, the clinician may have to switch to an entirely different drug class.

Dependence and Addiction

Another reaction associated with the repeated use of certain drugs is *physical dependence*. This occurs when an agent alters the physiological state of the body, and, to prevent the appearance of a *withdrawal syndrome*, the drug must continue to be administered. Physical dependence has been demonstrated with a number of drugs including opiates, barbiturates, alcohol, amphetamines, and nicotine (Jaffe, 1980). Because the symptoms that characterize the withdrawal syndrome are associated with the same area of the body that was initially altered by the drug and are often the complete opposite of the drug effect, they are sometimes referred to as *rebound effects*. For example, some hyperactive children become more hyperactive when their short-acting stimulant medication wears off than when they are off medication altogether.

Psychological dependence is a somewhat ambiguous term because it is used to refer to more than one concept and is often misapplied in the popular press. Increasingly it is becoming to signify a pattern of drug self-administration in which either the drug is perceived as a reinforcer, drug-taking behavior is considered a coping mechanism, or both. This definition is favored over others because it demystifies the term. When psychological dependence does not impair adaptive behavior (e.g., working, raising children), it is no different from any other behavioral pursuit (e.g., jogging). When drug-taking does interfere with social functioning or health, then it is of course bad, but no more so than any other activity that produced equivalent levels of disability or impairment. The fact that hundreds of millions of people throughout the world, children and adults alike, are psychologically dependent upon at least one substance (caffeine, alcohol, tobacco, hallucinogens, and so forth) suggests that habitual drug use is an integral part of the human experience. Unfortunately, excessive and even moderate use of substances such as alcohol and tobacco can lead to an inferior quality of life for family and friends, serious disability, and death, as can poor dietary intake, reckless driving, inadequate exercise, and overwork. When drug use becomes compulsive, the term *addiction* is often, but not always, applied. To be addicted, one must be psychologically dependent, but to be psychologically dependent, one does *not* have to be physically dependent.

The difference between physical dependence and *drug addiction* is not often made clear. Drug addiction refers to a "behavioral pattern of drug use, characterized by overwhelming involvement with the use of a drug (compulsive use), the securing of its supply, and a high tendency to relapse after withdrawal" (Jaffe, 1980, p. 536). It is important to note that one can be physically dependent upon a drug and *not* be addicted, or be addicted and *not* be physically dependent.

Parents and teachers often worry whether children receiving psychotropic medication for behavior or learning disorders will become addicted. They will not! Nor are they more apt to become drug abusers in later life. Followup studies of hyperactive children treated with medication, for example, show they are not remarkably different from their peers in illegal drug use patterns, and some may even use illicit and common substances to a lesser degree than nonhyperactive agemates.

DRUG INTERACTIONS

It is not unusual for children to receive two or more different drugs during the same day. Some behavior disorders may require more than one medicine to achieve a satisfactory therapeutic response, but this is rarely necessary. Children may also have more than one disorder that requires long-term drug treatment. Studies show that from 7 to 10% of the children on medication in special education programs receive drugs for both behavior and seizure disorders (Gadow, 1977; Gadow & Kalachnik, 1981). There are also tens of thousands of nonprescription products available to parents for the treatment of common childhood maladies such as colds, headaches, upset stomachs, and so forth. Although we do not always regard these products as "drugs," the concomitant administration of a prescription and a nonprescription medicine is a drug combination. Another situation for which a combination of drugs is used is the management of adverse reactions. For example, if a medicine causes serious side effects but cannot be stopped for therapeutic reasons, the physician may prescribe an additional drug specifically to control the side effects.

The terminology pertaining to multiple drug use is hopelessly muddled. The term *polypharmacy*, for example, is used by many to denote multiple drug use in general (regardless of the reason for treatment), and by others to mean the use of two or more drugs for the *same* disorder. There does not appear to be any special label for multiple drug use stemming from the concurrent treatment of two or more disorders (or different symptoms of the same disability). The distinction as to whether or not the drugs are being prescribed for the same or different disorders is very important because the treatment issues associated with each are only partially interrelated.

Using two different drugs for the same disorder (probably best referred to as *multiple-drug therapy*) is generally unwarranted and ill-advised unless the two agents (a) possess a different mechanism of action and (b) the clinical utility of the two in combination is clearly superior to either when used singly. Some classic examples of effective multiple-drug therapy based upon independent mechanisms of action can be found in antimicrobial therapy (see Sande & Mandell, 1980). The use of trimethoprim and sulfamethoxazole in combination to treat lower urinary tract infections is a case in point because these two drugs interact *synergistically* (the combination is more powerful than either agent used alone). Each interferes with a *different* step in the production of folic acid in certain bacteria. Because (a) there are few truly compelling examples of useful polypharmacy in either adult or pediatric psychopharmacology and (b) indiscriminate multiple neuroleptic drug use was once a common practice, the term *polypharmacy* now implies dumb clinical practice to many and has even been defined in terms of drugs with similar mechanisms of action (see Klein et al., 1980, p. 39).

Multiple drug use that arises out of the concurrent management of two or more disorders (or symptoms) has also generated international concern. Reports of multiple drug use in residential facilities, hospitals, and community care centers for the mentally retarded, elderly, and psychiatrically ill have led some clinicians to question the necessity for all of the drugs that are prescribed. Drug combinations in these settings are an important clinical consideration in that the effects of one agent may be significantly altered by the presence of another. When this does occur, it is referred to as a drug *interaction*.

One way in which drugs interact is an alteration in the absorption, distribution, biotransformation, or excretion of one agent by another (*pharmacokinetic interactions*). Changes in the rate at which these processes occur can result in an increase or decrease in the blood level of the altered drug. Several examples of drug interactions are presented here to better explain these processes.

If drug A slows down the rate at which drug B is absorbed into the blood, it will take longer for drug B to reach an effective level. This could be very important if it is necessary to obtain a high level of drug B in the bloodstream to be really effective for medical treatment. One example of this type of interaction is between milk and milk products and the antibiotic drug tetracycline. It is generally recommended that orally administered tetracycline be taken 1 hour before or 2 hours after meals because these foods can impair the absorption of tetracycline.

Once drug molecules have entered the bloodstream, another type of drug interaction becomes possible, and this involves plasma protein binding. If drug A is associated with a clinically significant degree of plasma protein binding, the addition of drug B to the treatment regimen could create problems if it also binds to plasma proteins and has greater affinity for the binding site than drug A. This situation could lead to a marked increase in the number of unbound (free) drug A molecules in the blood, which in turn could result in a rapid and dramatic increase in drug A effects (both therapeutic and adverse). Ironically, this heightened effect is typically short-lived because the free drug molecules are now also available for biotransformation and excretion (glomerular filtration), and the end result may be lower blood levels of drug A.

The rate at which drugs are broken down by the liver can also be altered. Say, for example, drug A is poorly soluble in water and must be transformed into water-soluble metabolites before it can be excreted by the kidney. Any drug that inhibited the metabolism of drug A would produce an increase in the blood level of the latter. Because there would now be more drug A molecules in general circulation, the effect would be greater. This could result in either unwanted side effects, a more pronounced therapeutic effect than when drug A was administered alone, or both. When one drug inhibits the biotransformation of another, the consequences of this interaction are typically experienced within hours or days after the addition of the offending medication.

In addition to being inhibited, biotransformation can also be made to occur more rapidly (*induced*). One way this can happen is for one drug (B) to cause an increase in the production of the microsomal enzymes that break down another drug (A). When drug B is added to the treatment regimen, the blood level of drug A may drop because it is being converted into metabolites for excretion at a faster rate. This is generally a more gradual process and may not become clinically significant until after weeks or months of concurrent drug use.

Another type of drug interaction occurs when two drugs with similar effects are given in combination. For example, alcohol and barbiturates both produce central nervous system depression ranging from mild sedation to coma, depending upon the amount consumed. When they are both used during the same period of time, their effects are *additive* and the outcome may be fatal. The combination of the two substances is similar to a much larger amount of either one ingested alone.

ROLE OF CAREGIVERS IN PHARMACOTHERAPY

The effectiveness of psychotropic drug therapy is dependent upon the efforts of a variety of care-providers. It is people, after all, who must recognize the child's problem, make the appropriate diagnosis, prescribe the appropriate medication, evaluate and adjust the medication, supervise its administration, monitor treatment effects, provide the necessary educational and psychological services, and terminate pharmacotherapy when it is either no longer warranted, ineffective, or detrimental. Even a casual consideration of these activities will generate an appreciation for the complexity of the treatment process. Whereas for many youngsters and their families taking medication is a fairly straightforward procedure, many others will experience some difficulty with one or more of these activities. Moreover, given the number of people who may become involved in making, or in some way influencing, treatment-related decisions, there are going to be disagreements as to what the appropriate course of action should be. Ways that care-providers can assist the physician are probably the most well documented in the treatment of hyperactivity (Sprague & Gadow, 1976), a few of which are discussed here. It must be emphasized, however, that they also apply to the pharmacological management of many other disorders and to all caregivers, not just school personnel.

The treatment process consists of three stages: diagnosis, dosage adjustment, and followup. There is a period prior to referral and diagnosis when caregivers and child cope with the problem, and a period following the termination of drug treatment when other approaches are used to maintain therapeutic gains. The predrug and postdrug periods have generally been excluded from most scientific investigations although there is no shortage of discussion on this matter, particularly with regard to the events that lead to referral.

The diagnostic phase of the treatment process begins with the decision that the child's behavior deviates enough from expected standards to warrant special attention. Because school underachievement is a common problem, and the classroom is uniquely stressful to the hyperactive child, learning and behavior problems inevitably come to the attention of teachers. They may try to cope with the child's behavior, make special adjustments in their demands, separate him or her from the rest of the class, have conferences with the parents, or provide special assistance. If these efforts fail, the child may undergo a psychological-educational evaluation by the school's assessment team, who in turn may request a medical, neurological, or psychiatric evaluation. If it is determined that the child has developmental delays, learning problems, or handicaps requiring special attention, he or she may then be scheduled for an academic (tutoring, remedial exercises, or special education), psychological, or medical intervention, or some combination of these. Survey studies of hyperactive children treated with a medication show that these youngsters often receive many different types of therapy.

The teacher can play an important role in the medical evaluation by supplying the physician with a characterization of the child's behavior. This is particularly important because the child may perform quite well in face-to-face interaction with the physician. In fact, many cases of hyperactivity may go undiagnosed if the physician relies solely on behavior during an office visit (Sleator & von Neumann, 1974; Sleator & Ullmann, 1981). The Abbreviated Teacher Rating Scale (Conners, 1973), which the physician can mail directly to the teacher, has proved to be particularly useful in diagnosing the disorder.

Caregiver ratings may differ, which presents a diagnostic problem for the physician (Klein & Gittelman-Klein, 1975). Multiple sources of information give the physician an opportunity to contrast evaluations and possibly to develop insights into the etiology of the child's problems. Identifying functional relationships between the environment and the child's behavior has direct bearing upon treatment strategy (Eisenberg, 1972; Freeman, 1970).

In addition to completing diagnostic evaluation forms, Slimmer and Brown (1985) have shown that school personnel can play an important role in explaining treatment options to parents and providing information about medication. This procedure can be effective by providing answers to questions so that parents are better able to decide what they want to do.

Once the decision has been made to initiate drug therapy, the child is typically administered a minimum initial dose that is gradually increased until the desired therapeutic effect is achieved. Through this process the dosage is said to be *titrated*. As in the diagnostic phase, the teacher can play an important role in monitoring medication by evaluating the effect of different dosage levels on the child's behavior and by reporting side effects. These evaluations can be conveniently phoned or mailed to the physician. Sleator and Sprague (1978) note that feedback from the teacher regarding the response to medication is essential:

> Remarkable sensitivity to drug effects on the part of the teacher has been replicated regularly in our laboratory. No other clinical measure even approaches this sensitivity [and] we recommend strongly that monitoring of drug effects must include reports from the teacher if the physician hopes to effectively treat school children with learning and/or behavior disorders. He must be in active communication with the child's teacher. The physician would not consider treating anemia, for example, without repeated laboratory tests. For the child with learning problems the teacher is the physician's clinical laboratory. (p. 579)

Initial adverse reactions may require withdrawal of the drug to be followed by a gradual reintroduction that provides the child with an opportunity to develop a tolerance for the side effects. If the response to medication is unsatisfactory, it may be necessary to try different drugs or even drugs in combination until the desired therapeutic effect is achieved.

If medication facilitates performance in the classroom, the consequences of therapy can be quite beneficial. There is, however, also the possibility that medication will retard classroom performance or alter behavior to the point of decreasing learning. Many side effects are self-limiting, can be managed with adjustments in dosage, or both. However, those that impair performance present serious questions in regard to the choice of therapeutic criteria. It should also be pointed out that not all children respond to medication, and some even develop a tolerance for a favorable response.

The last phase of treatment, followup, includes continual monitoring of medication to observe changes in therapeutic response and the possible development of side effects. Temporary breaks in medication (*drug-free periods*) provide caregivers with an opportunity to evaluate therapeutic progress and the physician a chance to assess the continued need for medication. For teachers who first interact with a child on medication, this may be crucial for the establishment of therapeutic objectives. Because drugs are an adjunct to the total therapeutic management of the child, the teacher is in a position to use other measures such as behavior modification techniques, which may permit the child to function without medication. In this regard, followup is the continued effort to facilitate the child's development toward stated therapeutic objectives. It would seem imperative that the reason for which the drug was prescribed—for example, conduct problems, academic underachievement, peer difficulties, or family crisis—be continually evaluated in terms of the child's progress toward identified behavioral goals.

The termination of drug therapy does not signal the end of followup efforts. Medication in and of itself teaches the child nothing, although changes in the child's behavior that are a function of pharmacotherapy may make him or her more responsive to natural contingencies, regular teaching efforts, or special education. Many children, however, will require continued ameliorative efforts long after drug treatment has been terminated.

We must, then, conclude from laboratory and clinical research that the teacher can play a valuable role in pharmacotherapy for hyperactivity. The teacher can supply the physician with characterizations of the child's behavior, either anecdotal or with standardized scales, before drug therapy is initiated, while dosage is titrated, during drug-free periods, and intermittently for the duration of therapy. Perhaps the teacher's most significant contribution is the continued effort to facilitate the child's development.

SUGGESTED READINGS

Campbell, M., Anderson, L. T., & Green, W. H. (1983). Behavior-disordered and aggressive children: New advances in pharmacotherapy. *Developmental and Behavioral Pediatrics*, 4, 265–271. (C, S)

Eisenberg, L. (1975). The ethics of intervention: Acting amidst ambiguity. *Journal of Child Psychology and Psychiatry, 16*, 93–104. (C)

Engel, G. L. (1977). The need for a new medical model: A challenge for biomedicine. *Science, 196*, 129–135. (C)

Gillman, A. G., Goodman, L. S., & Gilman, A. (Eds.). (1980). *The pharmacological basis of therapeutics* (6th ed.). New York: MacMillan. (C, S)

Gualtieri, C. T., Golden, R. N., & Fahs, J. J. (1983). New developments in pediatric psychopharmacology. *Developmental and Behavioral Pediatrics, 4*, 202–209. (C, S)

Klein, D. F., Gittelman, R., Quitkin, F., & Rifkin, A. (1980). *Diagnosis and drug treatment of psychiatric disorders: Adults and children* (2nd ed.). Baltimore: Williams & Wilkins. (C)

Leavitt, F. (1982). *Drugs and behavior* (2nd ed.). Philadelphia: Saunders. (C, S)

Silverman, M., & Lee, P. R. (1974). *Pills, profits, and politics*. Berkeley: University of California Press. (C, S)

Sprague, R. L., & Gadow, K. D. (1976). The role of the teacher in drug treatment. *School Review, 85*, 109–140. (S)

Werry, J. S. (Ed.). (1978). *Pediatric psychopharmacology: The use of behavior modifying drugs in children*. New York: Brunner/Mazel. (C)

REFERENCES

Abel, E. L. (1974). *Drugs and behavior: A primer in neuropsychopharmacology*. New York: Wiley.

Bevan, J. A. (Ed.). (1976). *Essentials of pharmacology* (2nd ed.). New York: Harper & Row.

Blackwell, B., & Currah, J. (1973). The psychopharmacology of nocturnal enuresis. In I. Kolvin, R. C. MacKeith, and S. R. Meadow (Eds.), *Bladder control and enuresis* (pp. 231–257). Philadelphia: Lippincott.

Bradley, C. (1937). The behavior of children receiving Benzedrine. *American Journal of Psychiatry, 94*, 577–585.

Briant, R. H. (1978). An introduction to clinical pharmacology. In J. S. Werry (Ed.), *Pediatric psychopharmacology: The use of behavior modifying drugs in children* (pp. 3–28). New York: Brunner/Mazel.

Burack, R. B., & Fox, F. J. (1975). *The new handbook of prescription drugs* (rev. ed.). New York: Ballantine Books.

Campbell, M., Anderson, L. T., & Green, W. H. (1983). Behavior-disordered and aggressive children: New advances in pharmacotherapy. *Developmental and Behavioral Pediatrics, 4*, 265–271.

Conners, C. K. (1973). Rating scales for use in drug studies with children. *Psychopharmacology Bulletin* (Special issue, Pharmacotherapy of children), 24–84.

Dodson, W. E. (1984). Antiepileptic drug utilization in pediatric patients. *Epilepsia, 25* (Suppl. 2), S 132–S139.

Eisenberg, L. (1972). Symposium: Behavior modification by drugs III. The clinical use of stimulant drugs in children. *Pediatrics, 49*, 709–715.

Eisenberg, L. (1975). The ethics of intervention: Acting amidst ambiguity. *Journal of Child Psychology and Psychiatry, 16*, 93–104.

Engel, G. L. (1977). The need for a new medical model: A challenge for biomedicine. *Science, 196*, 129–135.

Freeman, R. D. (1970). Use of psychoactive drugs for intellectually handicapped children. In N. R. Bernstein (Ed.), *Diminished people: Problems and care of the mentally retarded* (pp. 277–304). Boston: Little, Brown.

Fromm, G. H., Wessel, H. B., Glass, J. D., Alvin, J. D., & van Horn, G. (1978). Imipramine in absence and myoclonic-astatic seizures. *Neurology, 28*, 953–957.

Gadow, K. D. (1977). *Psychotropic and antiepileptic drug treatment with children in early childhood special education.* Champaign, IL: Institute for Child Behavior and Development, University of Illinois. (ERIC Document Reproduction Service No. ED 162 294)

Gadow, K. D., & Kalachnik, J. (1981). Prevalence and pattern of drug treatment for behavior and seizure disorders of TMR students. *American Journal of Mental Deficiency, 85*, 588-595.

Gadow, K. D., White, L., & Ferguson, D. G. (1986). Placebo controls and double-blind conditions: Placebo theory in experimental design. In K. D. Gadow & A. D. Poling (Eds.), *Advances in learning and behavioral disabilities* (Suppl. 1): *Methodological issues in human psychopharmacology.* Greenwich, CT: JAI Press.

Gilman, A. G., Goodman, L. S., & Gilman, A. (Eds.). (1980). *The pharmacological basis of therapeutics* (6th ed.). New York: Macmillan.

Gittelman-Klein, R. (1975). Pharmacotherapy and management of pathological separation anxiety. *International Journal of Mental Health, 4*, 255–271.

Gray, M. G., & Trowbridge, E. B. (1942). Methods for investigating the effect of drugs on psychological function. *Psychological Record, 5*, 127–148.

Gross, M. D., & Wilson, W. C. (1974). *Minimal brain dysfunction.* New York: Brunner/Mazel.

Gualtieri, C. T., Golden, R., Evans, R. W., & Hicks, R. E. (1984). Blood level measurement of psychoactive drugs in pediatric psychiatry. *Therapeutic Drug Monitoring, 6*, 127–141.

Gualtieri, C. T., Golden, R. N., & Fahs, J. J. (1983). New developments in pediatric psychopharmacology. *Developmental and Behavioral Pediatrics, 4*, 202–209.

Heuyer, G., Gerard, G., & Galibert, J. (1953). Traitement de l'excitation psychometrics chez l'enfant pare (le 4560 r.p.). *Archives Françaises de Pediatrie, 9*, 961.

Hollingworth, H. L. (1912). Psychological aspects of drug action. *Psychological Bulletin, 9*, 420–423.

Jaffe, J. H. (1980). Drug addiction and drug abuse. In A. G. Gilman, S. Goodman, & A. Gilman (Eds.), *The pharmacological basis of therapeutics* (6th ed.). New York: Macmillan.

Katz, S., Saraf, K., Gittelman-Klein, R., & Klein, D. F. (1975). Clinical pharmacological management of hyperkinetic children. *International Journal of Mental Health, 4*, 157–181.

Klein, D. F., Gittelman, R., Quitkin, F., & Rifkin, A. (1980). *Diagnosis and drug treatment of psychiatric disorders: Adults and children* (2nd ed.). Baltimore: Williams and Wilkins.

Lennox, W. G. (1942). Brain injury, drugs and environment as causes of mental decay in epilepsy. *American Journal of Psychiatry, 99*, 174–180.

Levy, L. L., & Fenichel, G. M. (1965). Diphenylhydantoin activated seizures. *Neurology, 15*, 716–722.

MacPhail, A. (1933). *The source of modern medicine*. Unpublished manuscript later presented as a paper to the meeting of the American College of Physicians, Montreal, February 8, 1939.

Rapoport, J. L., Quinn, P. O., Bradbard, G., Riddle, K. D., & Brooks, E. (1974). Imipramine and methylphenidate treatments of hyperactive boys. *Archives of General Psychiatry, 30*, 789–793.

Reynolds, E. H., Chadwick, D., & Galbraith, A. W. (1976). One drug (phenytoin) in the treatment of epilepsy. *Lancet, 1*, 923–926.

Sande, M. A., & Mandell, G. L. (1980). Antimicrobial agents: General considerations. In A. G. Gilman, L. S. Goodman, & A. Gilman (Eds.), *The pharmacological basis of therapeutics* (6th ed., pp. 1080–1105). New York: Macmillan.

Silverman, M., & Lee, P. R. (1974). *Pills, profits, and politics*. Berkeley: University of California Press.

Sleator, E. K., & Sprague, R. L. (1978). Pediatric pharmacotherapy. In W. G. Clark & J. del Guidice (Eds.), *Principles of psychopharmacology* (2nd ed., pp. 573–591). Orlando, FL: Academic Press.

Sleator, E. K., & von Neumann, A. (1974). Methylphenidate in the treatment of hyperkinetic children. *Clinical Pediatrics, 13*, 19–24.

Sleator, E. K., von Neumann, A. W., & Sprague, R. L. (1974). Hyperactive children: A continuous long-term placebo controlled follow-up. *Journal of the American Medical Association, 229*, 316–317.

Sleator, E. K., & Ullmann, R. K. (1981). Can the physician diagnose hyperactivity in the office? *Pediatrics, 67*, 13–17.

Slimmer, L. W., & Brown, R. T. (1985). Parents' decision-making process in medication administration for control of hyperactivity. *Journal of School Health, 55*, 221–225.

Sonnenreich, M. R., & Menger, J. M. (1977, April). State substitution laws: A lawyer's view. *U. S. Pharmacist*, pp. 18–23.

Sprague, R. L., & Gadow, K. D. (1976). The role of the teacher in drug treatment. *School Review, 85*, 109–140.

Sprague, R. L., & Sleator, E. K. (1975). What is the proper dose of stimulant drugs in children? *International Journal of Mental Health, 4*, 75–104.

Sprague, R. L., & Sleator, E. K. (1977). Methylphenidate in hyperkinetic children: Differences in dose effects on learning and social behavior. *Science, 198*, 1274–1276.

Sprague, R. L., & Werry, J. S. (1971). Methodology of psychopharmacological studies with the retarded. In N. R. Ellis (Ed.), *International review of research in mental retardation* (Vol. 5, pp. 147–219). Orlando, FL: Academic Press.

Swonger, A. K. (1978). *Nursing pharmacology: A systems approach to drug therapy and nursing practice*. Boston: Little, Brown.

Usdin, E. (1970). Classification of psychopharmaca. In W. G. Clark & J. del Guidice (Eds.), *Principles of psychopharmacology*. Orlando, FL: Academic Press.

Usdin, E., & Efron, D. H. (1972). *Psychotropic drugs and related compounds* (2nd ed., DHEW Publication No. 72-9074). Washington, DC: U.S. Government Printing Office.

Vesell, E., & Page, J. (1968). Genetic control of drug levels in man: Antipyrine. *Science, 161,* 72–73.

Weiss, G. (1981). Controversial issues of the pharmacotherapy of the hyperactive child. *Canadian Journal of Psychiatry, 26,* 385–392.

Werry, J. S., & Aman, M. G. (1975). Methylphenidate and haloperidol in children. *Archives of General Psychiatry, 32,* 790–795.

White, L., Tursky, B., & Schwartz, G. E. (Eds.). (1985). *Placebo: Theory, research, and mechanisms.* New York: Guilford.

Wittenborn, J. R. (1980). Behavioral toxicity of psychotropic drugs. *Journal of Nervous and Mental Disease, 168,* 171–176.

Zbinden, G. (1963). Experimental and clinical aspects of drug toxicity. In S. Garattini & P. A. Shore (Eds.), *Advances in pharmacology* (Vol. 2, pp. 1–112). Orlando, FL: Academic Press.

Chapter 2

Hyperactivity

In recent years, no other childhood disorder has received as much attention, generated more controversy, or left educators and parents in more confusion about what to do than the condition known as hyperactivity. The vagueness of the term has resulted in an ''epidemic'' of cases, causes, and cures (Freeman, 1976). Accusations have been made that teachers and physicians conspire to enslave boisterous school children in chemical straight jackets. It has been claimed that instead of accommodating our social institutions to the needs of these children, we take the easy way out—pills. Physicians, under pressure from parents and teachers, have been accused of capriciously ''doping kids up.'' Critics say that creating medical disorders out of socially unacceptable behavior is a most hideous form of social control.

The emotional anguish that often accompanies uncertainty about what is the right thing to do for our children is aggravated by a host of individuals proclaiming they have found the truth. Eisenberg (1964) observed that the less that is known about a particular aspect of drug treatment, the stronger the convictions about what is correct and about what should be done. Although differing views may provide a healthy competition in the search for effective techniques and explanations, it is often difficult for parents, teachers, and even clinicians to know where to begin.

The school is often in the middle of this controversy because it is (a) frequently the source of medical referral, (b) intimately involved in fostering academic achievement, and (c) one of the most challenging settings for the hyperactive child. This chapter is a sincere attempt to present an unbiased discussion of what is, to many care-providers, an emotionally charged topic: drug treatment of hyperactive behavior in children.

There is a voluminous literature on hyperactivity and its management, only a small portion of which is presented here. It is useful, therefore, to note several books that are worthy of special comment as sources of additional information. One is *Hyperactivity: Current Issues, Research and Theory* by Dorothea and Sheila Ross (1982), which is without peer as an extensive review of the scientific literature. Two additional books that are particularly useful for clinicians are Safer and Allen's (1976) earlier text, *Hyperactive Children: Diagnosis and Medical Management* and Barkley's (1981) more recent book, *Hyperactive Children: A Handbook for Diagnosis and Treatment*. There is also an excellent book for parents, Stewart and Old's (1973), *Raising a Hyperactive Child*. The primary focus of this discussion is on medication and its effect on child behavior.

Because there are age-related changes in the relative severity of the behavioral, cognitive, and social symptoms of hyperactivity as well as age-related medication issues, the treatment of this disorder appears in two different chapters. In the present chapter, the clear focus is on the elementary school years. Chapter 5 (Early Childhood) presents a detailed discussion of hyperactivity and its medical management in children under 6 years of age. Readers interested in the preschool age group will nevertheless benefit from the following discussion of diagnostic issues and stimulant drug effects because the great bulk of medical research on hyperactivity pertains to children between 6 and 12 years of age.

BASIC FEATURES

The term *hyperactivity* is somewhat confusing because it is used both as a diagnostic construct and as a behavioral characteristic. As a behavioral characteristic, hyperactivity refers to overactivity and motor restlessness. As a diagnostic construct, however, hyperactivity is a particular childhood disorder that is defined in a specific way and diagnosed according to a specific set of criteria. Confusion arises because some children who might be characterized as being hyperactive would not be diagnosed as having the disorder hyperactivity. For example, children who are severely emotionally disturbed and very overactive would probably be described as being hyperactive, but these same children would also be very different from the children we normally diagnose as having hyperactivity. The distinction is important because the two groups of children are probably very different with regard to the cause of their problems and often respond best to different types of treatment. The labeling problem is compounded by the fact that highly active normal children are sometimes called hyperactive in everyday speech.

Because there is, and always has been, controversy regarding exactly what a child had to do to be diagnosed as having the disorder hyperactivity, no definition of hyperactivity is going to satisfy even a simple majority of the clinicians and scientists who study this problem. While the American Psychiatric Association (1980) publishes guidelines on how to diagnose hyperactivity, these guidelines change periodically along with the diagnostic label. In addition, there are many who take exception to the specifics of the APA definition. Before going into this controversy in more detail, Safer and Allen's (1976) definition of hyperactivity is presented because it contains the essential elements of most diagnostic schemes:

> Hyperactivity is simply defined as a long term childhood pattern characterized by excessive restlessness and inattentiveness. It is a developmental disorder which begins in early to midchildhood (ages 2–6), and begins to fade during adolescence. . . . The only necessary feature . . . is developmental hyperactivity [which] . . . is best determined by history. It is a persistent pattern of excessive activity in situations requiring motor inhibition. Persistent means consistently, year after year. Excessive means extreme (i.e., the most restless 3–5%). (pp. 5–7)

One of the more important distinctions in this definition is the fact that hyperactivity just does not pop us as a reaction to emotional stress, tight underwear, or fluctuations in blood sugar levels (Walker, 1974). It is a developmental disorder with an early onset. As an infant, the hyperactive child may be fretful, colicky, and restless. Mothers who have more than one offspring may even comment that their hyperactive child was more restless than his or her siblings *in utero*. Hyperactivity is usually first manifested during the preschool years, kindergarten, or first grade and is particularly noticeable in settings that include peers (e.g., day care and public schools). Older children who develop conduct problems for the first time between the third and fifth grades should not be confused with children labeled hyperactive in this discussion (Safer & Allen, 1976).

Classroom situations that require sustained attention and sitting still typically differentiate the hyperactive child from his or her peers. However, in other school settings (e.g., playgrounds) the differences *may* not be as apparent. While some children are considered hyperactive in the school, the home, and the physician's office, others are perceived as hyperactive only at home or only in school (Lambert et al., 1978). This situational variability, which is due in part to the subjective nature of judgments about what constitutes "excessive" motor restlessness, creates opportunity for disagreement among parents, teachers, and physicians as to whether or not a child is hyperactive. It should not be inferred from this statement that child behavior is necessarily situation specific. Zentall (1985), for example, after conducting an extensive review of the literature, concluded that hyperactive children are clearly discernible from nonhyperactive peers (activity level, attention shifts, excessive talking) in home, school, and clinic settings, whether activity is restricted or unrestricted or whether the setting is social or nonsocial.

A recent study by Porrino et al. (1983) is worthy of special comment with regard to activity level because its findings underscore the importance of activity level as a diagnostic feature of hyperactivity. The motor activity of hyperactive and normal boys was assessed on a 24-hour basis for 1 week in both home and school settings. It was found that the hyperactive group was more active regardless of the time of day. (They were even more active during sleep!) However, the biggest differences were for the school day. An analysis of motor activity in various school settings showed that the hyperactive group was most different from normal control subjects during academic lessons (reading and arithmetic). The two groups did *not* differ, however, during lunch, recess, or physical education.

The hyperactive child usually has a number of other problems along with excessive motor restlessness. Inattentiveness, one of the most common problems, is defined by teachers as not being able to stay on a task for any length of time or follow directions. Parents state that when younger the hyperactive child cannot sit and watch television like other children, is difficult to read to, and does not pay attention to what they say. Hyperactive children are often impulsive (see Brown & Sleator, 1979; Milich & Kramer, 1984). They raise their hands in class in response to a question without first determining if they know the answer. Impulsive children rush into activities without thinking, and when younger, appear unable to keep themselves from doing things they clearly know are wrong. Teachers and parents alike report that the hyperactive child jumps from one activity to another in an erratic manner. Poor school performance is also common, but the majority of medicated hyperactive children are nevertheless maintained in the regular classroom (Safer & Krager,

1984). Not only do many of these children achieve less well than expected, but some have learning disabilities (Lambert & Sandoval, 1980) and are placed in special education programs for learning disabled children (Epstein et al., 1985).

Other common features associated with hyperactivity are conduct problems and immaturity. Behavior problems at school take the form of hitting other children, not following classroom rules, disturbing others, and noisiness. Parents complain that the child is unmanageable. Because many hyperactive children do not act their age, people think of them as being immature. Their best friends may be several years younger, and their interests may seem childish. Emotionally, they are easily frustrated and have temper tantrums when other children have outgrown that stage. If the conduct problems are severe and involve a relatively serious level of aggressive behavior, the child may well be labeled "emotionally disturbed," "behavior disordered," or some variant of these terms (see Bricklin & Gallico, 1984) and placed in a special education class (Epstein et al., 1985).

Some of the possible consequences of school failure and behavior problems are peer difficulties (see Pelham & Milich, 1984) and poor self-image. Immaturity, restlessness, and learning problems all contribute to the child's undesirability as a friend. One study of adults diagnosed and treated for hyperactivity as children reported that many considered their childhood to be unhappy (Weiss et al., 1979). As adults, they stated that family fights (usually concerning themselves), feeling different (inferior, dumb), and being criticized "made things worse" as a child.

At one time, it was believed that children simply "grew out" of hyperactivity during adolescence (Laufer et al., 1957). However, more recent studies have shown that many of the problems associated with the disorder persist into adolescence and even into adulthood (Bellak, 1979; Hechtman et al., 1984b; Hoy et al., 1978; Safer & Allen, 1975; Weiss et al., 1971, 1979). Although hyperactive children become less restless during their early teens, teachers still consider their activity patterns to be different from those of their classmates. For many, impulsivity and inattentiveness are still major problems. Even as high school seniors, teachers rate the performance of hyperactive students as inferior to that of their peers (Weiss et al., 1978). As adults, they are more apt to see themselves as being inferior in social interactions and may have lower self-esteem. Although they are still restless and impulsive, the level of education and degree of job satisfaction and job status is not significantly different from that of normal adults (Weiss et al., 1978).

A number of followup studies of hyperactive children have now been conducted (see Thorley, 1984, for a review). While we have a fairly accurate picture of what happens to these youngsters as they grow up, there is still some difference of opinion as to the seriousness of this disorder in terms of their outcome. Thorley (1984), for example, concluded that "the outcome for children diagnosed hyperactive when compared with normal controls is relatively poor" (p. 125). However, it must be emphasized that most of these children appear to experience adulthood in a fairly normal way. They graduate from high school, marry, have families, become economically self-sufficient, and so forth (e.g., Hechtman et al., 1984a, 1984b; Weiss et al., 1978, 1979). Although it is true that some individuals do experience psychological problems or get into trouble with the law, the same can be said for other groups of handicapped people, such as learning disabled, educable mentally retarded, severe language impaired, physically handicapped, and sensory impaired people. In the hyperactive group, it appears that conduct problems (aggressive-defiant behaviors), lower intellectual functioning (IQ) during middle childhood, and severe hyperactive symptoms are important predictors of antisocial behavior in adolescence and adulthood (Gittelman et al., 1985; Hechtman et al., 1984c; Loney et al., 1981a, 1983; Milich & Loney, 1979).

DIAGNOSIS

Some clinicians may take issue with Safer and Allen's definition of hyperactivity as being too broad. The problem lies not so much in the definition as in the ambiguities inherent in diagnosing the condition (Loney, 1983; Loney & Milich, 1982). Their definition does include three of the most widely accepted criteria for a diagnosis of hyperactivity: (a) severe motor restlessness and inattentiveness, (b) a consistent developmental pattern, and (c) an early onset of symptoms. The first can be determined with the use of a behavior rating scale. Children receiving scores above a certain level are considered to be in the hyperactivity range. A consistent developmental pattern and an early onset of symptoms can be established with school reports from both present and prior teachers and from the child's parents. Although behavioral ratings and developmental histories from both the home and the school are two of the most frequently cited pieces of diagnostic information in the medical literature, a variety of procedures and criteria are employed in real-world situations. What is diagnosed as hyperactivity by one physician may be considered emotional disturbance or "spoiled child syndrome" by another.

The use of the term *hyperactivity* as a diagnostic construct is currently undergoing change. This is due, in part, to the idea that poor attending skills rather than excessive motor restlessness may be the essence of the problem (Douglas, 1972; Douglas & Peters, 1979), a notion that has been discussed for a number of years (see, for example, Ounsted, 1955) and is now somewhat controversial (see, for example, Porrino et al., 1983). In keeping with this observation, the American Psychiatric Association has changed its label for these children from *hyperkinetic reaction of childhood* to *attention deficit disorder with (or without) hyperactivity*. Interestingly, the earlier term has not received anywhere near the notoriety that *attention deficit disorder* has. The acronym for *attention deficit disorder with hyperactivity* is commonly written ADD-H. The criteria for making a diagnosis of ADD-H are presented in Table 2–1. While there are many aspects of ADD-H that are genuinely controversial (see Loney, 1983, for example), it has, nevertheless, been very influential. Even the failure to use the label ADD-H when referring to hyperactive children can elicit sharp criticism (e.g., Baren & Swanson, 1982; see also Loney & Gadow, 1982). The term *hyperactivity* is used in this book for a number of reasons, not the least of which are the following: (a) it appears to be the most consistently used label (or some variant of it) in the medical literature to refer to this disorder (or its primary feature) for the past four decades, (b) most of the drug research in this area was conducted on samples of children identified as being hyperactive, and (c) the advantages of an alternate term remain to be clearly established.

Two other diagnostic labels that have been used somewhat interchangeably with hyperactivity in the past are *hyperkinetic syndrome* and *minimal brain dysfunction* (MBD). Safer and Allen (1976) made a distinction between MBD and hyperactivity in that not all MBD children are hyperactive, and not all hyperactive children have learning disabilities, an important feature of MBD. For educators, the distinction is also useful because the term *hyperactivity* focuses in on a behavioral characteristic of the disorder, whereas MBD denotes etiology (cause). MBD implies that a child has some form of minimal brain damage. Hyperkinetic syndrome suggests a collection of symptoms that are often found in association with one another. This expression has also lost favor because the symptoms associated with hyperactivity do not appear to fall into a closely knit cluster (Safer & Allen, 1976).

Table 2–1. DSM–III Diagnostic Criteria for Attention Deficit Disorder with Hyperactivity[a]

The child displays, for his or her mental and chronological age, signs of developmentally inappropriate inattention, impulsivity, and hyperactivity. The signs must be reported by adults in the child's environment, such as parents and teachers. Because the symptoms are typically variable, they may not be observed directly by the clinician. When the reports of teachers and parents conflict, primary consideration should be given to the teacher reports because of greater familiarity with age-appropriate norms. Symptoms typically worsen in situations that require self-application, as in the classroom. Signs of the disorder may be absent when the child is in a new or a one-to-one situation.

The number of symptoms specified is for children between the ages of eight and ten, the peak age range for referral. In younger children, more severe forms of the symptoms and a greater number of symptoms are usually present. The opposite is true of older children.

A. Inattention. At least three of the following:
 (1) Often fails to finish things he or she starts
 (2) Often doesn't seem to listen
 (3) Easily distracted
 (4) Has difficulty concentrating on schoolwork or other tasks requiring sustained attention
 (5) Has difficulty sticking to a play activity

B. Impulsivity. At least three of the following:
 (1) Often acts before thinking
 (2) Shifts excessively from one activity to another
 (3) Has difficulty organizing work (this not being due to cognitive impairment)
 (4) Needs a lot of supervision
 (5) Frequently calls out in class
 (6) Has difficulty awaiting turn in games or group situations

C. Hyperactivity. At least two of the following:
 (1) Runs about or climbs on things excessively
 (2) Has difficulty sitting still or fidgets excessively
 (3) Has difficulty staying seated
 (4) Moves about excessively during sleep
 (5) Is always "on the go" or acts as if "driven by a motor"

D. Onset before the age of seven

E. Duration of at least six months

F. Not due to schizophrenia, affective disorder, or severe or profound mental retardation

[a]American Psychiatric Association. (1980). *Diagnostic and statistical manual of mental disorders* (3rd ed.). Washington, DC: Author.

One final comment must be made with regard to the diagnosis of hyperactivity. There has been a tendency over the years to formulate assessment procedures that involve a multitude of tests. Although special university clinics or diagnostic centers may employ such practices, they are certainly not characteristic of typical treatment practices. Until more empirical data are available on the relative utility of various diagnostic procedures, particularly with regard to the use of medication, Safer and Allen's (1976) suggestions regarding diagnosis (caregiver evaluations and developmental history) are still sound. An extremely thoughtful analysis of the practical aspects of diagnosing hyperactivity from the pediatrician's perspective is available in a chapter by Esther Sleator (1982).

PREVALENCE OF HYPERACTIVITY AND DRUG TREATMENT

One of the most common reasons for psychiatric referral among children is hyperactivity. The actual prevalence figures of hyperactivity among elementary school children varies from study to study, but the generally agreed upon rate is between 5 and 10%. This would mean that in a classroom of 30 students, an average of 1 to 2 pupils could be characterized as hyperactive. All studies report that hyperactivity is much more common in boys than girls. Because hyperactivity is often associated with epilepsy, cerebral palsy, emotional disturbance, learning disabilities, brain damage, and mental retardation, the prevalence of this disorder in special education programs may be quite high.

Lambert et al. (1978) found that the prevalence of hyperactivity varied depending upon who was asked to make the evaluation: teachers, parents, or physicians. When the criterion for hyperactivity was agreed among all three, approximately 1 to 1 ½% of students in their sample of 5,000 elementary school children were considered hyperactive. However, the prevalence of hyperactivity was 5% when based on all children considered hyperactive by either teachers, parents, or physicians. Because the prevalence of hyperactivity is often determined from teacher ratings, they asked a sample of teachers to evaluate all the children in their class on a behavioral rating scale. A cutoff point for hyperactivity was determined from the scores of children considered hyperactive by all three sources. Approximately 12 to 13% of the children were scored as being in the hyperactivity range.

A number of scientists have used the Teacher Rating Scale (TRS) or the Abbreviated Teacher Rating Scale (ATRS) developed by Keith Conners (Conners, 1969, 1973) to measure behavioral symptoms associated with hyperactivity in school children around the world. While scores on these instruments should definitely *not* be considered the sole basis for a diagnosis of hyperactivity, they can tell us what percentage of students are behaviorally similar (at least in some ways) to children who have been diagnosed as having hyperactivity and successfully treated with medication. Interestingly, the figures are fairly similar for many countries: approximately 12 to 18% of the elementary school children in Italy (O'Leary et al., in press), New Zealand (Sprague et al., 1977), Spain (Arias & O'Leary, 1984), and United States (Ullmann et al., in press) obtain scores (15 or above on the ATRS) that are within the range for children who are diagnosed and treated for hyperactivity. This does *not* mean that all or even most of these children would or should be referred for medical evaluation. These figures do suggest, however, that hyperactivity symptoms are fairly common in elementary school children in many countries of the world.

More children receive psychotropic drugs for hyperactivity than for any other disorder. The best available data about the extent of drug use for hyperactivity among elementary school children comes from Baltimore County, Maryland. Krager and Safer (1974; Safer & Krager, 1984) reported that the prevalence of drug treatment in that area was 1.1% in 1971 and 3.6% in 1983. Ritalin (methylphenidate), by far the most frequently prescribed drug for hyperactivity, was administered to 90% of the children on medication in 1983. Approximately 5% were receiving Dexedrine (dextroamphetamine), 2% Cylert (pemoline), and 3% nonstimulant drugs. Teachers frequently ask if older children receive medication. These investigators reported that 1.5% of the students in middle and junior high schools were on medication for hyperactivity, or less than one-half the figure for elementary schools. Cylert was used more frequently with teenagers than with the elementary school population, presumably because physicians want a longer lasting drug (to avoid having to take medicine in school) for the older children. Prevalence of drug use as a function of school grade level is presented in Figure 2–1.

The findings from Baltimore County as well as from other areas of the country (see Table 2–2) suggest that approximately 1 to 2% of *all* elementary-age school children (including those enrolled in special education) receive medication for hyperactivity. On the basis of national school enrollment figures for 1977, it was estimated that between 300,000 and 550,000 school children in kindergarten through 8th grade were on medication for hyperactivity (Gadow, 1981). Although there are problems inherent in making national estimates from selected samples, it is certainly true that large numbers of school-aged children in the United States receive stimulant drugs for this disorder.

The use of medication for the treatment of hyperactivity is more extensive with children receiving special education services. As can be seen in Table 2–3, treatment prevalence rates vary depending upon the type of special education program. Moreover, there are also

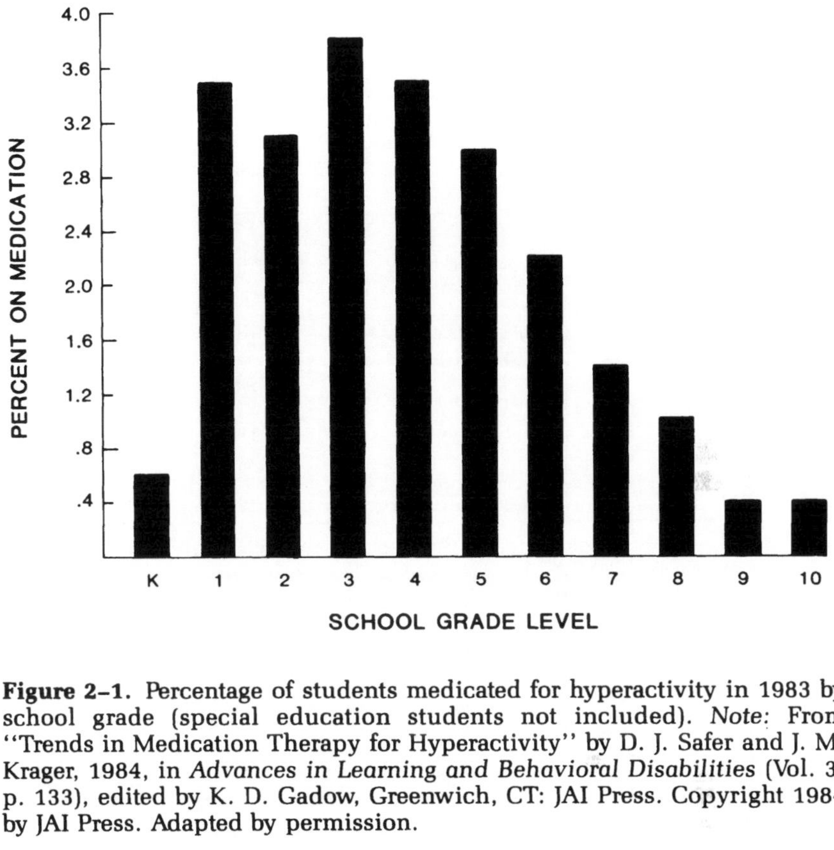

Figure 2–1. Percentage of students medicated for hyperactivity in 1983 by school grade (special education students not included). *Note:* From "Trends in Medication Therapy for Hyperactivity" by D. J. Safer and J. M. Krager, 1984, in *Advances in Learning and Behavioral Disabilities* (Vol. 3, p. 133), edited by K. D. Gadow, Greenwich, CT: JAI Press. Copyright 1984 by JAI Press. Adapted by permission.

considerable differences in drug use from one classroom to the next even though they may serve children with the same handicapping condition. In one study (Epstein et al., 1985) of learning disabled, educable mentally retarded, and emotionally disturbed children, it was reported that medication-treated children scored higher on ratings of hyperactivity (ATRS), were more socially deficient, and were more likely to be placed in special education programs that removed them from the mainstream of everyday educational experience. It is also noteworthy that although the stimulants were still the drugs of first choice for these children, a variety of other medications were also used, suggesting that some of these youngsters had other psychiatric disorders in addition to hyperactivity. Detailed descriptions of medication treatment practices for trainable mentally retarded and preschool-aged children are available in Chapters 4 and 5, respectively.

Table 2–2. Prevalence of Drug Treatment for Hyperactivity (District-Wide Surveys) in the United States

Study	Area	Year	Grades	Rate
Bosco & Robin (1980)	Grand Rapids, Michigan	1977	K–9	0.81
		1977	K–6	0.94
Conway (1976)	Mid-state New York	1975	K–6	2.56
Krager et al. (1979)	Baltimore county, Maryland	1975	K–6	2.03
Krager et al. (1979)	Baltimore county, Maryland	1977	K–6	2.12
		1977	7–9	0.66
Lambert et al. (1978)	East Bay area, California	1974	K–5	0.75
Ross (1979)	Queens, New York	1975	K–6	0.88

Note: From "Prevalence of Drug Treatment for Hyperactivity and Other Childhood Behavior Disorders" by K. D. Gadow in *Psychosocial Aspects of Drug Treatment for Hyperactivity* (pp. 44–45) by K. D. Gadow and J. Loney (Eds.), 1981, Boulder, CO: Westview Press. Copyright 1981 by the American Association for the Advancement of Science. Adapted by permission.

BEHAVIORAL EFFECTS OF STIMULANT DRUGS

Because stimulants are by far the most frequently prescribed agents for hyperactivity, they are the only group of drugs discussed in this chapter in any detail. The stimulants most commonly used are Ritalin, Dexedrine, and Cylert. Two other stimulants, Benzedrine (amphetamine sulfate) and Deaner (deanol), were also once prescribed for hyperactivity, but they are now rarely used.

Stimulant drugs have been administered to treat childhood behavior disorders for over 40 years, but one of the earliest reports on their use with children was for the treatment of *narcolepsy* (Prinzmetal & Bloomberg, 1935). Bradley (1937) was the first to record their effects on elementary school–aged children with behavior disorders. He noted that about half of the children in a residential school who were receiving Benzedrine showed a marked therapeutic improvement, and commented

> To see a single daily dose of benzedrine produce a greater improvement in school performance than the combined efforts of a capable staff working in a most favorable setting would have been all but demoralizing to the teachers, had not the improvement been so gratifying from a practical viewpoint. (p. 582)

Table 2–3. Prevalence of Drug Treatment for Hyperactivity in Special Education Programs

Study	Area	Special Education Category	Age (Years)	Treatment Rate (%)	Stimulants (% of Total)
Gadow (1977)	Illinois (State-wide)	Early childhood special education	3–5	7.9	70
Gadow & Kalachnik (1981)	Illinois (State-wide)	Trainable mentally retarded	3–21	6.7	51
Safer & Krager (1983, 1984)	Baltimore County, Maryland	Learning disabled (self-contained classes)	5–12	23.0	97
	Baltimore County, Maryland	Learning disabled (self-contained classes)	12–14	10.6	97
	Baltimore County, Maryland	Special schools for severely and multiply handicapped			
		Total	5–21	13.0	?
		LD and ED only	5–21	27.0	?
Epstein et al. (1985)	Northern Illinois	Learning disabled	6–18	7.4	83
	Northern Illinois	Educable mentally retarded	6–18	13.2	53
	Northern Illinois	Behavior disordered (emotionally disturbed)	6–18	14.2	55

A decade later, epileptologists discovered that Dexedrine was effective in the treatment of certain types of seizures (Livingston et al., 1948), and Bradley (1950) reported on the use of Dexedrine in the management of childhood behavior disorders. Ritalin has been used to treat behavior disorders since the 1950s (Carter, 1956; Zimmerman & Burgemeister, 1958) and is now the primary drug prescribed for hyperactivity. In 1975, the Food and Drug Administration approved a long-acting stimulant, Cylert, for use with hyperactive children. Considering how long these drugs have been on the market, literally millions of American children at one time or another have received stimulant medication for either hyperactivity, seizures, or drowsiness produced by some antiepileptic drugs (Gadow, 1981; Livingston et al., 1973; Safer & Krager, 1984).

Scores of studies have been published about the effects of drug treatment on hyperactive children (Winchell, 1975). Because a number of excellent reviews of stimulant drug therapy are available (Barkley, 1981; Cantwell & Carlson, 1978; Conners, 1971; Eisenberg & Conners, 1971; Ross & Ross, 1982; Safer & Allen, 1976; Sprague & Werry, 1974; Whalen, 1982), this discussion of the behavioral effects of stimulant drugs focuses on only some of the well-controlled studies. Changes in behavior that are the result of medication can be divided into six areas: activity level, motor performance, learning and cognitive performance, conduct problems, school achievement, and interpersonal relationships.

Activity Level

The effect of stimulants on activity level is not just a simple matter of slowing the child down. For example, there is no difference in the activity level of hyperactive children in a playroom whether they are on placebo (fake pill) or taking Ritalin (Ellis et al., 1974). However, these *same* children are perceived as being much less active by the classroom teacher (Sleator & von Neumann, 1974) and wiggle measurably less in their seats when asked to perform a task that requires concentration (Sprague & Sleator, 1973). Others have also found that stimulants reduce activity during laboratory testing (Rapoport et al., 1978) and during highly structured, task-oriented classroom situations (e.g., Whalen et al., 1979). Stimulant drug effects appear to be most apparent during tasks that require sitting still and paying attention. They help the child channel his or her activity to one event instead of flitting from one thing to another.

Motor Performance

A number of researchers have explored how stimulants alter fine and gross motor coordination and performance on perceptual motor tasks. Knights and Hinton (1969), for example, investigated the effect of Ritalin on motor steadiness. Children were asked to (a) move a stylus through a maze without touching the sides and (b) hold a stylus in the center of a hole without hitting the edge. On both tasks, medication improved fine motor performance (i.e., the children could hold the stylus longer without accidentally touching the sides of the cutout maze and circle). Ritalin also appears to facilitate the acquisition of gross motor skills. For example, Wade (1976) asked children to balance on a tilted 3- by 3-foot board that rotated on a central shaft. On medication, hyperactive children performed much better than when on placebo. More important, medication enabled hyperactive children to act more like their nonhyperactive peers. That is, they actually learned how to balance better over time (trials). Wade argued that Ritalin helps the hyperactive child learn motor skills in the same way it affects performance on cognitive tasks.

Ritalin can have a pronounced effect on handwriting (see also Chapter 3, Learning Disabilities). Lerer et al. (1977), for example, compared the effect of placebo and Ritalin on the handwriting of 50 children diagnosed as having MBD. All had serious problems with handwriting according to their teachers. Handwriting improved in 25 of the children on medication while improvement was reported for only one child on placebo. In general, handwriting deteriorated when children who showed improvement were taken off medication. However, gains in handwriting improvement were maintained for months in children who continued to receive Ritalin.

Cognition

There are scores of stimulant drug studies with hyperactive children that have used some type of cognitive task or test to assess treatment effects in a laboratory setting, but relatively little research has been conducted on classroom learning per se. There are at least three reasons for this. One, it has been generally believed that hyperactivity and learning disabilities are basically cognitive deficits and that an understanding of these processes will ultimately lead to the discovery of the etiology of these disorders and possibly to the formulation of effective interventions. Two, it is much easier for researchers to exercise control over studies with laboratory tasks than it is to manage data collection in a public school classroom. Third, few researchers involved in the study of drug therapy have training in the assessment of academic-related behaviors. While the research with cognitive tasks appears somewhat removed from clinical management concerns, with a little effort it is possible to think of a variety of classroom activities that involve these processes.

Douglas and her colleagues (1972; Douglas & Peters, 1979) have argued rather convincingly that the distinguishing characteristic of the hyperactive child is an inability to inhibit impulsive responding and to organize and sustain attention or, in other words, a deficiency in the ability to "stop, look, and listen" (Douglas, 1972) which may stem from a compulsion to seek out stimulation, particularly in nonstimulating situations (e.g., Zentall, 1977; Zentall & Zentall, 1983). The most commonly used measures of attention and impulsivity in pharmacological studies with hyperactive children have been reaction time tasks, vigilance tasks, and Kagan's (1966) Matching Familiar Figures test. More recently, much attention has focused on paired-associate learning tasks, in problem solving strategies (e.g., match-to-sample tasks), and complex cognition.

Reaction Time

The typical reaction time (RT) task requires the child to push a button or press a lever as quickly as possible after seeing or hearing a signal (e.g., a light flash or a brief sound). One variant of this task, the delayed reaction time task, consists of a warning signal (which alerts the child to the imminent occurrence of the reaction signal), a preparatory interval, and the reaction signal. Studies have shown that hyperactive children, compared with normal control subjects, take longer to respond to the target signal (slower mean RT) and that their reaction times were much more variable (e.g., Cohen & Douglas, 1972). Ritalin produces faster and less variable RTs in hyperactive children (Ackerman et al., 1982; Cohen et al., 1971; Reid & Borkowski, 1984).

Sustained Attention

The Continuous Performance Test (CPT), developed by Rosvold et al. (1956), is a vigilance task in which a series of letters is presented one at a time on a visual display. The subject is instructed to press a lever each time a target letter (e.g., X) appears or only when it follows another designated letter (e.g., A). The CPT has been modified in a variety of ways from one study to the next, and some investigators have presented the stimuli auditorily through earphones. Hyperactive children make more errors of omission (fewer correct detections) and more errors of commission (more incorrect responses) on the CPT than normal control subjects do (e.g., Sykes et al., 1971). In addition, the performance of the hyperactive group greatly deteriorates over time, whereas that of the control group does not. A number of investigators have shown that Ritalin, compared with placebo, reduces both errors of omission and errors of commission in hyperactive children (e.g., Conners & Rothschild, 1968; Michael et al., 1981; Rapport et al., in press; Sykes et al., 1971). There are some data to suggest that commission errors continue to decrease with increasing dosage and that omission errors do not (Rapport et al., in press).

Impulsivity

One of the most widely used measures of impulsivity in children is the Matching Familiar Figures test (MFF), but its status as an impulsivity measure is somewhat controversial (see Milich & Kramer, 1984). It contains 12 tasks, each of which consists of presenting a target figure and a separate array of six figures. Five of these six figures are variations of the target figure, and one is identical to the target figure. The child is asked to identify the identical figure (by pointing) and can choose until the correct one is selected. The MFF generates both an error score (total number of incorrect figures that were selected) and a latency score (amount of time required to make the first response), which are averaged over the 12 tasks. Hyperactive children receive a much higher error score than normal controls (Quay & Brown, 1980).

Brown and Sleator (1979) reported that Ritalin significantly lowered error scores as compared with a placebo. Of particular interest was the fact that this effect was dose-related (see Figure 2–2). Improved performance was observed with a moderate dose (0.3 mg/kg) but not with a high therapeutic dose (1.0 mg/kg). In fact, there was no significant difference in error scores between the placebo and the high-dose condition. Latency scores were unaffected by medication.

Several investigators (e.g., Douglas, 1972) have commented that commission errors on the CPT are an index of impulsivity, particularly when the child is asked to respond when the target letter follows a specific letter (e.g., A). Seeing the letter A, the impulsive child responds before the target letter appears on the screen. As noted previously, Ritalin reduces commission errors.

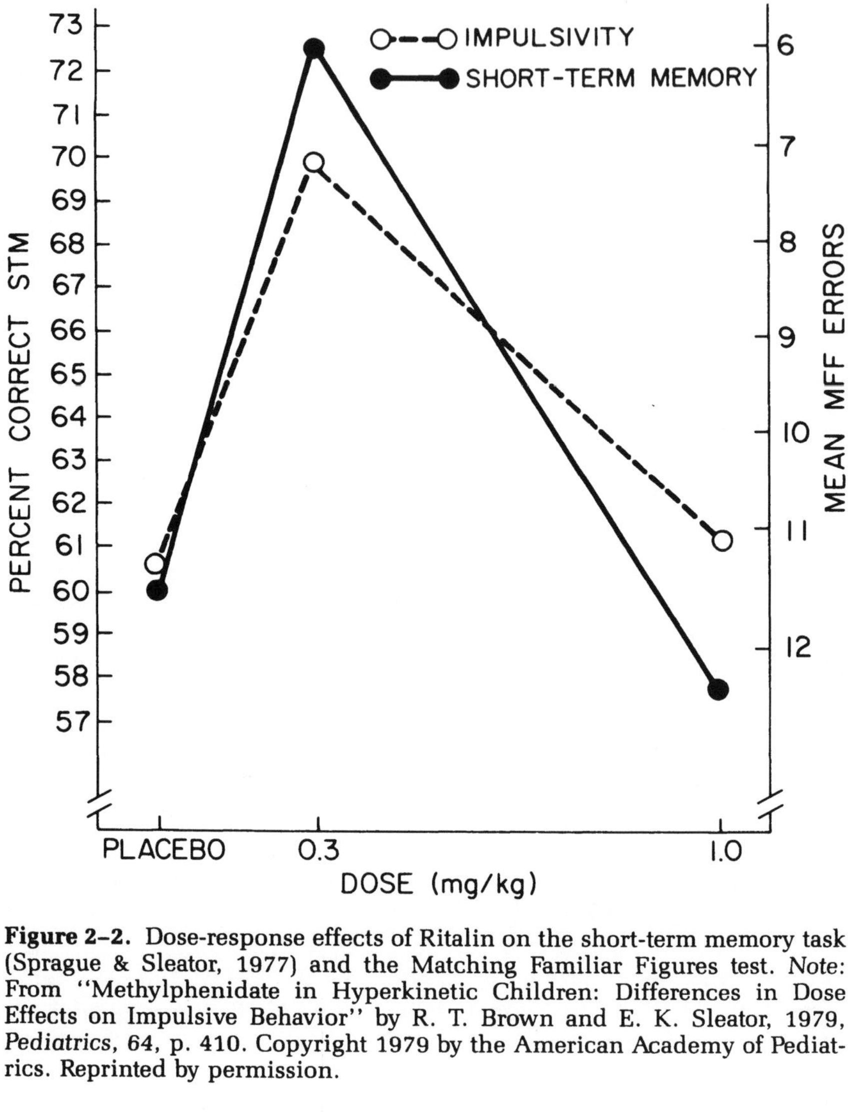

Figure 2–2. Dose-response effects of Ritalin on the short-term memory task (Sprague & Sleator, 1977) and the Matching Familiar Figures test. *Note:* From "Methylphenidate in Hyperkinetic Children: Differences in Dose Effects on Impulsive Behavior" by R. T. Brown and E. K. Sleator, 1979, *Pediatrics*, 64, p. 410. Copyright 1979 by the American Academy of Pediatrics. Reprinted by permission.

Memory

Researchers have employed memory tasks in a number of studies. One research team has used the Short-Term Memory task (STM) developed by Keith Scott (1970) to demonstrate stimulant drug effects on hyperactive children (Sprague & Sleator, 1977). For this task, the subject sits and watches what appears to be a television screen. An array of figures from children's books are flashed on the screen. Each array contains either 1, 3, 9, or 15 figures. The amount of viewing time for each array is based on the number of figures (e.g., 1 second for each). For an array of nine figures, the subject would have 9 seconds to watch and memorize. The screen momentarily becomes dark, and then a target figure (e.g., a fire truck) flashes on the screen. If the target was in the previous array, the child presses the "yes" or "same" lever; if not, he or she presses "no" or "different." A counter adds up the number of correct answers or points. The counter serves as an incentive because the points can be exchanged for items in the toy shop. Most children find this activity enjoyable and interesting. The STM task probably involves a number of mental processes, the most salient being short-term memory and sustained attention.

Studies that have compared the effects of a placebo and Ritalin in hyperactive children while they performed this task have repeatedly shown that medication significantly increases the percentage of correct answers (e.g., Sprague & Sleator, 1977). Interestingly, this effect was dose-related. Most, but certainly not all, hyperactive children perform their best when the dose of Ritalin is between 0.3 mg/kg and 0.5 mg/kg. If the dose is increased to anywhere from 0.7 mg/kg to 1.0 mg/kg, some children actually do worse on the short-term memory task. This simply indicates that if a child receives too much medication, it *may* not help him or her learn. As can be seen in Figure 2-2, the group accuracy score for the 1.0 mg/kg dose was not much different from the placebo score. In some children, a high dose may even impair cognitive performance.

Another interesting finding that emerged from the STM task research was that the effects of the medication became more pronounced as the task became more cognitively challenging (Sprague et al., 1969; Sprague & Sleator, 1977). In other words, the fact that a moderate dose was more effective than a high dose was more evident for the stimulus array with 15 pictures than for the array with 3 pictures (Figure 2-3). This suggests that simple, routine tasks such as the CPT *may* not be a very good way to study drug effects on more complex cognitive processes. More importantly, however, the adverse effects of higher therapeutic doses *may* be most detrimental when the child is learning a new complicated academic skill (e.g., learning long division) and least detrimental when the child is simply practicing a skill that is already learned (e.g., doing drill exercises).

Weingartner et al. (1980) conducted a study to differentiate between the attentional and cognitive effects of stimulant medication on hyperactive children and normal controls. They developed a word game that consisted of 20 sets of words, with three words in each set. In 10 of the sets, two of the three words were related in meaning, and in the remaining 10 sets, two of the three words rhymed. Subjects

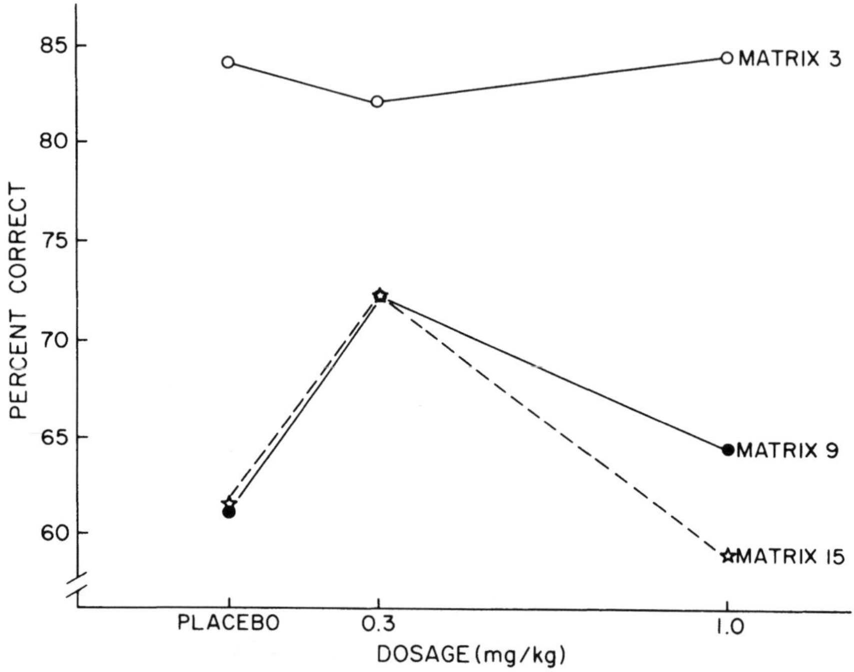

Figure 2–3. Dose-response effects of Ritalin on the short-term memory task obtained for differing levels of information load (matrix size) for hyperactive children. (Courtesy of Dr. Robert L. Sprague, Director, Institute for Child Behavior and Development, University of Illinois at Urbana-Champaign.)

were asked to identify the odd word in each set. Following the word game, each child engaged in a distractor task to prevent the rehearsal of word sets. After the distractor activity, subjects were asked to remember as many words as they could from the word game (free recall). Then, they were read one word from each word pair and were asked to recall the match word (cued recall). This activity involves the storage, processing, and retrieval of information. The hyperactive group did significantly poorer on the free recall of semantically related words than did the normal sample. Dexedrine (compared with a placebo) improved performance for semantically-related and rhyming words in both samples on free recall. For cued recall, both groups showed improvement in total recall scores. The data suggest that unlike normal children who show a preference for semantic information processing, hyperactive children rely more on acoustic processing, which may lead to weaker memory traces.

Paired-Associate Learning

A number of investigators have reported that stimulants facilitate paired-associate learning (PAL) in hyperactive children (e.g., Conners & Rothschild, 1968; Swanson & Kinsbourne, 1976). When students pair 7 + 5 with 12 in learning simple addition (e.g., flash card drill), they are engaging in paired-associate learning. Because PAL laboratory tasks more closely resemble classroom activities, they have been touted as superior to, and more meaningful than, vigilance and RT measures.

Swanson and Kinsbourne (1976, 1979) have employed a PAL task in a number of drug studies with hyperactive children. Their version of a PAL task consists of presenting a series of animal pictures. For each picture the subject is told to associate the animal with the name of a specific "zoo" labeled *north, south, east,* or *west.* The complete list of animal-zoo pairs is presented several times (trials). The actual stimulus items and the number of list presentations vary from one report to the next (Swanson & Kinsbourne, 1979). The child is praised for a correct response and is informed of the correct answer for an error. The score is the total number of errors on all trials. Using this task, Swanson and Kinsbourne reported that 30% of the hyperactive children and none of the normal controls showed improved performance (over a placebo) with Ritalin.

Interestingly, the relationship between cognitive performance and other measures of adaptive behavior such as amount of schoolwork completed accurately is not as straightforward as one would predict. A recent investigation by Rapport et al. (1985) demonstrates this point quite clearly. In this study, hyperactive children treated with stimulant medication and placebo (P) were assessed on academic performance, a PAL task, and the Abbreviated Teacher Rating. The results are presented in Figure 2-4. The "B" on the dose level scale stands for baseline (off medication). As is indicated in this figure, PAL improvement appears to level off at a dosage level below that for continuing academic improvement. The clinical implications of such findings are controversial at the present time.

Cognitive Strategies

Only recently have scientists begun to explore the effects of stimulants on problem solving behavior in hyperactive children. The tasks and skills required vary greatly and purportedly measure such things as search strategies (Dykman et al., 1980), flexible thinking (Dyme et al., 1982), information processing (Reid & Borkowski,

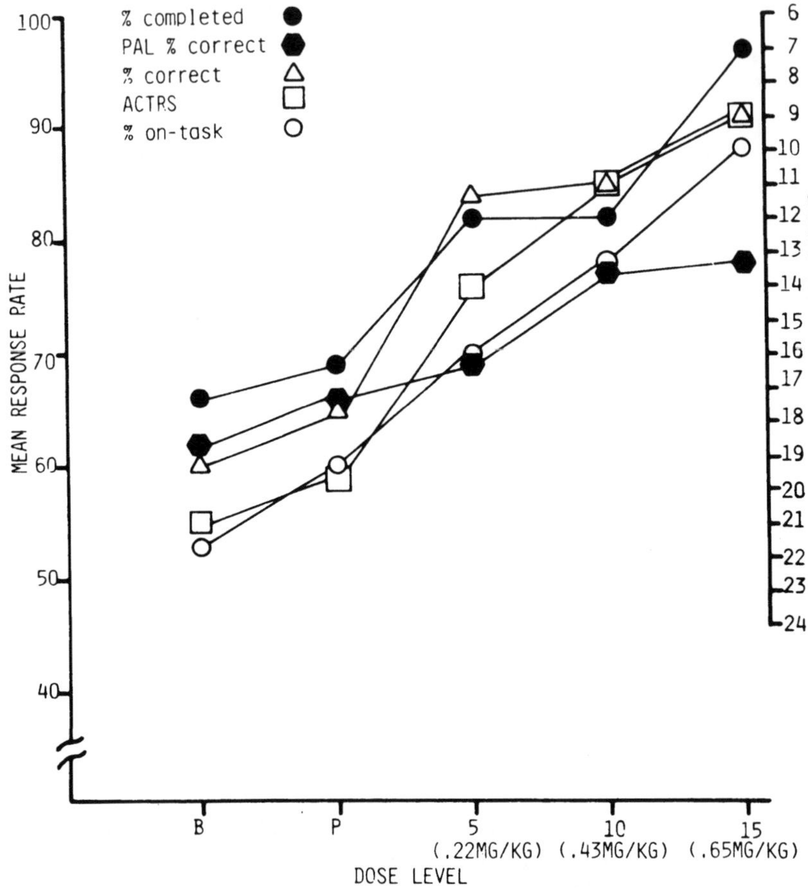

Figure 2–4. Dose-response effects of Ritalin on classroom academic assignments (% completed; % correct), classroom on-task behavior (% on task), cognitive performance (PAL % correct), and teacher ratings of classroom behavior (ACTRS). *Note:* "Methylphenidate in Hyperactive Children: Differential Effects of Dose on Academic, Learning, and Social Behavior" by M. D. Rapport et al., 1985, *Journal of Abnormal Child Psychology, 13*, p. 234. Copyright 1985 by Plenum Press. Reprinted by permission.

1984), visual scanning patterns (Flintoff et al., 1982), and inspection strategy (Sprague, 1984). It is very difficult to summarize the results from these and other studies of complex cognitive abilities, and it is probably accurate to say that much more will be known about this area in the coming years because it is a very active area of research. Nevertheless, two findings from this literature are particularly sobering and warrant special comment at the present time.

One, higher doses (1.0 mg/kg) of Ritalin may cause cognitive perseveration in some children (Dyme et al., 1982). In other words, it *may* impair problem solving ability. Two, this conclusion is reinforced in an exciting study conducted by Sprague (1984) and his coworkers using a computerized match-to-sample task that measures cognitive problem solving ability. An effective strategy for solving this task is to repeatedly inspect the sample, which can be measured as an inspection ratio. The higher the ratio, the more effective the child is in solving the problem. The results of this study are presented in Figure 2–5, which shows that the inspection ratio for a moderate dose (0.3 mg/kg) of Ritalin was much higher (4.7) than either the larger dose (0.7 mg/kg) or the placebo.

School Achievement

If stimulant medication produces such positive changes in sustained attention and paired-associate learning, what does it do for school achievement? One would guess that if stimulants can ameliorate attention deficits and improve learning ability, then children taking such medication should do better in school because they would be more able to focus on instruction. Unfortunately, after reviewing the relevant literature (17 short-term and 6 long-term studies), Barkley and Cunningham (1978) concluded that there was little support for the notion that stimulants improve academic performance. The findings from a number of more recently conducted studies, however, are causing us to rethink the drugs and achievement issue. Because school performance is so important and severe academic underachievement is a problem for some hyperactive children, an entire chapter has been devoted to this topic (see Chapter 3, Learning Disabilities).

Conduct Problems

Suppression of conduct problems is a fifth way in which stimulant drugs alter the behavior of hyperactive children. Conduct problems refer to a variety of antisocial behaviors such as noncompliance (not doing what you are told or expected to do), disturbing others, aggression, stealing, lying, and so forth. Although not all hyperactive children experience serious conduct problems, those who do are more likely to be referred for medical evaluations or placed in special education programs. Behavior rating scales are the usual means by which drug effects are documented. A number of rating instruments have been developed, but by far the most widely used is

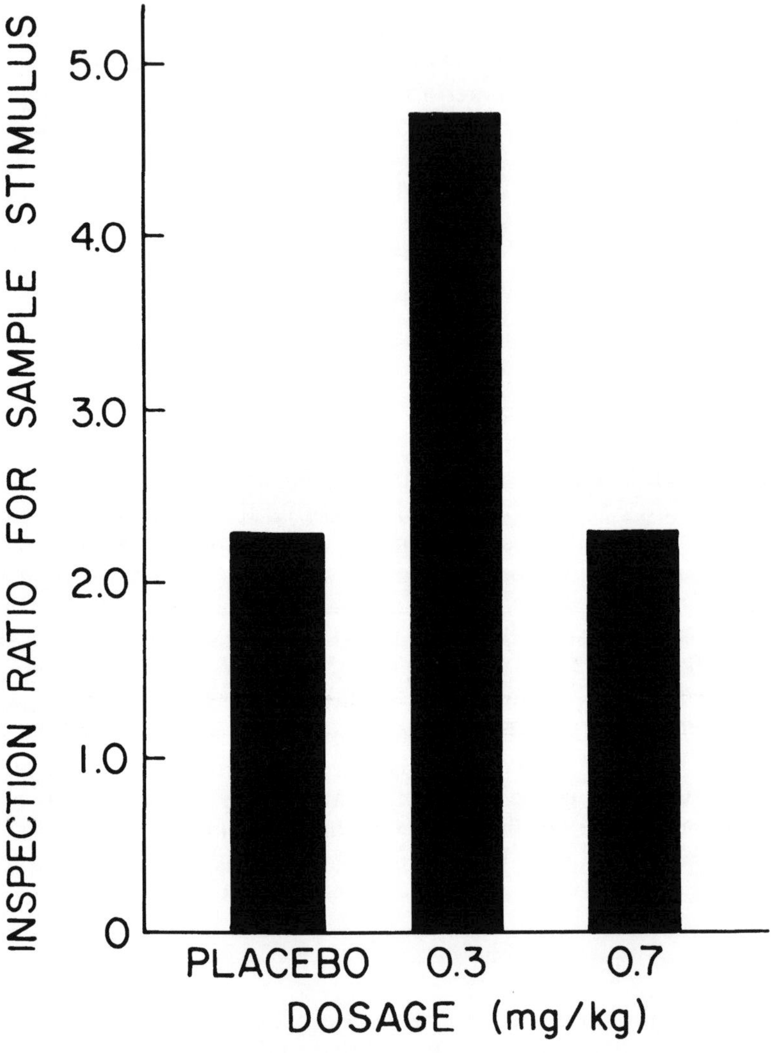

Figure 2–5. Dose-response effects of Ritalin on the inspection ratio for the sample stimulus (match-to-sample task). *Note:* From "Preliminary Report of Cross-Cultural Study and Cognitive Strategies of ADD Children" by R. L. Sprague, 1984, in *Attention Deficit Disorder: Diagnostic, Cognitive, and Therapeutic Understanding*, edited by L. M. Bloomingdale, New York: Spectrum. Copyright 1984 by Spectrum Publications. Adapted by permission.

the Teacher Rating Scale (TRS) developed by Keith Conners (Conners, 1969, 1973). An abbreviated version (Conners, 1973) of the original 39-item scale appears in Appendix B. The Abbreviated Teacher Rating Scale (ATRS) is easy to complete and takes only about 2 minutes. Each item is rated from 0 (never occurs) to 3 (occurs very often).

Unquestionably, one of the most serious conduct problems for caregivers is aggression, which can be manifested in a variety of ways: verbal aggression (e.g., cursing, name calling, malicious teasing), object aggression (e.g., breaking toys, destroying property, smashing things), symbolic aggression (e.g., feigning physical attack, making offensive gestures), and physical aggression (e.g., fighting). A number of studies have demonstrated that stimulant drugs can suppress these behaviors in hyperactive children. Allen et al. (1975), for example, found that stimulant drug treatment led to lower teacher ratings of aggressive behavior. Similarly, Amery et al. (1984) reported that the administration of Dexedrine resulted in lower parent and teacher ratings of aggressiveness as well as decreased levels fantasy and object aggression in a clinic playroom setting. Others have reported that stimulants produce a decrease in negative verbal statements and disruptiveness in the classroom (e.g., Abikoff & Gittelman, 1985; Whalen et al., 1979). Because acts of physical aggression are infrequent, particularly in classrooms (see Abikoff & Gittelman, 1985; Whalen et al., 1979) and laboratory playrooms, less is known about drug effects on this behavior. Nevertheless, given the documented evidence for other types of aggressive behavior, it seems reasonable to conclude that stimulant drugs probably decrease the frequency of acts of physical aggression as well.

Using the ATRS, teacher ratings have repeatedly shown that stimulant medication suppresses behavior problems in the classroom. Even when teachers are not told whether the child is on placebo or medication, they are very accurate evaluators of even small changes in dosage. Figure 2–6 shows teacher ratings for hyperactive children on placebo and on different doses of Ritalin. Moving from left to right, they score children the worst on placebo and best on the higher dose (0.7 mg/kg). Because certain school situations present special challenges for hyperactive children, it is not unusual for teachers to see big improvements in behavior. Parents will, of course, observe little or no change if medication is not administered on weekends or during after school hours.

When medication is effective in suppressing conduct problems, the impact on the child and family may be considerable. In clinical

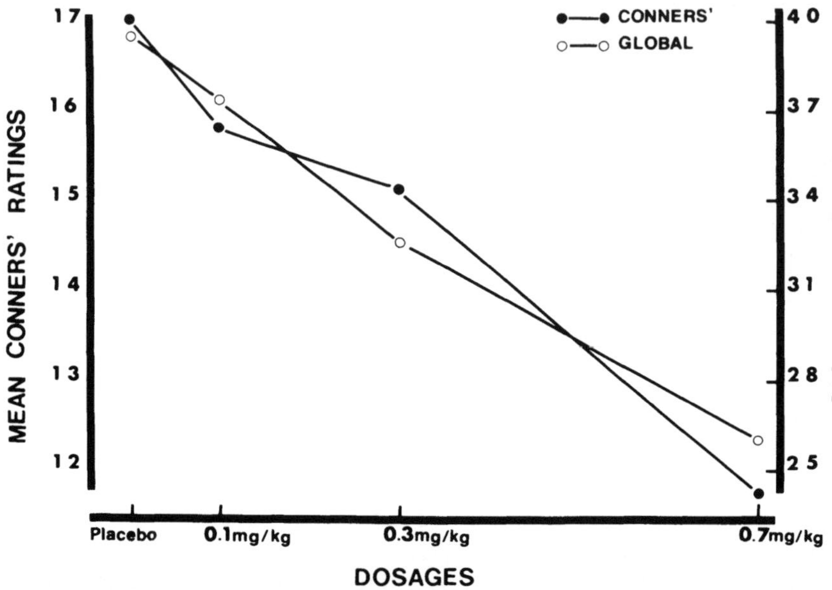

Figure 2–6. Dose-response effects of Ritalin on two different teacher rating scales. Numerical value of both scales decrease with improvement in classroom behavior. *Note:* From "Methylphenidate in the Treatment of Hyperkinetic Children" by E. K. Sleator and A. W. von Neumann, 1974, *Clinical Pediatrics, 13*, p. 23. Copyright 1974 by J. B. Lippincott Company. Reprinted by permission.

settings, it is not unusual to hear parents rejoice after receiving the first favorable report from school (E. K. Sleator, personal communication, March 13, 1978). The author can recall a father explaining how drug therapy had changed his son's ability to participate in Little League baseball. Prior to treatment, the child was unable to follow the rules, wait his turn at bat, or play cooperatively with the other children. With medication the child had become an effective member of the team. The father was very grateful, and the child was clearly pleased. Reductions in the amount of conflict at home with siblings and neighbors as well as between parents over their child's problems are also reported. After many interviews with hundreds of parents of children on medication, it is clear that drug therapy can have a significant effect on behavior outside of the classroom (Gadow, 1977). In the school, the impact of medication may appear even more dramatic. Bradley and Bowen (1941) described this reaction as follows:

> Many children began to walk and move quietly in contrast to previous noisy running and rushing about. A number spoke in a normal or lowered tone of voice instead of shouting raucously. Some of these same children, instead of quarrelling and arguing boisterously, began to avoid expressing differences of opinion or conducted their discussions in tones which were not offensive. In certain instances children appeared subdued because they began to spend their leisure time playing quietly or reading, whereas formerly they had wandered aimlessly about antagonizing and annoying others. (p. 95)

Interpersonal Relationships (Positive Social Interactions)

There are many ways in which drug-induced changes in a hyperactive child's behavior results in modifications in parent, teacher, and peer behavior. As hyperactive children become less disruptive and more compliant, others around them begin to react differently. In a certain sense, the effects of medication on appropriate social interaction is the opposite of of the coin with regard to conduct problems (negative social interactions). Changes in peer and caregiver behavior can probably be best summarized as a return to normalcy. Peers and caregivers react to the hyperactive child in ways that are more characteristic of their interactions with nonhyperactive youngsters. Unfortunately, the positive impact of medication can be limited in three ways. One, with short-acting stimulant drugs, treatment effects no doubt dissipate with time, which can make evenings a very difficult time for parents. Two, disliked children may develop bad reputations in school and in the neighborhood. While medication may make them less rejected by their peers, it does not necessarily make them loved. Third, caregivers sometimes forget to give medication regularly, and it is possible that a few "bad days" could wipe out weeks of good behavior in terms of the child being more liked by others.

Parent-Child Interactions

Much of our current knowledge about how stimulants alter parent-child interactions is found in a series of studies conducted by Russ Barkley and his colleagues. It has been shown that hyperactive children are more negative and noncompliant with their parents than nonhyperactive children (e.g., Campbell, 1975; Cunningham & Barkley, 1979). When the hyperactive youngster is administered Ritalin, mothers become less controlling and less negative in response to the improvement in their child's behavior (e.g., Barkley & Cunningham, 1979; Humphries et al., 1978). Moreover, changes in mother behavior appear to be dose-related (Barkley et al., 1984); that is, they were evident at a dose of 0.5 mg/kg administered twice a day but *not* at a low dose of 0.15 mg/kg twice a day. Barkley et al. also found evidence to support the idea that hyperactive children become more manageable as they grow older.

Teacher-Child Interactions

Just the presence of a hyperactive child in the classroom can increase disruptiveness in classmates and negative feedback in the teacher directed at the class as well as the hyperactive child (Campbell et al., 1977). Stimulant medication can alter this situation. At least one study has clearly shown that teachers react to hyperactive children receiving Ritalin much differently than when they are receiving placebo (Whalen et al., 1980). When the child is on medication, the teacher is less controlling (i.e., guidance, commands, and admonitions), less intense (i.e., vigor, loudness, rapidity, and emotionality), and less likely to call out the child's name. These findings are similar to those reported for parents.

Peer Interactions

Much has been written in recent years about the difficulties hyperactive children have getting along with other children (see Milich & Laundau, 1982; Pelham & Bender, 1982; Pelham & Milich, 1984; Whalen & Henker, 1985). Scientists and clinicians are concerned about peer relations because children who have serious difficulties interacting with other children are at much greater risk for problems in adulthood. Subsequently, peer relations and social skills training have become one of the most important topics in childhood psychopathology. Studies of stimulant drug effects on peer relations are somewhat discouraging. Bill Pelham and his colleagues (see Pelham & Bender, 1982) have conducted several studies of peer interactions, and they found that neither Ritalin nor Cylert seemed to improve peer relations that much. However, when the results were analyzed with regard to the child's level of aggressivity, a different pattern emerged. The high-aggression hyperactive children did become less aggressive and more prosocial on medication, while the low-aggression youngsters became less socially interactive. In spite of the more encouraging response to medication in the high-aggression children, Pelham and Milich (1984) suggest that both medication *and* social skills training are probably necessary to normalize peer relations in seriously disturbed youngsters.

Long-Term Therapeutic Outcome (Residual Benefits)

Because these drugs do effect striking behavioral changes in hyperactive children, it would be reasonable to conclude that treated children would do better years later than untreated children. If stimulants enhance the ability to pay attention, a child who followed rules better, got into mischief less often, and generally acted more "normal" would be expected to be better adjusted. Therefore, with treatment, one would expect a hyperactive child to have more friends, obtain better grades, and be more popular than those who are not treated.

There are a number of followup studies of hyperactive children who received medication (for reviews see Gadow, 1983; Hechtman, 1985; Ross & Ross, 1982), a few of which included a group that did not receive drug therapy. In general, research indicates that hyperactive children who were treated with medication are still different from their nonhyperactive classmates. That is, stimulant drugs do not "cure" all the behavioral concomitants of hyperactivity. Nevertheless, many clinicians who treat these children state they have had some patients who literally became "normal" while *on* medication. One should not infer that, over time, the effects of medication simply wear off. Even after several years of treatment, withdrawal of drug may lead to rapid behavioral deterioration (Sleator et al., 1974). Although medication appears to suppress deviant behavior, there is growing evidence that treated children are not significantly better off in the long run than hyperactive children who do not receive drug therapy.

It must be emphasized, however, that these results are preliminary and that much more research needs to be done. Moreover, some children may respond to treatment more favorably than others. Unfortunately, attempts to find variables that would predict a favorable response to treatment before therapy is begun have not been very successful (Barkley, 1976; Loney et al., 1978). Interestingly, there is some support for the notion that the nature and degree of hyperactivity symptoms at referral are generally unrelated to behavior at adolescence (Loney et al., 1981a). In other words, whether or not a hyperactive child will have severe problems during adolescence cannot be predicted from the severity of his or her restlessness, inattentiveness, or impulsivity when treatment first begins. However, others have found that youngsters with more severe hyperactivity symptoms are at greater risks for the development of conduct problems during adolescence (Gittelman et al., 1985), so this remains an open issue. Hyperactive adolescents who do have serious problems tend to be more aggressive, come from poorer homes, and have less controlling fathers when they were first referred for treatment (Loney et al., 1981a). If these environmental variables do play an important role in therapeutic outcome, this may explain, in part, why it is difficult to document long-term benefits from medication.

Perhaps one of the more thoughtful conclusions that can be drawn at this time is that caregivers should not become sanguine about the needs of the hyperactive child just because medication is suppressing behavior problems. Special efforts must be made to ameliorate learning problems and developmental delays and to facilitate the acquisition of social skills. In their followup study, Weiss et al. (1979) asked their hyperactive subjects " 'what had helped them most during their childhood.' The commonest responses regarded one parent (nearly always the mother) who believed in their final success, a teacher who seemed to turn the tide of failure, or discovering that they had some special talent" (p. 680).

General Comments

The findings from drug studies clearly indicate that stimulants diminish what Douglas (1972) referred to as an inability to "stop, look, and listen." In fact, the evidence is so compelling that Gittelman-Klein et al. (1976a) commented:

> No rational, knowledgeable individual can dispute the efficacy of short-term stimulant treatment in the management of hyperkinetic children. Of all the therapies in child psychiatry, it is the best documented. (p. 362)

Drug-induced changes in child behavior can be so dramatic that parents and teachers occasionally comment that "he's a different child" or "it's like night and day." Studies of hyperactive children on medication and normal children in regular classrooms show that stimulants do normalize many behaviors (e.g., Abikoff & Gittelman, 1985; Whalen et al., 1979, 1980).

Given the aforementioned list of ways in which stimulant medication can help hyperactive children, one might conclude that they are some type of miracle drug. For some children, they probably are. However, several notes of caution are warranted. First, there are many children for whom stimulants do not work at all. Figures vary, but approximately 30% of the hyperactive children who are scheduled for a trial of medication fail to show a clinically meaningful degree of improvement in their behavior. Some youngsters even become worse on medication! Unfortunately, there is no way to tell whether medication is going to work other than to have the child take it. Second, children who respond to medication do not experience the same degree of improvement in all of the academic, cognitive, and social behaviors described in this chapter. For some people this is a very difficult notion to come to grips with. Even back in the 1930s when scientists were studying the effects of Benzedrine in normal volunteers (e.g., Turner & Carl, 1939) and behavior disordered children (Bradley, 1937), it was realized that reaction to stimulants was variable and dependent upon the task the person was asked to do. Moreover, improvement in one area did not necessarily mean that there would be improvement in another, although some subjects did do better in both. Because scientists generally present their findings as *group* averages, these individual differences are often obscured in most drug studies with hyperactive children. One might well ask, "Why is response to medication so variable?"

At least two things are going on here. First, as we have already noted, the dose of medication is important. Low and high doses appear to produce different effects on different behaviors. Second, stimulants appear to affect different areas of the brain in different ways in different people. Put much more eloquently by Weingartner et al. (1982), "it is likely that amphetamine has multiple, possibly independent actions and that different children may benefit differentially" (p. 28).

Clinicians once believed that stimulants had a "paradoxical" calming effect on hyperactive children (Millichap, 1975). Because no one had ever studied the effects of these drugs in normal youngsters, it was unknown whether or not the decreased motor restlessness observed in hyperactive children receiving medication was truly "paradoxical." However, this question was resolved when a research team at the National Institute of Mental Health administered both Dexedrine and placebo to 14 normal prepubertal boys (Rapoport et al., 1978). The results showed that these nonhyperactive children responded to stimulants in much the same way as children diagnosed as hyperactive. On a dose of 0.5 mg/kg, nonhyperactive children were significantly less active than when on placebo. They also made fewer CPT errors and were able to learn and remember more words on a memory task. In addition, language performance, which was measured through picture descriptions, storytelling, and instructions to a listener, also improved. The drug seemed to help the child focus attention on these activities, as evidenced by increased task-related speech and decreased nontask-related speech. A sample of normal adults who were administered this drug showed a similar pattern of results (Rapoport et al., 1980). Only the adults, however, reported an elevation of mood or euphoric reaction to Dexedrine. These results with nonhyperactive students and normal adults are clearly contrary to the idea of a paradoxical effect of stimulant drugs for hyperactive children.

Some might infer that stimulants are unwarranted as a treatment because they do not affect hyperactive children in some special way. However, this situation is not unusual in medicine. For example, Rapoport et al. (1978) pointed out that diuretics are used in the treatment of congestive heart failure even though these drugs alter the bodily functions of normal adults and cardiac patients in the same manner.

SIDE EFFECTS OF STIMULANT DRUGS

At moderate doses, stimulant drugs produce few serious side effects and are generally considered to be quite safe. At the onset of drug treatment, the two most common adverse reactions are insomnia and anorexia (loss of appetite). Insomnia is typically not a problem if medication is administered only in the morning, but many children receive a dose at noon, and some even get medication late in the day. If such a schedule is necessary, the physician may prescribe an additional drug in the evening (e.g., Benadryl) to induce sleep (Arnold, 1973). Anorexia can usually be managed by taking the pill just before meals. Other minor side effects are also possible. These include headache, stomachache, nausea, moodiness, irritability, and increased talkativeness. Children typically develop a tolerance for these side effects, but the dose may have to be reduced and gradually increased to lessen the degree of discomfort.

Perhaps the most distressing side effects for parents and teachers are changes in appearance and mood and the suppression of adaptive behavior. Change in appearance has been described as an "amphetamine look" by Laufer et al. (1957):

> A pale, pinched, serious facial expression with dark hollows under the eyes. It is of no serious consequence but the parents must be prepared for adverse comment concerning the child's appearance. (p. 471)

They also report a marked decrease in activity:

> Sometimes, if too high a dosage [of Dexedrine] is given, the counteraction of the syndrome may go to the extreme of "freezing the patient" or fixating him to what he is doing, and may even put him to sleep. (p. 470)

Changes in activity level are not always appreciated if they are extreme. Parents sometimes comment that their child is "overly quiet," "stares into space," or "has a stillness about him that I don't like" (Gadow, 1977, p. 35). These extreme changes in activity level and mood prompt teachers and parents to describe some children treated with stimulants as looking like "zombies" (Sprague & Gadow, 1976). Interestingly, Rapoport et al. (1978) found in their study of normal boys that Dexedrine made them appear "unusually inactive, not simply less restless" (p. 562).

Changes in mood may give the appearance of depression. Schain and Reynard (1975) reported that 6.4% of the 6 to 12 year old children in their study became withdrawn, lethargic, and apathetic on Ritalin. The prevalance of these reactions is evidently higher among preschool-age children (see Chapter 5, "Early Childhood," for a detailed description of these reactions). Other changes in mood include weepiness, irritability, euphoria, and fearfulness.

Drowsiness, a side effect one would not ordinarily associate with stimulants, is sometimes reported by parents and teachers of young children (Gadow, 1982a). This effect of stimulants also appears in older children as well as in adults (Montagu & Swarbrick, 1975; Tecce and Cole, 1974).

The cognitive side effects of stimulant drugs have been demonstrated most clearly on tasks that require paired-associate learning (Swanson et al., 1978) and "flexibility in thinking" (Robbins & Sahakian, 1979). There are at least two types of reactions. One group of children does more poorly on cognitive tasks regardless of the dose of stimulant medication. A second group shows performance deterioration only when the dosage of medication is too high. It appears as if they get too much of a good thing. Medication improves attention span to the point where the child is "overfocused." On tasks that require problem-solving ability, the child exhibits perseverative errors (makes the same mistake over and over). Because these reactions are difficult to diagnose without the aid of an actual laboratory task, clinicians have generally recommended more conservative dosages in their suggested guidelines for treatment. Although there is little evidence that these drugs can impair classroom academic activities, the findings from two studies certainly suggest that higher doses of medication *may* suppress academic productivity in some children (see Rapport et al., 1982; Sulzbacher, 1972). Nevertheless, this possibility has yet to be proved.

The management of these reactions varies depending upon the clinician. Some believe that treatment should be discontinued when medication produces pronounced mood changes or suppression of adaptive behavior (Schain & Reynard, 1975; Schleifer et al., 1975), whereas others see this as an indication to decrease dosage (Safer &

Allen, 1976). Esther Sleator, research pediatrician at the Institute for Child Behavior and Development, stated that she observed these reactions in hyperactive children primarily on higher dosages of Ritalin (greater than 0.7 mg/kg). She also noted that reducing the dosage not only eliminates this side effect in most children but produces a more desirable therapeutic response from the standpoint of cognitive performance (Sleator, 1978).

Other possible side effects of stimulant medication do not occur very often but should be monitored nevertheless. One type is involuntary movements of muscles. They include a variety of actions such as protrusion of the mouth, grimacing, facial tics (*spasm* or twitching of the facial muscles), *choreo-athetoid* (jerking and writhing) movements of arms or legs, and twisting of the head and neck (e.g., Denkla et al., 1976; Gadow, 1982a; Husain et al., 1980; Mattson & Calverley, 1968; Robbins & Sahakian, 1979; Rapport et al., 1982). These drugs can cause stereotypies such as nail biting or lead to an increase in the frequency of stereotypies or tics in children who already have these problems prior to treatment (e.g., Robbins & Sahakian, 1979; Wulbert & Dries, 1977). In some cases, these side effects will abate by simple reduction of the dosage. In others, treatment may have to be discontinued or the child switched to a different drug.

There have been reports of stimulant-induced hallucinations (Lucas & Weiss, 1971) and psychosis (Greenberg et al., 1972), but this is considered a rare phenomenon. A child who experiences such a reaction may complain about "hearing things" or talk in a strange or bizzare manner. Discontinuation of medication is recommended.

It is reported that treatment with stimulant drugs can cause seizures in children who are brain-damaged, have abnormal EEGs, or are prone to develop a seizure disorder (e.g., Millichap, 1968, 1969, 1973). The package insert for Ritalin, for example, contains a warning to this effect. It is further recommended (Millichap, 1973) that youngsters who are suspected of being at risk should also be treated with Dilantin (phenytoin) as a *prophylactic measure* (i.e., to prevent the possibility of seizures occurring). While it is difficult to find evidence for this reaction, the author is familiar with a few purported cases of Ritalin-induced seizures. Nevertheless, the risk of seizure disorder subsequent to stimulant drug therapy is rare. Moreover, stimulants are used with apparent impunity with many children who receive pharmacotherapy for both seizure disorders and hyperactivity (see Gadow, 1982b).

Stimulant drugs also have an effect on the cardiovascular system. Ritalin, for example, has been shown to increase both blood pressure and heart rate (Ballard et al., 1976). Although there is considerable variability across children in terms of the degree of increase in heart rate and blood pressure, the higher the dose of Ritalin, the greater the effect. At lower dosages (0.3 to 0.5 mg/kg), these side effects are usually negligible and do not appear to have any adverse effect on the child even after long-term treatment (Hechtman et al., 1984b; Satterfield et al., 1980).

Parents are often concerned about the long-term side effects of stimulant drug use. Although the benign, short-term side effects of Ritalin and Dexedrine are well documented, only a few studies have investigated potential long-term adverse drug reactions. There are a number of problems inherent in conducting well-controlled follow-up studies, problems not peculiar to the area of stimulants and hyperactive children. For example, little is known about the long-term consequences of toxic blood levels of antiepileptic drugs (Reynolds, 1975). This is interesting because Dilantin (phenytoin), one of the most frequently prescribed antiepileptic drugs, was first reported in the treatment of epilepsy only 1 year after stimulants were discovered to have a therapeutic effect on children with behavior disorders (Bradley, 1937; Merritt & Putnam, 1938). The only long-term side effects of Ritalin or Dexedrine that have been reported so far are small changes in height and weight gain (Safer & Allen, 1973a). That is, children who receive Dexedrine or fairly high doses of Ritalin (e.g., Mattes & Gittelman, 1983), gain less height and weight than would have been expected had they not been placed on medication. When drug treatment is stopped, children show a *growth rebound*, an increase in growth rate that compensates for the slower rate while on medication (Safer et al., 1975). In contrast, well-controlled studies of hyperactive children receiving low and moderate doses of Ritalin have failed to demonstrate growth suspension (Kalachnik et al., 1982; McNutt et al., 1977).

The Pediatric Advisory Panel of the Food and Drug Administration reviewed the available literature about stimulants and growth suppression (Roche et al., 1979) and concluded that "stimulant drugs, particularly in the 'high normal' dose range, moderately suppress growth in weight . . . (but) early growth suppression during treatment is no longer evident in adulthood" (p. 849). A recent study of adults who were treated with stimulants when younger found no adverse effect on either weight or height (Hechtman et al., 1984b). Nevertheless, because some children may be affected to a greater degree than others, treatment should be carefully monitored and drug-free periods (summer vacation, holidays) should be scheduled when possible.

As for other biological processes, the research is limited. Nevertheless, at present there is no evidence that long-term treatment with Ritalin (approximately 0.25 mg/kg given twice a day) adversely affects the functioning of the liver, the endocrine system, or the cardiovascular system (Satterfield et al., 1980).

DRUG ABUSE

Perhaps one of the biggest concerns parents have about the use of stimulant (and other) medication for hyperactive children is the risk of drug abuse. They often want to know if their child (a) will become physically dependent upon stimulant medication and seek it out like a drug addict after the doctor decides that it is time to stop treatment, (b) will get into the habit of taking prescription medication to solve their problems, and (c) will become a drug addict as a teenager or adult because stimulants are one class of drug that are abused by adults. The answer to all of these questions is "no." Several studies have been conducted on this subject (see Kramer & Loney, 1982, for a review), and there is little evidence for such a risk. One study (Gadow & Sprague, 1980) of adolescents who were treated with stimulants for hyperactivity found few differences between them and a group of nonhyperactive adolescents in terms of regular substance use (see Figure 2–7). In fact, the two groups of youths were almost identical with regard to "regular" coffee, cigarette, and alcohol use and having used marijuana regularly at some time. While it is true that some studies show that hyperactive individuals, *as a group*, experiment with a wider array of substances (Hechtman et al., 1984a; Weiss et al., 1979), during any given year they are fairly similar to their peers with regard to substance use.

REBOUND EFFECT OF STIMULANT DRUGS

For parents, a most frustrating reaction to stimulant treatment is a transient increase in the severity of their child's behavior problems, which occurs when the therapeutic benefits of the drug wear off, usually in the late afternoon or early evening. This may also be a problem when drug-free periods are scheduled on weekends. Presumably, the level of the drug in the blood drops, and the child

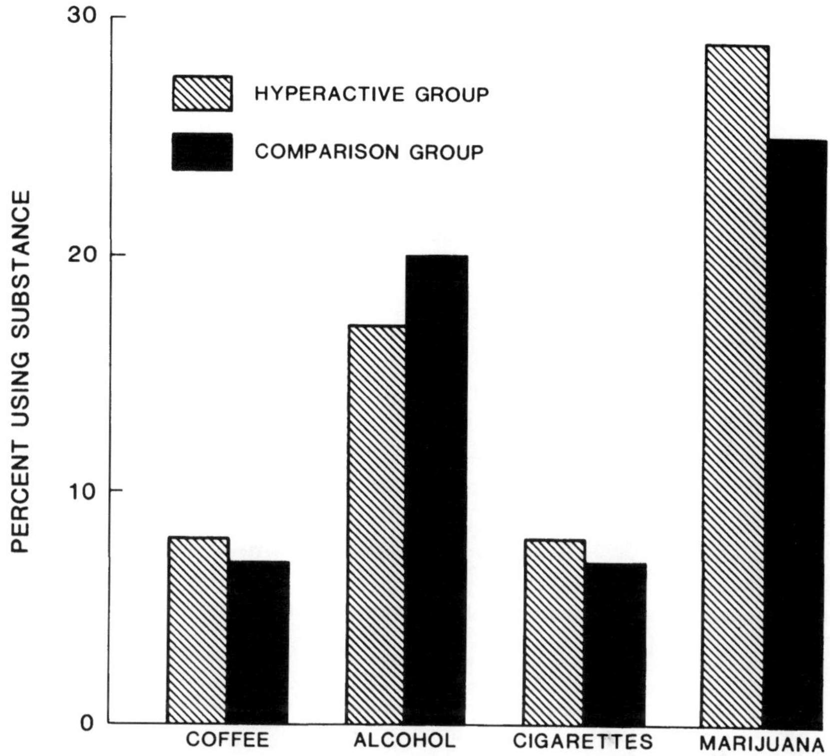

Figure 2–7. Use of substances on a regular basis as reported by adolescents treated at one time with stimulant medication for hyperactivity and classroom peers. *Note:* From "An Anterospective Follow-Up of Hyperactive Children into Adolescence: Licit and Illicit Drug Use" by K. D. Gadow and R. L. Sprague, 1980, paper presented at the meeting of the American Psychological Association, Montreal.

experiences a drug withdrawal reaction, which is referred to as a *rebound effect*. The child may become irritable and even more hyperactive than usual. In their study of the effects of Dexedrine on normal (nonhyperactive) boys, Rapoport et al. (1978) found that 10 of the 14 children demonstrated "behavioral overactivity" approximately 5 hours after taking medication. Other signs of a rebound effect were "excitability, talkativeness, and for three children apparent euphoria" (p. 562). Although there are reports in the literature describing this phenomenon in hyperactive children (Katz et al., 1975; Werry & Sprague, 1974), the problems this may cause the family or the school are not always emphasized.

PATTERN OF TREATMENT

Information from both the medical literature and various surveys indicate that stimulant drugs are prescribed for people of all ages who are diagnosed as hyperactive. They are used with infants, toddlers, and preschoolers (see Chapter 5), as well as elementary school children and adolescents. Others, too, have found these agents to be useful in the treatment of adults with MBD (Mann & Greenspan, 1976; Wender et al., 1985).

Duration of Effect

Stimulants are relatively short-acting drugs. Their behavioral effects can be observed within a half hour after the medicine is taken orally. A 10 mg tablet of Ritalin produces a therapeutic effect for approximately 3 to 4 hours, and a 20 mg tablet lasts for at least an hour longer (Carter, 1956; Safer & Allen, 1976). There is a time release form of Dexedrine (Dexedrine Spansule) that produces a longer lasting effect than the tablets, approximately 12 hours. Also, a long-lasting (8 hours) form of Ritalin called Ritalin-SR is now available. The SR stands for "sustained-release." According to one report, one 20 mg tablet of Ritalin-SR administered at breakfast produces a therapeutic effect equivalent to a 10 mg tablet of regular Ritalin given twice a day (Whitehouse et al., 1980). Children on amphetamine or Ritalin show their best performance approximately 2 hours after taking medication (Bradley & Bowen, 1941; Swanson et al., 1978). Four hours after ingestion of the drug, it has already lost half of its peak effectiveness.

Schedule

Using behavioral ratings, some researchers have demonstrated that one dose of medication in the morning may be adequate for an entire school day (Safer & Allen, 1973b; Sleator & von Neumann, 1974; Sprague et al., 1974). However, many hyperactive children treated with Ritalin or Dexedrine are given a dose in the morning, and between 60 to 80% receive an additional dose at noon (Gadow, 1981; Krager & Safer, 1974; Safer & Krager, 1984). Stimulants are also given late in the day. One survey of hyperactive preschoolers reported that 28% of the treated children received Ritalin or Dexedrine in the evening (Gadow, 1977). The parents of these children said the medication helped their child go to sleep at night. One study that used Dexedrine Spansules found that an evening dose was beneficial for sleep problems in elementary school–aged hyperactive children (Chatoor et al., 1983). Parents noted that medication made the children more cooperative at bedtime. What probably happens is that the rebound effect makes going to bed extremely difficult for some hyperactive children who receive their last dose of medication at noon or late afternoon (see also Kinsbourne, 1973). Interestingly, the findings from the preschool study suggest that the practice of administering evening medication has been going on for some time. Moreover, Livingston et al. (1973) have been treating nocturnal seizures with Dexedrine Spansules administered at bedtime for many years.

Cylert, which is a long-acting stimulant, is administered once each day in the morning. The dose is usually 37.5 mg at first, and it may be increased to 75 mg per day (Safer & Allen, 1976). The dosage ratio of Ritalin to Cylert ranges from 1:4 to 1:6 (Pelham, 1983; Stephens et al., 1984). In other words, the behavioral effect produced by 0.3 mg/kg of Ritalin administered twice a day is similar to the effect produced by 1.9 mg/kg of Cylert given once a day.

Dosage

There is some disagreement as to what is the best dose or dosage range for Ritalin and Dexedrine. Some clinicians (e.g., Sleator & von Neumann, 1974) have found that moderate dosages (0.3 mg/kg to 0.5 mg/kg) of Ritalin are quite effective, while other experts (e.g., Klein et al., 1980, p. 674) believe that low dosages, such as 0.3 mg/kg are *homeopathic* (subtherapeutic) and may account for cases of drug failure. Children do differ greatly in terms of optimal dosage. Some do quite well on a low dose, whereas others appear unchanged unless the dose is very high. For this reason, most clinicians start out with a small dose that is gradually increased until the desired effect is achieved. There are obviously general guidelines for maximal and minimal limits. The average *daily* dose of Ritalin is usually 20 to 30 mg, with a morning dose of 10 to 20 mg and a noon dose of 10 mg (Safer & Allen, 1976). Others have also found that the optimal dose (for paired-associate learning) of Ritalin is 10 to 15 mg for most, but certainly not all, elementary school–aged children (Swanson et al., 1978). It is not unusual, however, to find reports that state that the average *daily* dose of Ritalin is 60 mg or that some children are receiving as much as 120 to 140 mg per day (Gittelman-Klein & Klein, 1976; Renshaw, 1974).

It is common clinical lore that Dexedrine is twice as potent as Ritalin and, therefore, the average dose of Dexedrine is half that for

Ritalin (Safer & Allen, 1976). However, comparisons between the two drugs with regard to performance on a laboratory task suggest that dose effects may be fairly similar (Sprague & Sleator, 1976). In actual practice, the daily dosages of Ritalin and Dexedrine prescribed by physicians appear to be comparable (Gadow, 1981).

Multiple-Drug Therapy

Children on medication for hyperactivity rarely receive more than one type of drug per day for that condition. An additional drug may be administered in the evening to induce sleep, such as an antianxiety agent (Atarax, Vistaril, or Valium), Benadryl, or a hypnotic. Some children, however, are treated with a combination of (a) Ritalin and Mellaril, (b) Ritalin and Tofranil, or (c) Tofranil and Mellaril (Gittelman-Klein et al., 1976b; Katz et al., 1975), but these combinations are used infrequently in everyday practice (Gadow, 1981; Safer & Krager, 1984).

Dosage Issues

It is the opinion of some clinicians and scientists who work in this area that traditional approaches to the treatment of psychiatric disorders have overemphasized symptom suppression and overlooked the psychosocial implications of impairing adaptive behavior. One important series of studies, originally initiated in the late 1960s and continued up to the present time, has addressed this issue by studying the dose-response effects of Ritalin, Dexedrine, and neuroleptics on a variety of cognitive, academic, and behavioral measures (e.g., Sprague, 1984; Sprague et al., 1969; Sprague & Sleator, 1977). The findings from one study are presented here for purposes of discussion.

The relationship between dose of Ritalin and cognitive performance, classroom behavior, and heart rate is presented in Figure 2–8. Learning (solid black line) refers to the child's performance (percent of correct answers) on the STM task, which has already been described. Most (65%) hyperactive children gave more correct answers with a 0.3 mg/kg dose compared with placebo (10%) and a higher dose, 1.0 mg/kg (25%). It appears that if the dose is increased even more, Ritalin will significantly impair performance on the STM task. This same dose relationship also holds for *latency of response* (the amount of time that elapses before responding). In other words, hyperactive children take less time to answer and, therefore, appear less inattentive. Inappropriate classroom behavior, however, becomes less and less apparent as the amount of medica-

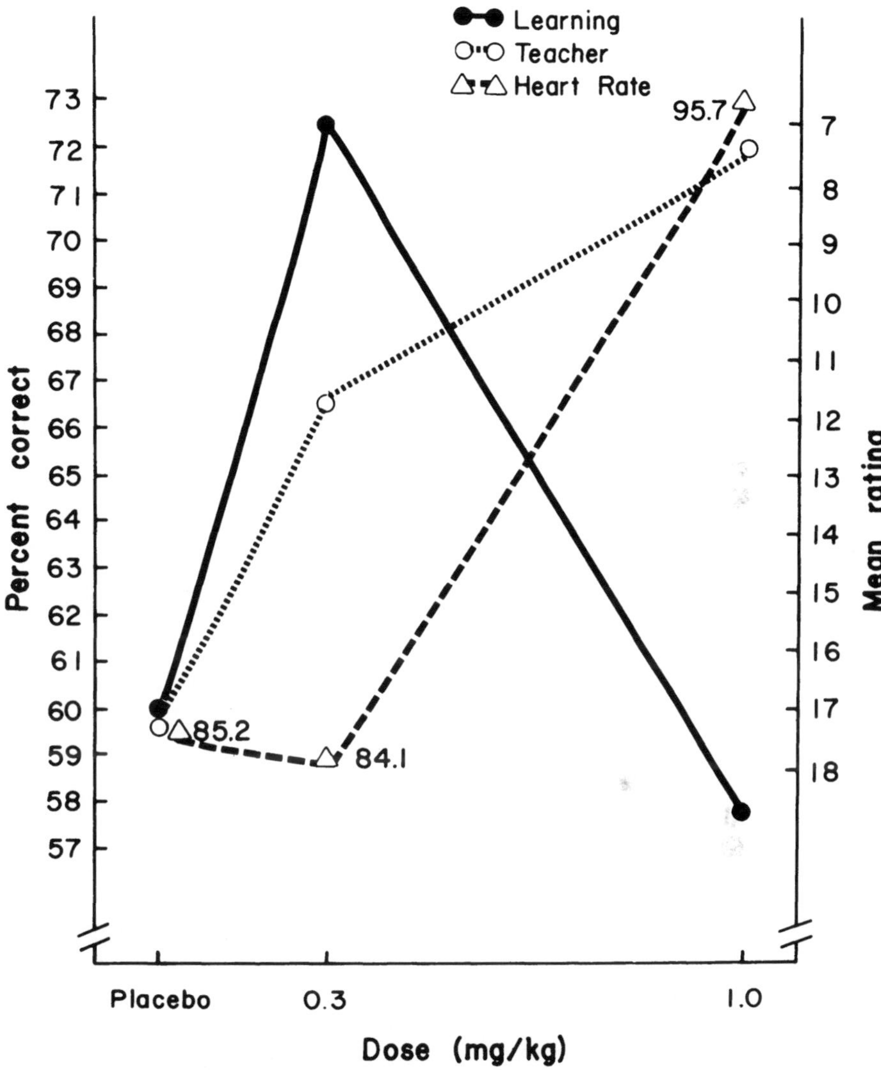

Figure 2–8. Dose-response effects of Ritalin on the short-term memory task with matrix size = 15 (learning), teacher ratings of classroom behavior (teacher), where smaller numbers indicate better behavior, and heart rate is in beats per minute. *Note:* From "Methylphenidate in Hyperkinetic Children: Differences in Dose Effects on Learning and Social Behavior" by R. L. Sprague and E. K. Sleator, 1977, *Science*, *198*, p. 1275. Copyright 1977 by the American Association for the Advancement of Science. Reprinted by permission.

tion is increased (dotted line). Using the ATRS, teachers rated 72% of the hyperactive children as behaving their best on the highest dose. Only 28% received their best ATRS scores on 0.3 mg/kg, and none of the children showed their greatest improvement in behavior on placebo. The optimal dose of Ritalin for certain classroom behaviors is, therefore, clearly different than that for concentrating on a laboratory memory task. Although the dosage differences for these two behaviors are significant in and of themselves, side effects are also important. As illustrated, heart rate (dashed line) increases as the dose becomes larger. (Although the degree of increase may not be clinically important, it must be remembered that these are group averages.) The point where teachers perceive the most improved classroom behavior is also associated with side effects. This does not mean that teachers actually preferred the higher dose. In many cases, although they rate the behavior as being better, they also often comment that the child's behavior is too controlled (e.g., overly quiet) by the higher dose.

The results of the Sprague and Sleator (1977) study imply that careful consideration should be given to dosage adjustment and to the selection of treatment objectives. If higher doses are required to control severe behavior problems, side effects should be carefully monitored. Caregivers should evaluate drug effects on positive behaviors as well such as appropriate social interaction, academic performance, and so forth. One may well wonder what dosages are typically used by physicians in everyday practice. Although data are limited, it appears that physicians prescribe conservatively, employing low and moderate doses of stimulant drugs (Gadow, 1981; Sprague & Sleator, 1975).

Duration of Treatment

The length of time a particular child is treated with medication depends upon many things. Because stimulants can ameliorate the problems associated with hyperactivity at any age, it is possible that drug treatment could last for many years with some children. Gittelman-Klein et al. (1976b) reported that 5% of the hyperactive children in their study no longer required medication after 3 months of treatment. Sleator et al. (1974), in a followup study of 42 hyperactive children, reported that 26% no longer required medication after 2 years of treatment. Solomons (1973) reported on a followup study of 97 hyperactive children who were treated by family physicians. In that study, the average duration of treatment was 39 months for children still on medication and 27 months for those no longer receiving drug treatment. It is clear that while some children require drug therapy for relatively short periods, others are maintained on medication either continuously or intermittently for many years. Pediatricians who treat relatively large numbers of hyperactive children have commented that some of their patients are maintained on medication through high school and into college if necessary.

Because there is no real way to tell if drug therapy is still necessary other than by a dosage reduction or, more typically, a temporary break in treatment, drug-free periods are an important aspect of followup care. Some clinicians have stated that by starting the child in school off medication, the continued need for treatment can be reassessed on a yearly basis (Arnold, 1973).

Termination of Medication

Although there is no shortage of discussion with regard to placing a child on medication or making diagnostic decisions, there has been little research about how to terminate treatment. O'Leary and Pelham (1978) conducted a study in which seven hyperactive children receiving stimulants were taken off medication and subsequently treated with behavior therapy. Before treatment was started, each child was placed on placebo for a short time to determine how bad his classroom behavior really was. When the study began, medication was either stopped immediately or terminated after gradual dosage reduction. For 4 months, the child's teacher and family were guided by a behavioral therapist while implementing behavior modification techniques. The main focus of the treatment program was the child's social behavior (conduct problems). The following month, both teacher and family carried out the program on their own. At the end of the fifth month, the children were reevaluated. The results showed dramatic improvement in social behavior to the point where the hyperactive children were not significantly different from their peers. The investigators noted that although the effects of their drug withdrawal and behavioral treatment program were encouraging, "behavior therapy is more expensive than drug treatment and should not be expected to benefit families who are not well motivated to attempt such an alternative to medication" (p. 216).

Very little information is available about how and why medication is terminated in real-world settings. Two studies in which the parents of hyperactive children were interviewed showed that therapeutic improvement was *not* the major reason for stopping drug therapy (Gadow, 1981). Parents often cite side effects, rebound effects, acquired tolerance for therapeutic response, and failure of the drug to work effectively as reasons for taking their child off medication. One of the major reasons why medication is stopped during adolescence is that teenagers often refuse to take pills because it sets them apart from their peers and contributes to feelings of being "different" (Safer & Allen, 1975; Sleator et al., 1982).

NONSTIMULANT DRUGS

As previously stated, not all hyperactive children respond favorably to stimulant medication. In such cases, the physician may give an alternative agent for a trial period. A wide variety of nonstimulant drugs have been used, including neuroleptics, antidepressants, antianxiety agents, antiepileptics, and others. These alternative agents are more likely to be used with children who have severe problems or multiple handicaps, or both (Gadow, 1981). For children who are severely overactive and aggressive or who are mentally retarded or emotionally disturbed and have serious behavior problems (which may be accompanied by motor restlessness, impulsivity, and short attention span), neuroleptics are sometimes given when stimulant drugs fail to be clinically useful. In fact, the neuroleptics are the second most frequently prescribed drugs for these children (Gadow, 1985a). Even children who are considered to be "typically" hyperactive appear to respond favorably to neuroleptic medication (e.g., Gittelman-Klein et al., 1976b). The three most commonly prescribed neuroleptics for childhood behavior disorders are Mellaril (thioridazine), Thorazine (chlorpromazine), and Haldol (haloperidol), and a detailed discussion of their use with children and adolescents appears in Chapter 4 (Mental Retardation) and in the companion volume, respectively. In general, neuroleptics are prescribed only when necessary because they are associated with a greater risk of side effects (compared with stimulants), and do not appear to improve cognitive performance except at very low dosages (see Werry et al., 1980).

Tofranil (imipramine) is a tricyclic antidepressant drug that has been used to treat behavior disorders in children since 1965 (Rapoport, 1965), and was once considered the drug of second choice for the treatment of hyperactivity on the basis of findings from several studies (e.g., Rapoport et al., 1974; Werry et al., 1980). The total daily dose ranges from 50 to 180 mg, usually divided into three doses of 50 mg or 75 mg per day (Winsberg et al., 1976). In terms of body weight, the usual starting dose for a hyperactive child is 1 mg/kg with an upper maximum limit of 5 mg/kg per day (Hayes et al., 1975). The major side effects are drowsiness, dizziness, dry mouth, profuse sweating, nausea, increased appetite, weight gain, and weight loss. Many children appear to develop a tolerance to the therapeutic response (Quinn & Rapoport, 1975). Some serious side effects have been reported. For example, Tofranil may lower the seizure threshold, especially in brain damaged children (Brown et al., 1973). Also, one death, possibly due to a cardiotoxic reaction, has been reported in the case of a 6-year-old girl who was administered 300 mg (14 mg/kg) of Tofranil in one dose before bed for the treatment of school phobia (Saraf et al., 1974). A major use of tricyclic antidepressants (particularly Tofranil) with children and adolescents is in the treatment of enuresis and depression, respectively, which is discussed in the companion volume.

The antihistamine Benadryl (diphenhydramine) is sometimes used with hyperactive children. Fish (1971) found the drug particularly effective with children who had severe behavior problems. It is also administered at bedtime to calm a child down (Arnold, 1973). The dose to induce sleep is 50 to 100 mg, and, for daytime use, 100 to 200 mg per day (Safer & Allen, 1976).

Two antianxiety agents, Atarax (hydroxyzine hydrochloride) and Vistaril (hydroxyzine pamoate), are used infrequently. Their effectiveness in the management of hyperactivity is questionable, but they may be used in the evening to induce sleep (Gadow, 1977; Greenberg et al., 1972).

WHEN IS MEDICATION APPROPRIATE?

One of the more troubling aspects of drug therapy for hyperactivity is deciding when medication is the right thing to do. While there are no hard and fast rules regarding this situation, a number of clinicians have expressed their ideas on the topic. None, however, are more thoughtful or compelling than those of Gabrielle Weiss (1981), who has treated, counseled, and interviewed hundreds of hyperactive children, youth, and adults. Some of her reflections regarding the treatment decision-making process are presented here:

> It is common practice in medicine to use medication for a condition either in an attempt to cure the condition (for example, antibiotics for bacterial infections) or to ameliorate the prognosis (treatment for moderate hypertension) or to reduce symptomatology (for example, antipertussants for cough or analgesics for pain) when symptoms are sufficiently unpleasant or disabling. Stimulants for the hyperactive child syndrome do not cure, but have not yet been demonstrated to affect the prognosis of the disorder and are, therefore, used to reduce behaviour problems when they are sufficiently upsetting to the child, his parents, and teachers.

> Unfortunately, the above does not address itself to all the problems regarding whether or not to use stimulants for a given child. The hyperactive child syndrome is a behaviour disorder complained about more commonly by others than by the child himself. Parents and teachers, however, as all clinicians treating these children know, vary greatly in their degree of tolerance of difficult children. This influences physicians in their choice as to whether to use medication. For example, if a hyperactive child has an experienced, tolerant teacher who manages well with him, the physician is less likely to use stimulants than if that same child had a teacher who was threatening expulsion or placement in a special class. Similarly, if a parent calls a pediatrician daily, complaining about a hyperactive child's behaviour and indicates that the child is threatening family life or the marriage, the pediatrician is more likely to prescribe stimulants than if that same child were in a family which handled the difficult behaviour well and was not unduly disrupted by it. It is because the hyperactive child syndrome is defined mainly by its social consequences that treatment should focus not only on the child, but also on his environment, for example changing some aspect of the school setting if appropriate and/or helping the parents deal as well as possible with their youngster.
>
> It seems to this author that no definitive statement can be made in the present state of our knowledge whether or not stimulants should be prescribed for an individual hyperactive child as part of a total treatment plan. This question is left up to the clinical judgment of the treating physician. Most clinicians will weigh various factors in the balance, such as the severity of the problem, the therapeutic response to stimulants of the child in question, the degree of side effects, and the possibility of other treatments (such as counselling, behaviour modification) being sufficiently effective without the use of medication. Certainly for hyperactive children with severe behaviour problems the use of stimulants facilitates other treatment techniques such as remedial education and behaviour modification. (p. 390)

OTHER TREATMENTS

Alternatives to medication for the treatment of hyperactivity are important for at least three reasons: (a) not all youngsters respond to drug therapy; (b) medication is not always appropriate; and (c) there are often additional treatment needs that cannot be adequately met with medication alone. In a perceptive discussion of their early clinical experience with stimulant medication for behavior disorders, Bradley and Bowen (1941) noted the following:

> The use of pharmacological agents, such as amphetamine sulfate, offers a supplementary and relatively untried approach to the treatment of children's psychiatric problems. This approach in no sense replaces that of modifying a child's surroundings and so removing the source of conflict. Neither can it offer the same assurance of mental

> health as do forms of psychotherapy which enable a child to work out his emotional problems, or which train him to deal with future difficulties. However, distressing surroundings cannot always be altered, and lack of facilities frequently make effective psychotherapy impossible. In such situations the simple administration of a drug that produces an improved social adjustment or accelerated school progress may offer considerable assistance to some children. (p. 102)

A variety of nondrug treatments have been proposed for the management of hyperactivity. These include the use of coffee (caffeine), megavitamins, special diets, and behavior therapy.

Coffee (Caffeine)

Ross and Ross (1982) reviewed 11 studies in which coffee or caffeine was used as a treatment of hyperactivity and found the results were contradictory. While some researchers found therapeutic benefit, others showed that coffee was no better than placebo and certainly not as effective as conventional stimulants in controlling hyperactive behavior. At this point, there is no clear evidence that coffee suppresses behavior problems and enhances the ability to pay attention in hyperactive children, at least to any clinically meaningful degree. Nevertheless, there is of course a possibility that some youngsters *may* respond more favorably than others, but this notion requires further research (see Rapoport et al., 1984).

Megavitamins

Cott (1972) has argued that megavitamins should be used to treat hyperactive children. To date, there have been no well-controlled studies that support this claim. What is frustrating about the megavitamin area is that you can read one article that states megavitamins are just great for some hyperactive children (e.g., Brenner, 1982) and another that shows megavitamins are *worse* than placebo (Haslam et al., 1984). With such discrepant findings, caution is generally indicated. Moreover, megavitamins can exacerbate a child's problems, can cause both uncomfortable as well as serious side effects (depending upon the vitamins), and are associated with marked parental misconceptions about efficacy in some cases (see Haslam et al., 1984).

Special Diets

Perhaps the most hotly debated treatment for hyperactivity is the Kaiser-Permanente (K-P) diet, also called the Feingold diet

(Feingold, 1974). The diet consists of eliminating foods that contain artificial food coloring (especially red and yellow dyes); BHT (butylated hydroxytoluene), a food preservative; and natural salicylates (in foods such as apricots, prunes, raspberries, tomatoes, and cucumbers). Although Feingold never conducted well-controlled studies that documented the effectiveness of the diet, he claimed that 30 to 50% of the hyperactive children would experience marked behavioral improvement on an additive-free diet. Surveys show that between 20 and 35% of the hyperactive children who are on medication have also been placed on this diet (Gadow, 1981; Lambert et al., 1981).

In order to test the diet hypothesis scientifically, a research team at the University of Wisconsin conducted one of the first well-controlled large scale studies with children diagnosed as hyperactive (Harley et al., 1978). They purchased all the groceries for the participating families during the 8-week study and also bought snacks for special activities at school (e.g., birthday parties, holidays). To control for any biases, the family received the K-P diet for 4 weeks and a fake (placebo) diet for 4 weeks. In addition, the K-P diet was disguised by using specially prepared commercial foods that normally contained additives but were really additive-free. After collecting numerous measures on behavior at home, school, and in the laboratory, the researchers did *not* find that the K-P diet helped hyperactive elementary school children.

Feingold has also stated that if a child who is placed on the K-P diet and who responds well eats food containing artificial food colors or flavors, his or her hyperactivity will reappear within a few hours after the dietary infraction. Investigations into this hypothesis using children who responded favorably to the diet are inconclusive. While the results of some studies support this claim, others do not.

There are currently dozens of studies and case reports on the K-P diet or some variation of it. Reviews of this literature generally conclude that this dietary treatment is *not* effective for most hyperactive children (e.g., Conners, 1980; Kavale & Forness, 1983; Mattes, 1983; Prinz, 1985). Perhaps the best advice that can be given about the Feingold diet, particularly in severe cases of hyperactivity that do require help, is *caveat emptor* (let the buyer beware).

To date, there are few reports on the effectiveness of the K-P diet in comparison with another treatment. In one study (Williams et al., 1978), it was found that stimulant drugs were more effective in controlling the behavioral symptoms of hyperactivity than a diet free of artificial food colors and flavors.

People often ask, "What harm does it do to try a particular unproven treatment?" The primary problem with this point of view is that the use of a worthless method only denies the child a meaningful approach to his or her therapeutic needs. One might wonder, "What's wrong with at least giving it a try?" The problem here lies in the expectancy effect. If we want or expect something to happen, it is not unusual to *perceive* events as being the way we think they should be, or want them to be. Therefore, a useless approach may appear to be a cure. If the remedy is associated with a strong "placebo effect" that benefits the child, one might ask, "What's wrong with that?" If there really is an improvement in the child's condition for whatever reason, so much the better. However, if problems persist, using a worthless "therapy" is not a solution, and its use may also serve to divert the therapist's attention away from more germane remedies. The essence of the problem is that it is very difficult for caregivers to assess the effectiveness of any treatment appropriately because they generally do not know how to go about it. The irony is, with the school's support, it is really very easy. All that is needed are some baseline (before treatment is begun) and treatment assessments. The ATRS (see Appendix B) will do well as a starting point. It is better if the person doing the rating does not know whether the child is in a regular diet week or a special diet week. Now all that is needed is someone to help coordinate this effort. This is where you come in; that is why this book was written.

Another purported dietary cause of hyperactivity is processed sugar. While there is no evidence for this, it remains a popular and strongly held belief in many societies (see Milich, in press). For example, in a recently conducted, well-designed set of studies, Wolraich et al. (1985) compared the behavior of clinically diagnosed hyperactive children after they had drunk a beverage with a high sugar content and an identical beverage without sugar. There were no differences in behavior under either condition, except for a tendency for behavior to be *better* following the sugar beverage. While these studies do not address the question of whether or not sugar makes nonhyperactive children more active, it does cast serious doubt on the notion that sugar is a major cause of hyperactivity, at least as it is defined here. Moreover, Satterfield et al. (1980) found no evidence of *hypoglycemia* (abnormally low level of glucose in the blood) in medically treated hyperactive children.

Behavior Therapy

Another approach to managing hyperactive children and one for which there is considerable clinical and research support is behavior modification (e.g., Ayllon et al., 1975; O'Leary et al., 1976; Rapport et al., 1982). Because behavioral techniques can be used successfully with these children, many have argued that they should be tried *before* medication. In terms of educational programming, behavior modification is perceived by some as a "less restrictive" approach than drugs to the amelioration of learning and behavior problems. Research into the relative effectiveness of these two treatments is therefore considered to be an important scientific priority.

A fairly large number of studies have now been conducted comparing medication and behavioral interventions, and in some cases combinations of the two (see Brown et al., 1985; Gadow, 1985b; Pelham & Murphy, 1985). The findings from all these studies are difficult to summarize even when one specifies a particular target symptom (e.g., conduct problem, academic underachievement, and so forth). Because academic underachievement is discussed in the chapter on learning disabilities, we focus attention here on conduct problems and prosocial behavior. While medication appears to be clearly superior to some types of behavioral intervention (e.g., Abikoff & Gittelman, 1984, 1985; Gittelman-Klein et al., 1976a), there is also evidence that some behavioral interventions, such as response cost, are just as effective as stimulant drug therapy (e.g., Rapport et al., 1982). Pelham (1983; Pelham & Murphy, 1985) has emphasized, however, that the idea of "superiority" probably misses the point because the two types of treatment often *complement* each other if implemented appropriately. In fact, most studies in which conduct problems and social behavior were targeted for intervention show that the combination treatment is superior to each alone. A good example of this is a study by Pelham and coworkers (see Pelham & Bender, 1982) in which hyperactive children were assigned to one of three groups: Ritalin, social skills training, and a combination of the two. The results are presented in Figure 2–9. At pretest (before treatment began), all three groups were similar. At midtreatment, however, the combination of medication and behavior therapy was *more* effective than just behavior therapy alone. It is important to note that the behavior therapy program was, nevertheless, effective in its own right when compared with the contrast group. At posttreatment, when the medication group was no longer taking stimulant medication, the combination treatment was no better than the behavior therapy alone. This suggests that medication produced few lasting changes in child behavior. At least this was the case in the present study.

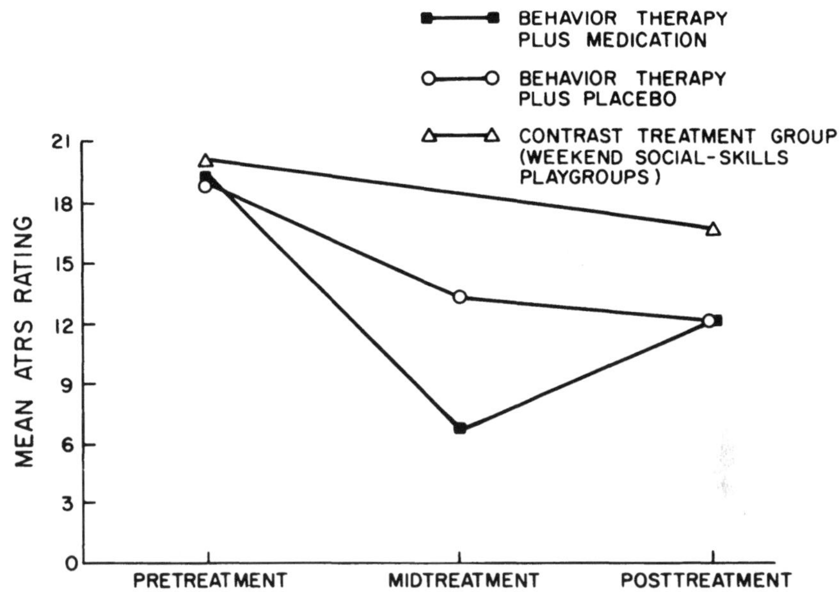

Figure 2–9. Comparison of the effectiveness of three different interventions on reducing negative classroom behavior as measured by teacher ratings. *Note:* From "Peer Relationships in Hyperactive Children: Description and Treatment" by W. E. Pelham and M. E. Bender, 1982, in *Advances in learning and behavioral disabilities* (p. 423), edited by K. D. Gadow and I. Bialer, Greenwich, CT: JAI Press. Copyright 1982 by JAI Press. Adapted by permission.

SUMMARY

A growing number of investigators are demonstrating that special training programs (Douglas et al., 1976), classroom organization (Flynn & Rapoport, 1976), and modifications in teaching methods (Zentall, 1977) can either effect changes in the behavior of hyperactive children or create an environment more suitable to the child's style of learning. Much research has yet to be done in these areas. After effective techniques are developed, questions similar to those posed about drug therapy will remain: Do these new methods make a difference in long-term outcome with hyperactive children? How effective are they in comparison with other therapeutic measures (including medication)? And, are the differences among children, families, schools, and physicians important in deciding which treatment approach is most appropriate? In recent years, hyperactivity has been one of the most heavily investigated topics in pediatric medicine, child psychology, and education. It is hoped that the products of these efforts and future research will provide insight into the care of these often unhappy children who frequently encounter frustration and failure in an environment poorly adapted to their needs.

SUGGESTED READINGS

Barkley, R. A. (1981). *Hyperactive children: A handbook for diagnosis and treatment*. New York: Guilford Press. (C, S, P)

Becker, W. C. (1971). *Parents and teachers*. Champaign, IL: Research Press. (P)

Bradley, C., & Bowen, M. (1941). Amphetamine (Benzedrine) therapy of children's behavior disorders. *American Journal of Orthopsychiatry*, 11, 92–103. (C, S)

Brown, R. T., Borden, K. A., & Clingerman, S. R. (1985). Pharmacotherapy in ADD adolescents with special attention to multimodality treatments. *Psychopharmacology Bulletin*, *21*, 192–211. (C, S)

Cantwell, D. P., & Carlson, G. A. (1978). Stimulants. In J. S. Werry (Ed.), *Pediatric psychopharmacology: The use of behavior modifying drugs in children* (pp. 171–207). New York: Brunner/Mazel. (C, S)

Conners, C. K. (1971). Drugs in the management of children with learning disabilities. In L. Tarnopol (Ed.), *Learning disorders in children: Diagnosis, medication, education* (pp. 253–301). Boston: Little, Brown. (C, S)

Douglas, V. I., & Peters, K. G. (1979). Toward a clearer definition of the attention deficit of hyperactive children. In G. A. Hale & M. Lewis (Eds.), *Attention and cognitive development* (pp. 173–247). New York: Plenum. (C, S)

Gadow, K. D. (1983). Pharmacotherapy for behavior disorders: Typical treatment practices. *Clinical Pediatrics*, *22*, 48–53. (C)

Hechtman, L. (1985). Adolescent outcome of hyperactive children treated with stimulants in childhood: A review. *Psychopharmacology Bulletin*, *21*, 178–191. (C, S)

Loney, J. (1983). Research diagnostic criteria for childhood hyperactivity. In S. B. Guze, F. J. Earls, & J. E. Barrett (Eds.), *Childhood psychopathology and development* (pp. 109–137). New York: Raven Press. (C)

Milich, R., & Landau, S. (1982). Socialization and peer relations in hyperactive children. In K. D. Gadow & I. Bialer (Eds.), *Advances in learning and behavioral disabilities* (Vol. 1, pp. 283–339). Greenwich, CT: JAI Press. (C)

O'Leary, K. D., & O'Leary, S. G. (1977). *Classroom management: Successful use of behavior modification* (2nd ed.). New York: Pergamon. (S)

Patterson, G. R. (1975). *Families: Application of social learning to family life* (Rev. ed.). Champaign, IL: Research Press. (P)

Patterson, G. R. (1976). *Living with children: New methods for parents and teachers* (Rev. ed.). Champaign, IL: Research Press. (P, S)

Pelham, W. E., & Bender, M. E. (1982). Peer relationships in hyperactive children: Description and treatment. In K. D. Gadow & I. Bialer (Eds.), *Advances in learning and behavioral disabilities* (Vol. 1, pp. 365–436). Greenwich, CT: JAI Press. (C)

Pelham, W. E., & Milich, R. (1984). Peer relations in children with hyperactivity/attention deficit disorder. *Journal of Learning Disabilities, 17*, 560–567. (C, S)

Ross, D. M., & Ross, S. A. (1982). *Hyperactivity: Research theory, and action* (2nd. ed.). New York: Wiley. (C, S)

Safer, D. J., & Allen, R. P. (1976). *Hyperactive children: Diagnosis and management*. Baltimore: University Park Press. (C, S)

Sleator, E. K. (1982). Office diagnosis of hyperactivity by the physician. In K. D. Gadow & I. Bialer (Eds.), *Advances in learning and behavioral disabilities* (Vol. 1, pp. 341–364). Greenwich, CT: JAI Press. (C)

Sprague, R. L., & Gadow, K. D. (1976). The role of the teacher in drug treatment. *School Review, 85*, 109–140. (S)

Sprague, R. L., & Werry, J. S. (1974). Psychotropic drugs and handicapped children. In L. Mann & D. A. Sabatino (Eds.), *The second review of special education* (pp. 1–50). Philadelphia: JSE Press. (C, S)

Stewart, M. A., & Olds, S. W. (1973). *Raising a hyperactive child*. New York: Harper & Row. (P)

Weiss, G. Controversial issues of the pharmacotherapy of the hyperactive child. *Canadian Journal of Psychiatry*, 1981, *26*, 385–392. (C)

Whalen, C. K. (1982). Hyperactivity and psychostimulant treatment. In J. R. Lachenmeyer & M. S. Gibbs (Eds.), *Psychopathology in childhood*. New York: Gardner Press. (C, S)

REFERENCES

Abikoff, H., & Gittelman, R. (1984). Does behavior therapy normalize the classroom behavior of hyperactive children? *Archives of General Psychiatry, 41*, 449–454.

Abikoff, H., & Gittelman, R. (1985). The normalizing effects of methylphenidate on the classroom behavior of ADDH children. *Journal of Abnormal Child Psychology, 13*, 33–44.

Ackerman, P. T., Dykman, R. A., Holcomb, P. J., & McCray, D. S. (1982). Methylphenidate effects on cognitive style and reaction time in four groups of children. *Psychiatry Research, 7*, 199–213.

Allen, R. P., Safer, D., & Covi, L. (1975). Effects of psychostimulants on aggression. *Journal of Nervous and Mental Disease, 160*, 138–145.

American Psychiatric Association. (1980). *Diagnostic and statistical manual of mental disorders* (DSM III). Washington, DC: Author.

Amery, B., Minichiello, M. D., & Brown, G. L. (1984). Aggression in hyperactive boys: Response to d-amphetamine. *Journal of the American Academy of Child Psychiatry, 23*, 291–294.

Arias, I., & O'Leary, K. D. (1984). *Prevalence rates of hyperactivity across cultures*. Unpublished manuscript, State University of New York, Department of Psychology, Stony Brook.

Arnold, L. E. (1973). The art of medicating hyperkinetic children. *Clinical Pediatrics, 12,* 35–41.

Ayllon, T., Layman, D., & Kandel, H. J. (1975). A behavioral-educational alternative to drug control of hyperactive children. *Journal of Applied Behavior Analysis, 8,* 137–146.

Ballard, J. E., Boileau, R. A., Sleator, E. K., Massey, B. H., & Sprague, R. L. (1976). Cardiovascular responses of hyperactive children to methylphenidate. *Journal of the American Medical Association, 236,* 2870–2874.

Baren, M., & Swanson, J. (1982). Drug management of hyperactivity. *Journal of Learning Disabilities, 15,* 132–133.

Barkley, R. A. (1976). Predicting the response of hyperkinetic children to stimulant drugs: A review. *Journal of Abnormal Child Psychology, 4,* 327–348.

Barkley, R. A. (1981). *Hyperactive children: A handbook for diagnosis and treatment.* New York: Guilford Press.

Barkley, R. A., & Cunningham, C. E. (1978). Do stimulant drugs improve the academic performance of hyperkinetic children? *Clinical Pediatrics, 17,* 85–92.

Barkley, R. A., & Cunningham, C. E. (1979). The effects of methyphenidate on the mother-child interactions of hyperactive children. *Archives of General Psychiatry, 36,* 201–208.

Barkley, R. A., Karlsson, J., Strzelecki, E., & Murphy, J. V. (1984). Effects of age and Ritalin dosage on the mother-child interactions of hyperactive children. *Journal of Consulting and Clinical Psychology, 52,* 750–758.

Bellak, L. (Ed.). (1979). *Psychiatric aspects of minimal brain dysfunction in adults.* Orlando, FL: Grune & Stratton.

Bosco, J. J., & Robin, S. S. (1980). Hyperkinesis: Prevalence and treatment. In C. K. Whalen & B. Henker (Eds.), *Hyperactive children: The social ecology of identification and treatment* (pp. 173–187). Orlando, FL: Academic Press.

Bradley, C. (1937). The behavior of children receiving Benzedrine. *American Journal of Psychiatry, 94,* 577–585.

Bradley, C. (1950). Benzedrine and dexedrine in the treatment of children's behavior disorders. *Pediatrics,* 5, 24–37.

Bradley, C., & Bowen, M. (1941). Amphetamine (Benzedrine) therapy of children's behavior disorders. *American Journal of Orthopsychiatry,* 11, 92–103.

Brenner, A. (1982). The effects of megadoses of selected B complex vitamins on children with hyperkinesis: Controlled studies with long-term follow-up. *Journal of Learning Disabilities,* 15, 258–264.

Bricklin, P. M., & Gallico, R. (1984). Learning disabilities and emotional disturbance: Critical issues in definition, assessment, and service delivery. *Learning Disabilities,* 3, 141–156.

Brown, D., Winsberg, B. G., Bialer, I., & Press, M. (1973). Imipramine therapy and seizures: Three children treated for hyperactive behavior disorders. *American Journal of Psychiatry, 130,* 210–212.

Brown, R. T., Borden, K. A., & Clingerman, S. R. (1985). Pharmacotherapy in ADD adolescents with special attention to multimodality treatments. *Psychopharmacology Bulletin, 21,* 192–211.

Brown, R. T., & Sleator, E. K. (1979). Methylphenidate in hyperkinetic children: Differences in dose effects on impulsive behavior. *Pediatrics, 64,* 408–411.

Campbell, S. B. (1975). Mother-child interaction: A comparison of hyperactive, learning disabled, and normal boys. *American Journal of Orthopsychiatry, 45,* 51–57.

Campbell, S. B., Endman, M. W., & Bernfeld, G. (1977). A three-year follow-up of hyperactive preschoolers into elementary school. *Journal of Child Psychology and Psychiatry, 18,* 239–249.

Cantwell, D. P., & Carlson, G. A. (1978). Stimulants. In J. S. Werry (Ed.), *Pediatric psychopharmacology: The use of behavior modifying drugs in children* (pp. 171–207). New York: Brunner/Mazel.

Carter, C. H. (1956). The effects of reserpine and methylphenidate (Ritalin) in mental defectives, spastics, and epileptics. *Psychiatric Research Reports, 4,* 44–48.

Chatoor, I., Wells, K. C., Conners, C. K., Seidel,W. T., & Shaw, D. (1983). The effects of nocturnally administered stimulant medication on EEG sleep and behavior in hyperactive children. *Journal of the American Academy of Child Psychiatry, 22,* 337–342.

Cohen, N. J., & Douglas, V. I. (1972). Characteristics of the orienting response in hyperactive and normal children. *Psychophysiology, 9,* 238–245.

Cohen, N. J., Douglas, V. I., & Morgenstern, G. (1971). The effect of methylphenidate on attentive behavior and autonomic activity in hyperactive children. *Psychopharmacologia, 22,* 282–294.

Conners, C. K. (1969). A teacher rating scale for use in drug studies with children. *American Journal of Psychiatry, 126,* 884–888.

Conners, C. K. (1971). Drugs in the management of children with learning disabilities. In L. Tarnopol (Ed.), *Learning disorders in children: Diagnosis, medication, education* (pp. 253–301). Boston: Little, Brown.

Conners, C. K. (1973). Rating scales for use in drug studies with children. *Psychopharmacology Bulletin* (Special issue, Pharmacotherapy of children), 24–84.

Conners, C. K. (1980). *Food additives and hyperactive children.* New York: Plenum.

Conners, C. K., & Rothschild, G. H. (1968). Drugs and learning in children. In J. Hellmuth (Ed.), *Learning disorders* (Vol. 3). Seattle, WA: Special Child.

Conway, A. (1976). An evaluation of drugs in the elementary schools: Some geographic considerations. *Psychology in the Schools, 13,* 442–444.

Cott, A. (1972). Megavitamins: The orthomolecular approach to behavioral disorders and learning disabilities. *Academic Therapy, 7,* 245–258.

Cunningham, C. E., & Barkley, R. A. (1979). The interactions of normal and hyperactive children with their mothers in free play and structural task. *Child Development, 50,* 217–224.

Denkla, M. B., Bemporad, J. R., & McKay, M. D. (1976). Tics following methylphenidate administration. *Journal of the American Medical Association, 235,* 1349–1351.

Douglas, V. I. (1972). Stop, look, and listen: The problem of sustained attention and impulse control in hyperactive and normal children. *Canadian Journal of Behaviour Science, 4,* 259–282.

Douglas, V. I., Parry, P., Marton, P., & Garson, C. (1976). Assessment of a cognitive training program for hyperactive children. *Journal of Abnormal Child Psychology, 4,* 389–410.

Douglas, V. I., & Peters, K. G. (1979). Toward a clearer definition of the attention deficit of hyperactive children. In G. A. Hale & M. Lewis

(Eds.), *Attention and cognitive development* (pp. 173–247). New York: Plenum.

Dykman, R. A., Ackerman, P. T., & McCray, D. S. (1980). Effects of methylphenidate on selective and sustained attention in hyperactive, reading-disabled, and presumably attention-disordered boys. *Journal of Nervous and Mental Disease, 168*, 745–752.

Dyme, I. Z., Sahakian, B. J., Golinko, B. E., & Rabe, E. F. (1982). Perseveration induced by methylphenidate in children: Preliminary findings. *Progress in Neuropsychopharmacology & Biological Psychiatry, 6*, 269–273.

Eisenberg, L. (1964). Role of drugs in treating disturbed children. *Children, 11*, 167–173.

Eisenberg, L., & Conners, C. K. (1971). Psychopharmacology in childhood. In N. B. Talbot, J. Kagan, & L. Eisenberg (Eds.), *Behavioral science in pediatric medicine* (pp. 397–423). Philadelphia: Saunders.

Ellis, M. J., Witt, P. A., Reynolds, R., & Sprague, R. L. (1974). Methylphenidate and the activity of hyperactives in the informal setting. *Child Development, 45*, 217–220.

Epstein, M. H., Cullinan, D., & Gadow, K. D. (1985). *Prevalence of psychotropic drug use with learning disabled, emotionally disturbed, and mentally retarded children*. Unpublished manuscript, Northern Illinois University, Department of Learning, Development, and Special Education, DeKalb.

Feingold, B. F. (1974). *Why your child is hyperactive*. New York: Random House.

Fish, B. (1971). The "one child, one drug" myth of stimulants in hyperkinesis. *Archives of General Psychiatry, 25*, 193–203.

Flintoff, M. M., Barron, R. W., Swanson, J. M., Ledlow, A., & Kinsbourne, M. (1982). Methylphenidate increases selectivity of visual scanning in children referred for hyperactivity. *Journal of Abnormal Child Psychology, 10*, 145–161.

Flynn, N. M., & Rapoport, J. L. (1976). Hyperactivity in open and traditional classroom environments. *Journal of Special Education, 10*, 285–290.

Freeman, R. D. (1976). Minimal brain dysfunction, hyperactivity, and learning disorders: Epidemic or episode? *School Review, 85*, 5–30.

Gadow, K. D. (1977). *Psychotropic and antiepileptic drug treatment with children in early childhood special education*. Champaign, IL: University of Illinois, Institute for Child Behavior and Development.

Gadow, K. D. (1981). Drug therapy for hyperactivity: Treatment procedures in natural settings. In K. D. Gadow & J. Loney (Eds.), *Psychosocial aspects of drug treatment for hyperactivity* (pp. 13–76). Boulder, CO: Westview Press.

Gadow, K. D. (1982a). School involvement in pharmacotherapy for behavior disorders. *Journal of Special Education, 16*, 385–399.

Gadow, K. D. (1982b). School involvement in the treatment of seizure disorders. *Epilepsia, 23*, 215–224.

Gadow, K. D. (1983). Pharmacotherapy for learning disabilities. *Learning Disabilities, 2*, 127–140.

Gadow, K. D. (1985a). Prevalence and efficacy of stimulant drug use with mentally retarded children and youth. *Psychopharmacology Bulletin, 21*, 291–303.

Gadow, K. D. (1985b). Relative efficacy of pharmacological, behavioral, and combination treatments for enhancing academic performance. *Clinical Psychology Review, 5,* 513–533.

Gadow, K. D., & Kalachnik, J. (1981). Prevalence and pattern of drug treatment for behavior and seizure disorders of TMR students. *American Journal of Mental Deficiency, 85,* 588–595.

Gadow, K. D., & Sprague, R. L. (1980, September). *An anterospective followup of hyperactive children into adolescence: Licit and illicit* drug use. Paper presented at the meeting of the American Psychological Association, Montreal.

Gittelman, R., Mannuzza, S., Shenker, R., & Bonagura, N. (1985). Hyperactive boys almost grown up: I. Psychiatric status. *Archives of General Psychiatry, 42,* 937–947.

Gittelman-Klein, R., & Klein, D. F. (1976). Methylphenidate effects in learning disabilities. *Archives of General Psychiatry, 33,* 655–664.

Gittelman-Klein, R., Klein, D. F., Abikoff, H., Katz, S., Gloisten, A. C., & Kates, W. (1976a). Relative efficacy of methylphenidate and behavior modification in hyperkinetic children: An interim report. *Journal of Abnormal Child Psychology, 4,* 361–379.

Gittelman-Klein, R., Klein, D. F., Katz, S., Saraf, K., & Pollack, E. (1976b). Comparative effects of methylphenidate and thioridazine in hyperkinetic children. *Archives of General Psychiatry, 33,* 1217–1231.

Greenberg, L. M., Deem, M. A., & McMahon, S. (1972). Effects of dextroamphetamine, chlorpromazine, and hydroxyzine on behavior and performance in hyperactive children. *American Journal of Psychiatry, 129,* 532–539.

Harley, J. P., Ray, R. S., Tomasi, L., Eichman, P. L., Matthews, C. G., Chun, R., Cleeland, C. S., & Traisman, E. (1978). Hyperkinesis and food additives: Testing the Feingold hypothesis. *Pediatrics, 61,* 818–828.

Haslam, R. H. A., Dalby, J. T., & Rademaker, A. W. (1984). Effects of megavitamin therapy on children with attention deficit disorders. *Pediatrics, 74,* 103–111.

Hayes, T. A., Panitch, M. L., & Barker, E. (1975). Imipramine dosage in children: A comment on "Imipramine and electrocardiographic abnormalities in hyperactive children." *American Journal of Psychiatry, 132,* 546–547.

Hechtman, L. (1985). Adolescent outcome of hyperactive children treated with stimulants in childhood: A review. *Psychopharmacology Bulletin, 21,* 178–191.

Hechtman, L., Weiss, G., & Perlman, T. (1984a). Hyperactives as young adults: Past and current substance abuse and antisocial behavior. *American Journal of Orthopsychiatry, 54,* 415–425.

Hechtman, L., Weiss, G., & Perlman, T. (1984b). Young adult outcome of hyperactive children who received long-term stimulant treatment. *Journal of the American Academy of Child Psychiatry, 23,* 261–269.

Hechtman, L., Weiss, G., Perlman, T., & Amsel, R. (1984c). Hyperactives as young adults: Initial predictors of adult outcome. *Journal of the American Academy of Child Psychiatry, 23,* 250–260.

Hoy, E., Weiss, G., Minde, K., & Cohen, N. (1978). The hyperactive child at adolescence: Cognitive, emotional, and social functioning. *Journal of Abnormal Child Psychology, 6,* 311–324.

Humphries, T., Kinsbourne, M., & Swanson, J. (1978). Stimulant effects on cooperation and social interaction between hyperactive children and their mothers. *Journal of Child Psychology and Psychiatry, 19,* 13–22.

Husain, A., Chapel, J., & Malek-Ahmadl, P. (1980). Methylphenidate, neuroleptics and dyskinesia-dystonia. *Canadian Journal of Psychiatry, 25,* 254–258.

Kagan, J. (1966). Reflection-impulsivity: The generality of dynamics of conceptual tempo. *Journal of Abnormal Psychology, 71,* 17–24.

Kalachnik, J. E., Sprague, R. L., Sleator, E. K., Cohen, M. N., & Ullmann, R. K. (1982). Effect of methylphenidate on stature in hyperactive children. *Developmental Medicine and Child Neurology, 25,* 586–595.

Katz, S., Saraf, K., Gittelman-Klein, R., & Klein, D. F. (1975). Clinical pharmacological management of hyperkinetic children. *International Journal of Mental Health, 4,* 157–181.

Kavale, K. A., & Forness, S. R. (1983). Hyperactivity and diet treatment: A meta-analysis of the Feingold hypothesis. *Journal of Learning Disabilities, 16,* 324–330.

Kinsbourne, M. (1973). Stimulants for insomnia (correspondence). *New England Journal of Medicine, 288,* 1129.

Klein, D. F., Gittelman, R., Quitkin, F., & Rifkin, A. (1980). *Diagnosis and drug treatment of psychiatric disorders: Adults and children* (2nd ed.). Baltimore: Williams & Wilkins.

Knights, R. M., & Hinton, G. G. (1969). The effects of methylphenidate (Ritalin) on the motor skills and behavior of children with learning problems. *Journal of Nervous and Mental Disease, 148,* 643–653.

Krager, J. M., & Safer, D. J. (1974). Type and prevalence of medication used in the treatment of hyperactive children. *New England Journal of Medicine, 291,* 1118–1120.

Krager, J. M., Safer, D. J., & Earhart, J. (1979). Type and prevalence of medication used to treat hyperactive school children: Follow-up survey results. *Journal of School Health, 49,* 317–321.

Kramer, J., & Loney, J. (1982). Childhood hyperactivity and substance abuse: A review of the literature. In K. D. Gadow and I. Bialer (Eds.), *Advances in learning and behavioral disabilities* (Vol. 1, pp. 225–259). Greenwich, CT: JAI Press.

Lambert, N., & Sandoval, J. (1980). The prevalence of learning disabilities in a sample of children considered hyperactive. *Journal of Abnormal Child Psychology, 8,* 33–50.

Lambert, N. M., Sandoval, J., & Sassone, D. (1978). Prevalence of hyperactivity in elementary school children as a function of social system definers. *American Journal of Orthopsychiatry, 48,* 446–463.

Lambert, N. M., Sandoval, J., & Sassone, D. M. (1981). Prevalence of hyperactivity and related treatments among elementary school children. In K. D. Gadow & J. Loney (Eds.), *Psychosocial aspects of drug treatment for hyperactivity* (pp. 249–291). Boulder, CO: Westview Press.

Laufer, M. W., Denhoff, E., & Riverside, R. I. (1957). Hyperkinetic behavior syndrome in children. *Journal of Pediatrics, 50,* 463–474.

Lerer, R. J., Lerer, P. M., & Artner, J. (1977). The effects of methylphenidate on the handwriting of children with minimal brain dysfunction. *Journal of Pediatrics, 91,* 127–132.

Livingston, S., Berman, W., & Pauli, L. L. (1973). Stimulant drugs for problem children. *New England Journal of Medicine, 289,* 1375–1376.

Livingston, S., Kajdi, L., & Bridge, E. M. (1948). The use of Benzedrine and Dexedrine sulfate in the treatment of epilepsy. *Journal of Pediatrics, 32,* 490–494.

Livingston, S., & Pauli, L. L. (1975). Dextroamphetamine for epilepsy. *Journal of the American Medical Association, 233,* 278–279.

Loney, J. (1983). Research diagnostic criteria for childhood hyperactivity. In S. B. Guze, F. J. Earls, & J. E. Barrett (Eds.), *Childhood psychopathology and development* (pp. 109–137). New York: Raven Press.

Loney, J., & Gadow, K. D. (1982). *Hyperactivity* a nonprofessional term? *Contemporary Psychology, 27,* 483.

Loney, J., Kramer, J., & Kosier, T. (1981b, August). *Medicated vs. unmedicated hyperactive adolescents: Academic, delinquent and symptomatological outcome.* Paper presented at the meeting of the American Psychological Association, Los Angeles.

Loney, J., Kramer, J., & Milich, R. (1981a). The hyperactive child grows up: Predictors of symptoms, delinquency, and achievement at follow-up. In K. D. Gadow & J. Loney (Eds.), *Psychosocial aspects of drug treatment for hyperactivity* (pp. 381–415). Boulder, CO: Westview Press.

Loney, J., & Milich, R. (1982). Hyperactivity, inattention, and aggression in clinical practice. In M. Wolraich & D. K. Routh (Eds.), *Advances in developmental and behavioral pediatrics* (Vol 3, pp. 113–147), Greenwich, CT: JAI Press.

Loney, J., Prinz, R. J., Mishalow, J., & Joad, J. (1978). Hyperkinetic/aggressive boys in treatment: Predictors of clinical response to methylphenidate. *American Journal of Psychiatry, 135,* 1487–1491.

Loney, J., Whaley-Klahn, M. A., Kosier, T., & Conboy, J. (1983). Hyperactive boys and their brothers at 21: Predictors of aggressive and antisocial outcomes. In K. T. Van Dusen & S. A. Mednick (Eds.), *Prospective studies of crime and delinquency* (pp. 181–207). Boston: Kluwer-Nijhoff.

Lucas, A., & Weiss, M. (1971). Methylphenidate hallucinosis. *Journal of the American Medical Association, 217,* 1079–1081.

Mann, H. B., & Greenspan, S. I. (1976). The identification and treatment of adult brain dysfunction. *American Journal of Psychiatry, 133,* 1013–1017.

Mattes, J. A. (1983). The Feingold diet: A current reappraisal. *Journal of Learning Disabilities, 16,* 319–323.

Mattes, J. A., & Gittelman, R. (1983). Growth of hyperactive children on maintenance regimen of methylphenidate. *Archives of General Psychiatry, 40,* 317–321.

Mattson, R. H., & Calverly, J. R. (1968). Dextroamphetamine-sulfate–induced dyskinesias. *Journal of the American Medical Association, 204,* 400–402.

McNutt, B. A., Boileau, R. A., Cohen, M. N., Sprague, R. L., & von Neumann, A. (1977). The effects of long-term stimulant medication on the growth and body composition of hyperactive children: II. Report on two years. *Psychopharmacology Bulletin, 13,* (2), 36–41.

Merritt, H. H., & Putnam, T. J. (1938). Sodium diphenyl hydantoinate in the treatment of convulsive disorders. *Journal of the American Medical Association, 111,* 1068–1073.

Michael, R. L., Klorman, R., Salzman, L. F., Borgstedt, A. D., & Dainer, K. B. (1981). Normalizing effects of methylphenidate on hyperactive children's vigilance performance and evoked potentials. *Psychophysiology, 18,* 665–667.

Milich, R. (in press). The behavioral effects of sugar: A comment on Buchanan. *American Psychologist.*

Milich, R., & Kramer, J. (1984). Reflections on impulsivity: An empirical investigation of impulsivity as a construct. In K. D. Gadow (Ed.), *Advances in learning and behavioral disabilities* (Vol. 3, pp. 57–94). Greenwich, CT: JAI Press.

Milich, R., & Landau, S. (1982). Socialization and peer relations in hyperactive children. In K. D. Gadow & I. Bialer (Eds.), *Advances in learning and behavioral disabilities* (Vol. 1, pp. 283–339). Greenwich, CT: JAI Press.

Milich, R., & Loney, J. (1979). The role of hyperactive and aggressive symptomatology in predicting adolescent outcome among hyperactive children. *Journal of Pediatric Psychology, 4,* 93–112.

Millichap, J. G. (1968). Drugs in management of hyperkinetic and perceptually handicapped children. *Journal of the American Medical Association, 206,* 1527–1530.

Millichap, J. G. (1969). Management of hyperkinetic behavior in children with epilepsy. *Modern Treatment, 6,* 1233–1246.

Millichap, J. G. (1973). Drugs in management of minimal brain dysfunction. *Annals of the New York Academy of Sciences, 205,* 321–334.

Millichap, J. G. (1975). The paradoxical effects of CNS stimulants on hyperkinetic behavior. *International Journal of Neurology, 10,* 241–251.

Montagu, J. D., & Swarbrick, L. (1975). Effect of amphetamines in hyperkinetic children: Stimulant or sedative. *Developmental Medicine and Child Neurology, 17,* 293–298.

O'Leary, K. D., Pelham, W. E., Rosenbaum, A., & Price, G. H. (1976). Behavioral treatment of hyperkinetic children. *Clinical Pediatrics, 15,* 510–515.

O'Leary, K. D., Vivian D., & Nisi, A. (in press). Hyperactivity in Italy. *Journal of Abnormal Child Psychology.*

O'Leary, S. G., & Pelham, W. E. (1978). Behavior therapy and withdrawal of stimulant medication in hyperactive children. *Pediatrics, 61,* 211–217.

Ounsted, C. (1955). The hyperkinetic syndrome in epileptic children. *Lancet, 2,* 303–311.

Pelham, W. E. (1983). The effects of psychostimulants on academic achievement in hyperactive and learning-disabled children. *Thalamus, 3,* 1–49.

Pelham, W. E., & Bender, M. E. (1982). Peer relationships in hyperactive children: Description and treatment. In K. D. Gadow & I. Bialer (Eds.), *Advances in learning and behavioral disabilities* (Vol. 1, pp. 365–436). Greenwich, CT: JAI Press.

Pelham, W. E., & Milich, R. (1984). Peer relations in children with hyperactivity/attention deficit disorder. *Journal of Learning Disabilities, 17,* 560–567.

Pelham, W. E., & Murphy, H. A. (1985). Behavioral and pharmacological treatment of attention deficit and conduct disorders. In M. Hersen (Ed.), *Pharmacological and behavioral treatment: An integrative approach.* New York: Wiley.

Porrino, L. J., Rapoport, J. L., Behar, D., Sceery, W., Ismond, D. R., & Bunney, W. E. (1983). A naturalistic assessment of the motor activity of hyperactive boys. *Archives of General Psychiatry, 40,* 681–687.

Prinz, R. J. (1985). Diet-behavior research with children: Methodological and substantive issues. In K. D. Gadow (Ed.), *Advances in learning and behavioral disabilities* (Vol. 4, pp. 181–199). Greenwich, CT: JAI Press.

Prinzmetal, M., & Bloomberg, W. (1935). The use of Benzedrine for the treatment of narcolepsy. *Journal of the American Medical Association, 105*, 2051–2054.

Quay, L. C., & Brown, R. T. (1980). Hyperactive and normal children and the error, latency and double median split scoring procedures for the Matching Familiar Figures Test. *Journal of School Psychology, 18*, 12–16.

Quinn, P. O., & Rapoport, J. L. (1975). One-year-follow-up of hyperactive boys treated with imipramine or methylphenidate. *American Journal of Psychiatry, 132*, 241–245.

Rapoport, J. (1965). Childhood behavior and learning problems treated with imipramine. *International Journal of Neuropsychiatry, 1*, 635–642.

Rapoport, J. L., Berg, C. J., Ismond, D. R., Zahn, T. P., & Neims, A. (1984). Behavioral effects of caffeine in children. *Archives of General Psychiatry, 41*, 1073–1079.

Rapoport, J. L., Buschbaum, M., Weingartner, H., Zahn, T. P., & Ludlow, C. (1980). Dextroamphetamine: Cognitive and behavioral effects in normal and hyperactive boys and normal men. *Archives of General Psychiatry, 37*, 933–943.

Rapoport, J. L., Buschbaum, M. S., Zahn, T. P., Weingartner, H., Ludlow, C., & Mikkelsen, E. J. (1978). Dextroamphetamine: Cognitive and behavioral effects in normal prepubertal boys. *Science, 199*, 560–563.

Rapoport, J. L., Quinn, P. O., Bradbard, G., Riddle, K. D., & Brooks, E. (1974). Imipramine and methylphenidate treatments of hyperactive boys. *Archives of General Psychiatry, 30*, 789–793.

Rapport, M. D., DuPaul, G. J., Stoner, G., & Jones, J. T. (in press). Comparing classroom and clinic measures of attention deficit disorder: Differential, diosyncratic, and dose-response effects of methylphenidate. *Journal of Consulting and Clinical Psychology.*

Rapport, M. D., Murphy, H. A., & Bailey, J. S. (1982). Ritalin vs. response cost in the control of hyperactive children: A within-subject comparison. *Journal of Applied Behavior Analysis, 15*, 205–216.

Rapport, M. D., Stoner, G., DuPaul, G. J., Birmingham, B. K., & Tucker, S. (1985). Methylphenidate in hyperactive children: Differential effects of dose on academic, learning, and social behavior. *Journal of Abnormal Child Psychology, 13*, 227–244.

Reid, M. K., & Borkowski, J. G. (1984). Effects of methylphenidate (Ritalin) on information processing in hyperactive children. *Journal of Abnormal Child Psychology, 12*, 169–185.

Renshaw, D. C. (1974). *The hyperactive child.* Chicago: Nelson-Hall.

Reynolds, E. H. (1975). Chronic antiepileptic toxicity: A review. *Epilepsia, 16*, 319–352.

Robbins, T. W., & Sahakian, B. J. (1979). "Paradoxical" effects of psychomotor stimulant drugs in hyperactive children from the standpoint of behavioral pharmacology. *Neuropharmacology, 18*, 931–950.

Roche, A. F., Lipman, R. S., Overall, J. E., & Hung, W. (1979). The effects of stimulant medication on the growth of hyperkinetic children. *Pediatrics, 63*, 847–850.

Ross, D. M., & Ross, S. A. (1982). *Hyperactivity: Research, theory, and action* (2nd ed.). New York: Wiley.

Ross, R. P. (1979). Drug therapy for hyperactivity: Existing practices in physician-school communication. In M. J. Cohen (Ed.), *Drugs and the special child* (pp. 99–109). New York: Gardner Press, 1979.

Rosvold, H. E., Mirsky, A. F., Sarason, I., Bransome, E. D., & Beck, L. H. (1956). A continuous performance test of brain damage. *Journal of Consulting Psychology, 20,* 343–350.

Safer, D. J., & Allen, R. P. (1973a). Factors influencing the suppressant effects of two stimulant drugs on the growth of hyperactive children. *Pediatrics, 51,* 660–667.

Safer, D. J., & Allen, R. P. (1973b). Single daily dose methylphenidate in hyperactive children. *Diseases of the Nervous System, 34,* 325–328.

Safer, D. J., & Allen, R. P. (1975). Stimulant drug treatment of hyperactive adolescents. *Diseases of the Nervous System, 36,* 454–457.

Safer, D. J., & Allen, R. P. (1976). *Hyperactive children: Diagnosis and management.* Baltimore: University Park Press.

Safer, D., Allen, R., & Barr, E. (1975). Growth rebound after termination of stimulant drugs. *Pediatrics, 86,* 113–116.

Safer, D. J., & Krager, J. M. (1984). Trends in medication treatment of hyperactive school children. In K. D. Gadow (Ed.), *Advances in learning and behavioral disabilities* (Vol. 3, pp. 125–149). Greenwich, CT: JAI Press.

Saraf, K. R., Klein, D. F., Gittelman-Klein, R., & Groff, S. (1974). Imipramine side effects in children. *Psychopharmacologica, 37,* 265–274.

Satterfield, J. H., Schell, A. M., & Barb, S. D. (1980). Potential risk of prolonged administration of stimulant medication for hyperactive children. *Developmental and Behavioral Pediatrics, 1,* 102–107.

Schain, R. J., & Reynard, C. L. (1975). Observations on effects of central stimulant drug (methylphenidate) in children with hyperactive behavior. *Pediatrics, 55,* 709–716.

Schleifer, M., Weiss, G., Cohen, N., Elman, M., Cvejic, H., & Kruger, E. (1975). Hyperactivity in preschoolers and the effect of methlyphenidate. *American Journal of Orthopsychiatry, 45,* 38–50.

Scott, K. G. (1970). A multiple-choice audio-visual discrimination apparatus with quick interchange display and response panels. *Journal of Experimental Child Psychology, 9,* 43–50.

Sleator, E. K. (1978). Personal communication, March 13.

Sleator, E. K. (1982). Office diagnosis of hyperactivity by the physician. In K. D. Gadow & I. Bialer (Eds.), *Advances in learning and behavioral disabilities* (Vol. 1, pp. 341–364). Greenwich, CT: JAI Press.

Sleator, E. K., & von Neumann, A. (1974). Methylphenidate in the treatment of hyperkinetic children. *Clinical Pediatrics, 13,* 19–24.

Sleator, E. K., von Neumann, A. W., & Sprague, R. L. (1974). Hyperactive children: A continuous long-term placebo controlled follow-up. *Journal of the American Medical Association, 229,* 316–317.

Sleator, E. K., & Sprague, R. L. (1978). Pediatric pharmacotherapy. In W. G. Clark & J. del Guidice (Eds.), *Principles of psychopharmacology* (2nd ed., pp. 573–591). Orlando, FL: Academic Press.

Sleator, E. K., Ullmann, R. K., & von Neumann, A. (1982). How do hyperactive children feel about taking stimulants and will they tell the doctor? *Clinical Pediatrics, 21,* 474–479.

Solomons, G. (1973). Drug therapy: Initiation and follow-up. *Annals of the New York Academy of Sciences, 205,* 335–344.

Sprague, R. L. (1984). Preliminary report of cross-cultural study and cognitive strategies of ADD children. In L. M. Bloomingdale (Ed.), *Attention deficit disorder: Diagnostic, cognitive, and therapeutic understanding* (pp. 211–219). New York: Spectrum.

Sprague, R. L., Christensen, D. E., & Werry, J. S. (1974). Experimental psychology and stimulant drugs. In C. K. Conners (Ed.), *Clinical use of stimulant drugs in children* (pp. 141–164). Amsterdam: Excerpta Medica.

Sprague, R. L., Cohen, M. N., & Eichlseder, W. (1977, August). *Are there hyperactive children in Europe and the South Pacific?* Paper presented at the meeting of the American Psychological Association, San Francisco.

Sprague, R. L., & Gadow, K. D. (1976). The role of the teacher in drug treatment. *School Review, 85,* 109–140.

Sprague, R. L., & Sleator, E. K. (1973). Effects of psychopharmacologic agents on learning disorders. *Pediatric Clinics of North America, 20,* 719–735.

Sprague, R. L., & Sleator, E. K. (1975). What is the proper dose of stimulant drugs in children? *International Journal of Mental Health, 4,* 75–104.

Sprague, R. L., & Sleator, E. K. (1976). Drugs and dosages: Implications for learning disabilities. In R. M. Knights & D. J. Bakker (Eds.), *Neuropsychology of learning disorders: Theoretical approaches.* Baltimore: University Park Press.

Sprague, R. L., & Sleator, E. K. (1977). Methylphenidate in hyperkinetic children: Differences in dose effects on learning and social behavior. *Science, 198,* 1274–1276.

Sprague, R. L., & Werry, J. S. (1974). Psychotropic drugs and handicapped children. In L. Mann & D. A. Sabatino (Eds.), *The second review of special education* (pp. 1–50). Philadelphia: JSE Press.

Sprague, R. L., Werry, J. S., Greenwold, W. E., & Jones H. (1969, November). *Dosage effects of methylphenidate on learning of children.* Paper presented at the meeting of the Psychonomic Society, St. Louis.

Stephens, R. S., Pelham, W. E., & Skinner, R. (1984). The state-dependent and main effects of methylphenidate and pemoline on paired-associates learning and spelling in hyperactive children. *Journal of Consulting and Clinical Psychology, 523,* 104–113.

Stewart, M. A., & Olds, S. W. (1973). *Raising a hyperactive child.* New York: Harper & Row.

Sulzbacher, S. I. (1972). Behavior analysis of drug effects in the classroom. In G. Semb (Ed.), *Behavior analysis and education* (p. 37–52). University of Kansas.

Swanson, J. M., & Kinsbourne, M. (1976). Stimulant-related state-dependent learning in hyperactive children. *Science, 192,* 1354–1357.

Swanson, J. M., & Kinsbourne, M. (1979). The cognitive effects of stimulant drugs on hyperactive children. In G. A. Hale & M. Lewis (Eds.), *Attention and cognitive development* (pp. 249–274). New York: Plenum.

Swanson, J., Kinsbourne, M., Roberts W., & Zucker, K. (1978). Time-response analysis of the effect of stimulant medication on the learning ability of children referred for hyperactivity. *Pediatrics, 61,* 21–29.

Sykes, D. H., Douglas, V. I., Weiss, G., & Minde, K. K. (1971). Attention in hyperactive children and the effect of methylphenidate (Ritalin). *Journal of Child Psychology and Psychiatry, 2,* 129–139.

Tecce, J. J., & Cole, J. O. (1974). Amphetamine effects in man: Paradoxical drowsiness and lowered electrical brain activity (CNV), *Science, 185,* 451–453.

Thorley, G. (1984). Review of follow-up and follow-back studies of childhood hyperactivity. *Psychological Bulletin, 96,* 116–132.
Turner, W. D., & Carl, G. P. (1939). Temporary changes in affect and attitude following ingestion of various amounts of Benzedrine sulfate (amphetamine sulfate). *Journal of Psychology, 8,* 415–482.
Ullmann, R. K., Sleator, E. K., & Sprague, R. L. (in press). A change of mind: Conners Abbreviated Teacher Rating Scale reconsidered. *Journal of Abnormal Child Psychology.*
Wade, M. G. (1976). Effects of methylphenidate on motor skill acquisition of hyperactive children. *Journal of Learning Disabilities, 9,* 443–447.
Walker, S. (1974, December). Drugging the American child: We're too cavalier about hyperactivity. *Psychology Today,* pp. 43–48.
Weingartner, H., Langer, D., Grice, J., & Rapoport, J. L. (1982). Acquisition and retrieval of information in amphetamine-treated hyperactive children. *Psychiatry Research, 6,* 21–29.
Weingartner, H., Rapoport, J. L., Buschbaum, M. S., Bunney, W. E., Ebert, M. H., Mikkelsen, E. J., & Caine, E. D. (1980). Cognitive processes in normal and hyperactive children and their response to amphetamine treatment. *Journal of Abnormal Psychology, 89,* 25–37.
Weiss, G. (1981). Controversial issues of the pharmacotherapy of the hyperactive child. *Canadian Journal of Psychiatry, 26,* 385–392.
Weiss, G., Hechtman, L., & Perlman, T. (1978). Hyperactives as young adults: School, employer, and self-rating scales obtained during ten-year follow-up evaluation. *American Journal of Orthopsychiatry, 48,* 438–445.
Weiss, G., Hechtman, L., Perlman, T., Hopkins, J., & Wener, A. (1979). Hyperactive children as young adults: A controlled prospective 10 year follow-up of the psychiatric status of 75 hyperactive children. *Archives of General Psychiatry, 36,* 675–681.
Weiss, G., Minde, K., Werry, J. S., Douglas, V., & Nemeth, E. (1971). Studies on the hyperactive child VIII: Five-year follow-up. *Archives of General Psychiatry, 24,* 409–414.
Wender, P. H., Reimherr, F. W., Wood, D., & Ward, M. (1985). A controlled study of methylphenidate in the treatment of attention deficit disorder, residual type, in adults. *American Journal of Psychiatry, 142,* 547–552.
Werry, J. S., Aman, M. G., & Diamond, E. (1980). Impramine and methylphenidate in hyperactive children. *Journal of Child Psychology and Psychiatry, 21,* 27–35.
Werry, J. S., & Sprague, R. L. (1974). Methylphenidate in children—Effect of dosage. *Australian and New Zealand Journal of Psychiatry, 8,* 9–19.
Whalen, C. K. (1982). Hyperactivity and psychostimulant treatment. In J. R. Lachenmeyer and M. S. Gibbs (Eds.), *Psychopathology in childhood* (pp. 375–402). New York: Gardner Press.
Whalen, C. K., & Henker, B. (1985). The social worlds of hyperactive (ADDH) children. *Clinical Psychology Review.*
Whalen, C. K., Henker, B., Collins, B. E., Finck, D., & Dotemoto, S. (1979). A social ecology of hyperactive boys: Medication effects in structured classroom environments. *Journal of Applied Behavior Analysis, 12,* 65–81.
Whalen, C. K., Henker, B., & Dotemoto, S. (1980). Methylphenidate and hyperactivity: Effects on teacher behaviors. *Science, 208,* 1280–1282.

Whitehouse, D., Shah, U., & Palmer, F. B. (1980). Comparison of sustained-release and standard methylphenidate in the treatment of minimal brain dysfunction. *Journal of Clinical Psychiatry, 41*, 282–285.

Williams, J. I., Cram, D. M., Tausig, F. T., & Webster, E. (1978). Relative effects of drugs and diet on hyperactive behaviors: An experimental study. *Pediatrics, 61*, 811–817.

Winchell, C. A. (1975). *The hyperkinetic child: A bibliography of medical, educational, and behavioral studies*. Westport, CT: Greenwood Press.

Winsberg, B. G, Yepes, L. E., & Bialer, I. (1976). Pharmacologic management of children with hyperactive/aggressive/inattentive behavior disorders. *Clinical Pediatrics, 15*, 471–477.

Wolraich, M. L., Milich, R., Stumbo, P., & Schulz, F. (1985). The effects of sucrose ingestion on the behavior of hyperactive boys. *Journal of Pediatrics, 106*, 675–682.

Wulbert, M., & Dries, R. (1977). The relative efficacy of methylphenidate (Ritalin) and behavior-modification techniques in the treatment of a hyperactive child. *Journal of Applied Behavior Analysis, 10*, 21–31.

Zentall, S. S. (1977). Environmental stimulation model. *Exceptional Children, 43*, 502–510.

Zentall, S. S. (1985). A context for hyperactivity. In K. D. Gadow (Ed.), *Advances in learning and behavioral disabilities* (Vol. 4, pp. 273–343). Greenwich, CT: JAI Press.

Zentall, S. S., & Zentall, T. R. (1983). Optimal stimulation: A model of disordered activity and performance in normal and deviant children. *Psychological Bulletin, 94*, 446–471.

Zimmerman, F. T., & Burgemeister, B. B. (1958). Action of methylphenidylacetate (Ritalin) and reserpin in behavior disorders in children and adults. *American Journal of Psychiatry, 115*, 323–328.

Chapter 3

Learning Disabilities

The term *learning disability* is generally applied to children who are doing poorly in school despite average or above average ability level. The latter is generally assessed with an individually administered IQ test. There are, of course, many children who have below average ability and who are doing poorly in school. Whether or not they will be placed in a special education program (which means the child will have to be officially labeled learning disabled); receive only remedial help, usually in reading or arithmetic (which means the child is not officially labeled learning disabled); or is not provided with any special services at all is pretty much up to the local school district. Because many parents and school administrators find the terms *emotionally disturbed* and *mentally retarded* unpalatable, children who could be diagnosed as having one or both of these handicaps are sometimes labeled learning disabled. Students who have above average IQs but who are performing at or only moderately below grade level are often not placed in special education at all. While many educators simply agonize over this somewhat sloppy system of identification and treatment prescription, an investigation into the diagnostic uncertainties of various types of complex partial seizures or the maze of psychosocial variables that lead to pharmacotherapy could relieve some of their stress. The fact that our culture equates academic competence with self-worth does not help matters and often causes much heartache for parents.

The study of learning disabilities is a relatively new area from the standpoint of political (e.g., federal legislation), scientific (e.g., professional journals), and educational (e.g., labeling, teacher training, program development) recognition. Nevertheless, children with the types of problems that are now referred to as learning disabilities have, of course, always been with us, and they have been the subject of study under a legion of labels. The historical bases for our current conceptualizations about learning disabilities have been discussed in some detail by the many reviewers of this literature (e.g., Wiederholt, 1974). As previously noted, the essential characteristic or criterion for a diagnosis of learning disability is a marked discrepancy between ability and school achievement. Why children should experience such problems is very puzzling, but the list of hypothesized causes is unending (Mayron, 1978) and ranges from the laughable (or pathetic, depending upon one's perspective) to the scientifically praiseworthy. The fact that there are probably multiple causes complicates matters considerably, as does the horde of charlatans and dilettantes who prey on parental fears with bogus therapies and meaningless assessments. While the seriousness of learning disabilities as an impediment to personal happiness requires thoughtful consideration (Snyder, 1979, 1983), there is clear evidence that in severe cases that are refractory to treatment, the inability to adequately use written or verbal communication can have an extraordinary effect on psychosocial development and even on the ability to achieve economic self-sufficiency. In such instances, it is almost always the case that an inability to negotiate some academically related hurdle (e.g., job application form), rather than an inability to do the job, prevents access to opportunity.

The term *learning disability* as it is currently used can be traced to the first edition of Sam Kirk's introductory textbook in special education, *Educating Exceptional Children* (Kirk, 1962). He stated:

> A learning disability refers to a retardation, disorder, or delayed development in one or more of the processes of speech, language, reading, spelling, writing, or arithmetic resulting from a possible cerebral dysfunction and/or emotional or behavioral disturbance and not from mental retardation, sensory deprivation, or cultural or instructional factors . . . . These disabilities refer to a discrepancy between the child's learning capacity (as indicated by aptitude tests) and his achievement, without reference to the cause of the discrepancy between capacity and achievement. (p. 263)

Kirk's description contains the two essential characteristics of learning disability that have survived intact for two decades. They are (a) discrepancy between ability and achievement and (b) specification of appropriate (e.g., neurological dysfunction) and inappropriate (e.g., other handicapping conditions) causal mechanisms. The latter is not clinically useful because, as Kirk (1962) notes, "Since in many cases it is difficult to determine whether or not there is a cerebral dysfunction except by inference from the behavior, the educator is interested chiefly in the behavior deficits rather than in the location or extent of brain damage" (p. 264).

Learning disability became a legislative reality in the United States in 1969 with the passage of the Children with Specific Learning Disabilities Act. A slightly modified version of the definition that was formulated for this piece of legislation appears in Public Law 94–142, which states:

> "Specific learning disability" means a disorder in one or more of the basic psychological processes involved in understanding or in using language, spoken or written, which may manifest itself in an imperfect ability to listen, think, speak, read, write, spell, or to do mathematical calculations. The term includes such conditions as perceptual handicaps, brain injury, minimal brain dysfunction, dyslexia, and developmental aphasia. The term does not include children who have learning problems which are primarily the result of visual, hearing, or motor handicaps, of mental retardation, of emotional disturbance, or of environmental, cultural, or economic disadvantage. (U.S. Office of Education, 1977, p. 65083)

This chapter differs somewhat from the others, both in style and format, for a very important reason. Namely, learning disability is *not* an indication for drug therapy. In other words, as a society we have yet to conclude that academic underachievement is a legitimate reason for prescribing medication. Once a highly effective and safe drug is discovered, however, this situation will probably change, but certainly not without some controversy. This chapter, therefore, focuses on how drugs (primarily the stimulants) affect academic performance, and in this sense it is more of a review of the medical literature than a description of recommended treatment practices. Given the importance that we attach to academic achievement, it seemed appropriate to treat this as a separate topic.

DIAGNOSIS

The most important criterion for a diagnosis of learning disability as implied by the identification criteria in Public Law 94-142 is a discrepancy between expected and attained achievement (U.S. Office of Education, 1977). Several formulas have been developed to quantify the severity of the disability: (a) deviation from grade level, (b) expectancy formula, (c) standard-score comparison, and (d) regression analysis (Berk, 1984; Cone & Wilson, 1981). Unfortunately, objections have been raised over the use of each of these formulas, which means that there is no nationally agreed-upon method for measuring the severity of academic underachievement.

At the present time, there is a considerable degree of dissatisfaction with our current notion of learning disabilities (see the February 1983 issue of the *Journal of Learning Disabilities*). Part of the problem stems from the fact that many children who are labeled learning disabled by the public schools and federally funded facilities (see Mann et al., 1983) bear little resemblance to the children originally conceptualized as learning disabled. In many situations, learning disability has become synonymous with academic underachievement. Subsequently, many programs for learning disabled students have disproportionately large numbers of poor and minority group children and slow learners (those with IQs between 70 and 85).

TYPES OF ACADEMIC SKILLS

To better understand the learning disabilities area, particularly research about medication, it is useful to have a fundamental understanding of the various types of academic skills. There are basically four groups of skills recognized by Public Law 94-142: reading, arithmetic, written communication, and oral communication. Although Public Law 94-142 states that "thinking" and "listening" disorders are included, we really do not test, diagnose, or label children according to these problem areas. Unquestionably the most common problem, and probably the most important, is reading disability.

In addition to recognizing major skill areas and their component subskills, educators in the learning disabilities area also draw distinctions between various stages of learning. For example, Smith (1981) lists five stages of learning to describe a student's level of skill development prior to the onset of instruction: acquisition (learn how to perform skill accurately), proficiency (perform task accurately and quickly), maintenance (retention of learning), generalization (skill used in appropriate settings), and adaptation (application of prior learning in problem solving situations). It is important to consider these aspects of the learning process when trying to evaluate exactly how medication alters academic performance.

Reading

Although reading is conceptualized in a variety of ways, and task analyses of component skills vary, there are, nevertheless, a group of reading skills that are generally recognized. Reading can be divided into two major groups of skills: word recognition and comprehension. Word recognition skills are necessary for fluent reading. The reader must be able to recognize a large number of known words as well as determine new words through sound analysis and context cues. There are three fundamental word recognition skills: phonetic analysis (the ability to sound out words), structural analysis (the ability to recognize meaningful units of written language such as prefixes, root words, and suffixes), and context analysis (the ability to use the meaning of a sentence or preceding sentences to determine an unknown word). Phonetic analysis can be further subdivided into letter-sound correspondence, phonetic generalization (the ability to identify words by using rules for sounding out similar letter combinations in similar ways), and syllabication (the ability to analyze sound units to identify unknown words). The second major skill area, comprehension, refers to the ability to conceptualize, classify, and determine relationships between concepts. It is often assessed by asking the reader to answer factual questions about or draw inferences from what is read.

Arithmetic

Arithmetic skills can be sorted into five content areas: numeration, computation, measurement, problem solving, and survival mathematics (see Smith, 1981, for a review). *Numeration* refers to basic number concepts and usage and includes such things as recognizing geometric shapes, classifying objects into sets, recognizing numbers, counting, and writing numbers. The mastery of these skills is usually assessed by the teacher by calculating the percentage of correct answers. *Computation* refers to arithmetic processes (addition, subtraction, multiplication, and addition) and fractions. The arithmetic processes can be further subdivided into facts and process problems. Facts are number relationships that are committed to memory (e.g., 7 + 5 = 12), and process problems are solved by utilizing facts and following specific rules (e.g., long division). Proficiency in the latter is generally associated with proficiency (accuracy and speed) in arithmetic facts. Many learning disabled students encounter difficulty in becoming proficient in arithmetic calculation and subsequently end up spending a great deal of time during the course of their academic careers performing drill activities. However, the development of the hand calculator has almost eliminated proficiency deficits in this area from the list of serious disabilities. Fractions, specifically the use of fractions in computations, can be extremely difficult for the learning disabled child. Fortunately, the ability to be able to do complex fractional calculations has little bearing on adult adjustment. The learning of *measurement* skills is one of the more practical aspects of the mathematics curriculum and concerns such things as linear and liquid measurement, money concepts, and time. The latter may be particularly deficient in learning disabled children (Forer & Keogh, 1971). Perhaps the most typical example of a *problem solving* skill is solving story problems that have a mathematical base. These problems can be particularly difficult for the learning disabled child because they also involve reading skills.

Written Communication

Although being able to express one's thoughts on paper is a very important skill for academic success (e.g., taking lecture notes), particularly in college (e.g., writing term papers), it is almost totally irrelevant to success in adult life. Moreover, with the development of economically affordable typewriters and tape recorders (for class lectures) and the growing availability of word processors, illegible handwriting should not prevent anyone from experiencing academic success. Nevertheless, most people master basic written communication skills without too much difficulty; it is convenient and requires no electronic gadgetry; and it remains a very important component of public education. Written communication skills (see Smith, 1981) can be conceptually divided into the following components: foundation skills (formation of letters), mechanical skills (spelling, capitalization, grammar), composition (functional and creative writing), and survival skills (e.g., signature, checks, and various forms such as job applications). In the foundation skill area, interest in learning disabilities has focused on poor motor skills, letter reversals, and the disadvantages of learning manuscript. Many learning disabled children encounter difficulty with the traditional group method for teaching spelling, but a number of alternative strategies do exist. Grammar and punctuation often present problems, and it is unrealistic to expect some learning disabled students to master all but the most basic of these skills. Composition is important in today's society only because it is much easier for a teacher to read about what a student knows than it is to conduct a personal interview. However, some educators would argue that survival skills should be the focus of instruction for students encountering severe problems in this area.

Oral Communication

Many learning disabled students are language disabled (i.e., they experience difficulty understanding or using language effectively). Numerous studies of children who are now considered to be learning disabled exhibit language problems (see Wiig & Semel, 1976, for a review). Language disturbances are many and varied and generally pertain to children's difficulties in understanding what is said to them and expressing their own thoughts. In the auditory area, learning disabled students are more likely to experience difficulty making sound discriminations. They may have difficulty identifying similar speech sounds, blending speech sounds, and locating sound sources. Many also encounter auditory memory problems and have difficulty recalling certain things. In the linguistic sphere, they may show delays in the acquisition of morphological and syntactic rules (e.g., understanding word meaning or problems making plural words). While the child may be able to say all of the words in a sentence and know what each means, he or she may not understand their meaning when arranged in a sentence. The cognitive deficits exhibited by some learning disabled children also make oral communication a problem. They may experience difficulty in concept formation, which makes understanding spoken language, such as following directions, a challenge.

Prevalence

Given the diagnostic uncertainties surrounding the term *learning disabilities*, it is somewhat senseless to talk about the "true" prevalence of these disorders. There are, however, fairly accurate data on the total number of children in the United States who are diagnosed as being learning disabled because the reporting of such information is a requirement of Public Law 94-142. Figure 3–1 shows the number of learning disabled children and the total number of handicapped children reported annually for the past 7 years. It should be evident from this figure that learning disabilities is a rapidly growing diagnostic category. The significance of this trend is difficult to evaluate.

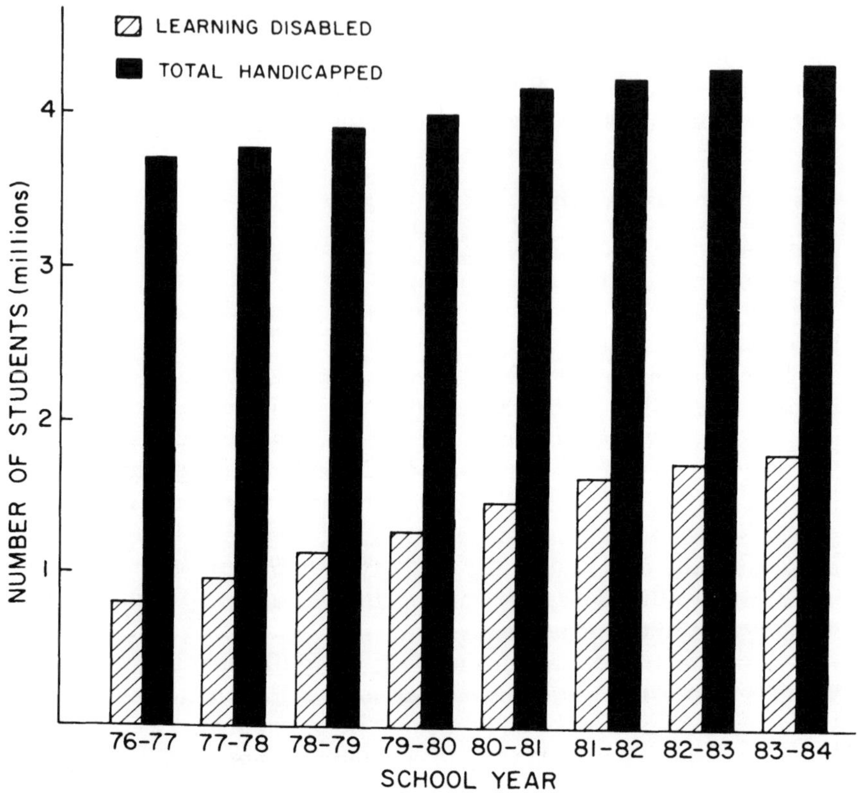

Figure 3–1. Number of children diagnosed as learning disabled in the United States between 1977 and 1983.

PHARMACOTHERAPY

It is not really accurate to say that there is a literature on the use of psychotropic drugs for learning disabilities per se because medication is rarely prescribed for academic underachievement. More accurately, medication is often prescribed for hyperactive children who are doing poorly in school and much less frequently for inattentive children with academic difficulties. More often than not, an underlying behavior disorder is creating enough stress for caregivers to seek help. The situation is complicated by the fact that some hyperactive children who refuse to do their work in school (as well as homework) actually test at or near grade level at the end of the school year when standardized achievement tests are generally administered. In other words, while they appear to be off-task and paying little attention to classroom learning, they manage to pick up enough knowledge and skills to successfully proceed from one grade level to the next. Although they may not be star students, they get by. Nevertheless, their reputation generally precedes them. Such is not the case for the nonhyperactive learning disabled student who may feel put upon by teachers, parents, and peers for years only to discover in adolescence that the world provides more than adequate reinforcers for people who are not academically oriented.

Research on pharmacotherapy for learning disabilities consists primarily of investigations into the effects of stimulant drugs on hyperactive children. In that the majority of the subjects in most of these studies experienced school achievement problems, it is accurate to say that over the past four and a half decades we have acquired a considerable body of information about stimulant drugs and learning disabilities. There are, however, only three published studies of stimulant drug research with nonhyperactive learning disabled children (Aman & Werry, 1982; Gittelman-Klein & Klein, 1976; Gittelman et al., 1983). In general, researchers in the field of hyperactivity have done a relatively poor job of describing learning disabilities in their treatment samples, and the converse is true for studies of learning disabled children (i.e., an assessment of hyperactivity is generally omitted). Unquestionably, the most serious and extensive inquiry into differences among groups of hyperactive, learning disabled, and hyperactive learning disabled children has been made by Dykman and his colleagues at the University of Arkansas (see, for example, Dykman et al., 1980).

As noted, academic underachievement is a common problem in clinic-identified samples of hyperactive children. Comparisons between hyperactive and normal peers have repeatedly shown higher rates of academic failure (e.g., failed grades, retentions [held back], special class placement, and so forth) in the former group (e.g., Borland & Heckman, 1976; Cantwell & Satterfield, 1978; Minde et al., 1971). Although academic deficits are common in hyperactive samples, (a) figures vary greatly from one study to the next; (b) few investigators have documented the prevalence of learning disabilities per se (cf. Lambert & Sandoval, 1980); and (c) the percentage who are labeled learning disabled and scheduled for special education services is generally not reported. One large survey study found that approximately 30% of all the students receiving medication for hyperactivity were classified as special education students (Safer & Krager, 1984).

In his seminal paper on Benzedrine (amphetamine sulfate) in behavior disordered children, Bradley (1937) observed that stimulant drugs enhanced academic performance. Although his treatment period lasted only 1 week, improvement in schoolwork was demonstrated by increased productivity, comprehension, and accuracy, which was attributed to a " 'drive' to accomplish as much work as possible during the school period' " (p. 578). Bradley conducted additional research and concluded that the drug did accelerate academic progress by increasing the number of pages of arithmetic "thoroughly learned" during a 1 month period (Bradley & Bowen, 1940). However, the effect upon the number of lists of spelling words thoroughly learned was less dramatic. Although they did not formally analyze their findings, they did present their raw data, so it is possible to graph their results (see Figure 3–2) and perform statistical analyses. Only in arithmetic were differences between medication and no medication statistically significant. Another important finding from this study is the fact that response to stimulants is quite variable. Some children showed vast improvement on medication, whereas others actually became worse. On the basis of the outcome of another study (Bradley & Green, 1940), Bradley concluded that amphetamine influenced "intellectual performance by altering the emotional attitude of the individual toward his task" (p. 787).

Bradley prepared an exquisite summary of his early clinical experience (Bradley & Bowen, 1941) in which he noted two additional findings relevant to the learning disability topic. One, and most important, drug-induced improvement in academic performance was observed in four children diagnosed as having "specific reading disability." Second, improvement in academic work was not always associated with better overall behavior.

In the same year that Bradley's astute clinical observations first appeared in print, Molitch and Sullivan's (1937) investigation of the effects of a single dose of Benzedrine on juvenile delinquents who were housed in a state-operated residential facility was also published. This was the first stimulant drug study to employ a standardized achievement test. While their data were not analyzed statistically, Molitch and Sullivan concluded that the drug group clearly outperformed the placebo group in enhancing academic achievement test performance and that the higher dose, which was given to poor responders, produced gain scores in 92% of the cases so treated. The mean number of points gained (or lost) for each group is plotted in Figure 3–3.

While Charles Bradley and, to a much lesser extent, Matthew Molitch are rightly recognized as the primary historical figures in stimulant drug therapy for behavior disorders and learning disabilities, Prinzmetal and Bloomberg (1935) published one of the first

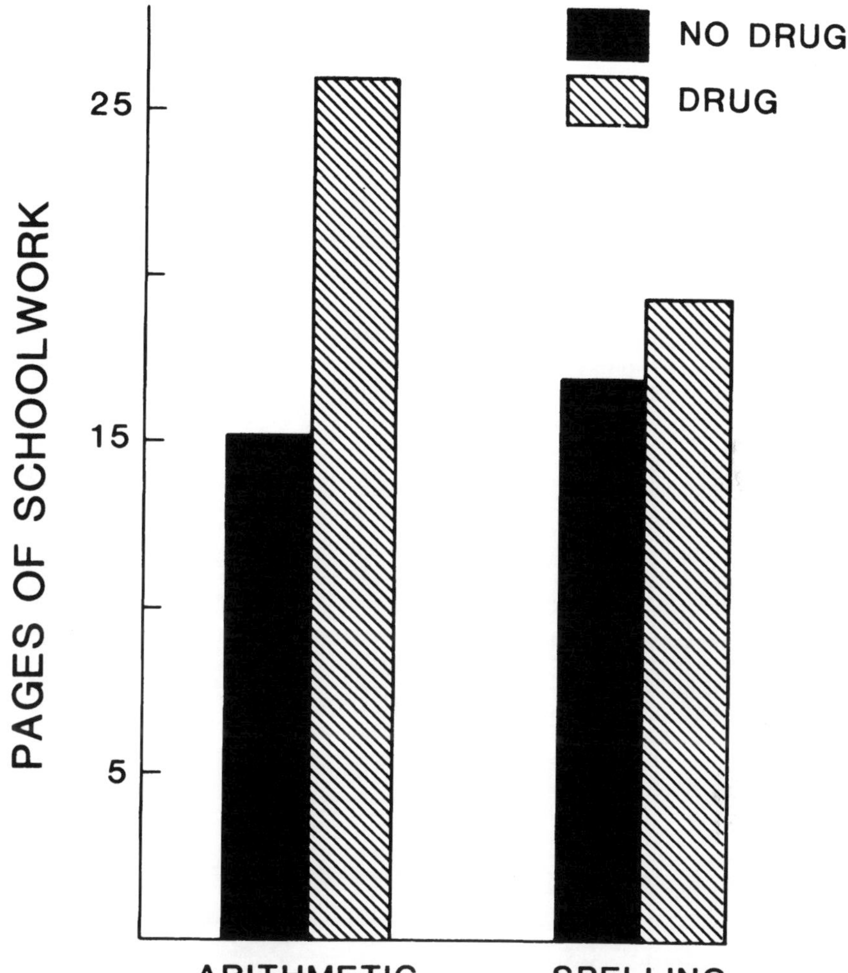

Figure 3–2. Mean number of pages of schoolwork completed under drug (amphetamine sulfate) and no-drug conditions. From data reported in "School Performance of Children Receiving Amphetamine (Benzedrine) Sulfate" by C. Bradley and M. Bowen, 1940, *American Journal of Orthopsychiatry, 10,* 782–788.

papers on the use of Benzedrine for a childhood disorder. The study included four adolescents and one 11 year old child, all of whom suffered from *narcolepsy* (a disorder characterized by an uncontrolled desire for sleep or attacks of sleep during normal waking hours). What is so interesting about this paper is that the 11 year old was failing school because he could not stay awake. Benzedrine helped him stay awake and ultimately allowed him to be promoted

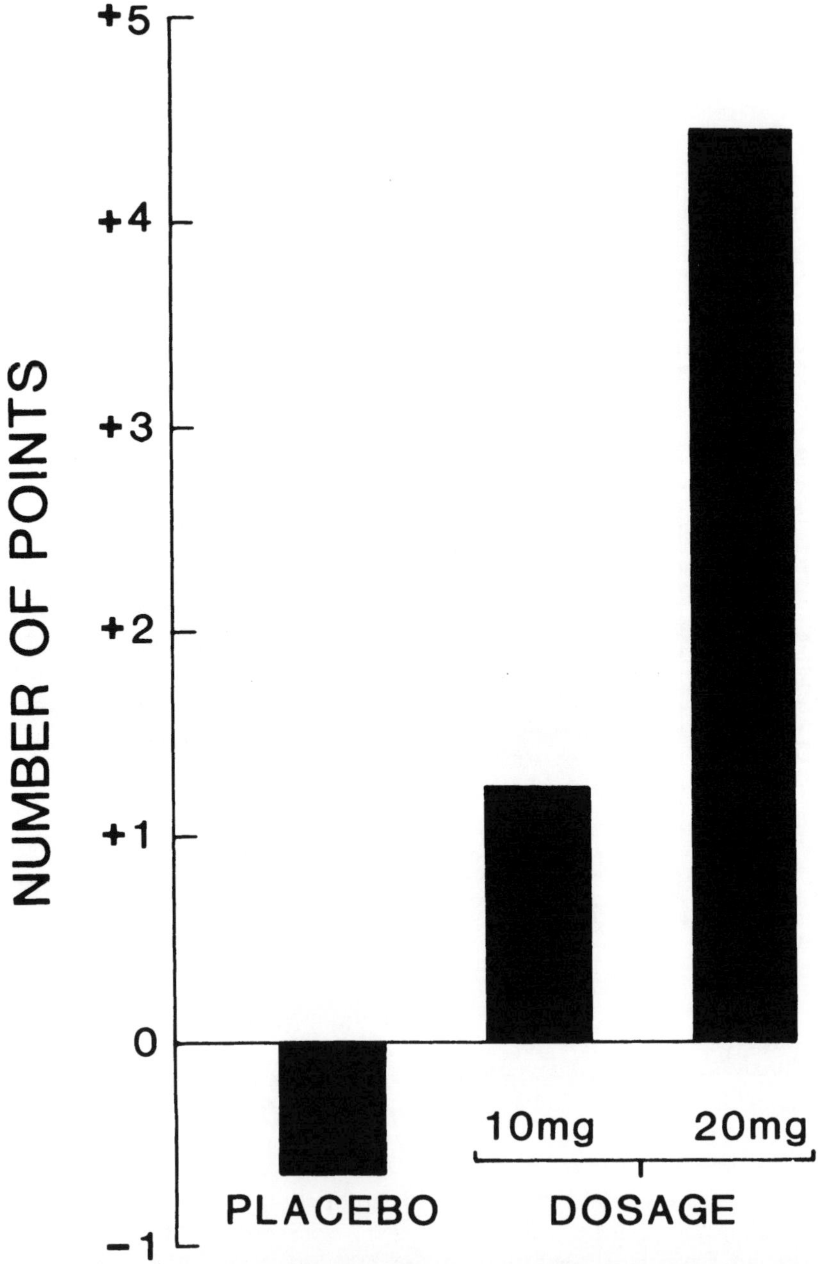

Figure 3–3. Mean number of points on the New Stanford Achievement Test gained (or lost) at retest for placebo and drug (amphetamine sulfate) groups. From data reported in "Effect of Benzedrine Sulfate on Children Taking New Stanford Achievement Test" by M. Molitch and J. P. Sullivan, 1937, *American Journal of Orthopsychiatry, 7*, 519–522.

to the next higher grade at the end of the school year. This may be the earliest published report in which stimulant drug therapy purportedly alleviated a learning disability in a perpubertal child.

The usefulness of stimulant drugs as a treatment for academic problems was also reinforced by case studies that appeared to demonstrate treatment effects. Bender and Cottington (1942), for example, describe the reaction of a boy treated with Benzedrine as follows:

> Case 4. - A. F., an eight-year-old negro boy with intelligence quotient of 94, was referred to the hospital for truancy. . . . Failing at school, and punished by the mother for his failure, he played truant, his reading disability unrecognized. Two years of failure, and ridicule had conditioned him against learning to read. With benzedrine he received a strong impetus to achievement, and made rapid progress with a reading tutor, gaining thereby in personal security. This we have found to be a frequent occurrence in the less complicated cases of reading disability. (p. 118)

Bender and Cottington describe additional cases in which medication was successful for severe reading disability and concluded that "Benzedrine is of great benefit in stimulating interest and drive in learning in the child with a *learning disability*" (italics added, p. 120), but that this was certainly not true for all childhood disorders associated with learning difficulties (e.g., severe emotional disturbance).

Another example of an early case study that suggested a therapeutic effect on academic performance is provided by Ginn and Hohman (1953):

> Case 1. - A seven-year-old child of average intelligence was brought to our clinic because she had not learned to read in the first and second grades. The mother, a teacher, attempted remedial reading at home, using kinesthetic methods under the clinic's direction. Concentration was very poor, attention span extremely short, and there was marked restlessness. Many months of training, both by the mother and a remedial reading teacher, resulted in practically no progress. Dextroamphetamine immediately cut down the restlessness and increased the attention span and concentration. Progress was rapid, and within months she was up to grade level in reading. (p. 1125)

The belief that stimulant medication was useful for the treatment of learning disabilities as they are now currently defined can be traced to a variety of sources. First, several investigations showed that teachers rated hyperactive children as having completed more school work when they were receiving medication (Comly, 1971; Conners, 1972; Conners et al., 1967; Rapoport et al., 1974). Others found that report card grades even improved (e.g., Comly, 1971). Moreover, many no doubt found the notion that medication was being prescribed to facilitate academic performance to be a much more acceptable justification for treatment than the suppression of conduct problems to the benefit of teachers and parents. Second, there are numerous studies of how stimulant drugs improve performance on a variety of psychological tests and cognitive tasks that measured important components of the learning process (see Chapter 2, *Hyperactivity*). In some instances it was reasoned that if stimulants improve mental abilities such as attention span, they must also improve learning. Others thought that because these drugs actually improved the very cognitive abilities that were believed to be the cause of learning disabilities (e.g., perceptual-motor skills, attention span, short-term memory), stimulants were a treatment for reading and arithmetic problems. Third, at one time both learning disabilities and hyperactivity were considered symptoms of the same disorder, minimal brain dysfunction, or MBD (Clements & Peters, 1962; see also Bradley, 1957). Consequently, the findings from drug studies with MBD samples were occasionally generalized to both hyperactive and learning disabled children. Lastly, some clinicians actually stated that stimulants were an effective treatment for nonhyperactive learning disabled children (e.g., Clements & Peters, 1962).

Optimism that stimulant treatment was beneficial for academic deficits began to wane in the mid 1970s with the publication of better-designed studies that failed to demonstrate treatment effects, and an influential review article by Barkley and Cunningham (1978) all but closed the case. The latter was an analysis of the results of 17 short-term (2 to 6 weeks) investigations of academic achievement in extremely varied samples of children that showed that of the 52 dependent measures (usually achievement test scores, the WRAT being the most popular) employed in these studies, 82.6% were not improved by stimulant treatment. Moreover, there was no consistent pattern in those measures that were drug sensitive. Barkley and Cunningham (1978) also evaluated the findings from six followup studies and failed to find any support for an achievement enhancement effect. Although these short- and long-term studies are very diverse (Barkley & Cunningham, 1978) and methodologically inadequate from the standpoint of generating a definitive answer (Cantwell & Carlson, 1978), Barkley (1981) notes that the burden of proof remains with those who maintain that a treatment effect does exist.

Just when it seemed that the academic achievement issue had finally been resolved, a series of investigations conducted primarily by Bill Pelham (Pelham, 1985; Pelham et al., 1985) and his colleagues at Florida State University and by Mark Rapport (e.g., Rapport et al., 1982, 1985) and his coworkers at the University of Rhode Island began to raise new questions about the role of medication in the management of learning disabilities. The findings from their studies suggested that stimulant medication can greatly increase on-task behavior, leading to greater academic output without a loss of accuracy. In fact, accuracy also improved in some cases. In other words, some hyperactive children on medication completed more schoolwork and appeared to learn more.

We have come full circle, then, and returned to the point of Bradley's initial observations. However, it is not exactly that simple because drug-induced improvement in academic achievement test performance has still not been compellingly demonstrated, at least in terms of clinically meaningful gains. It is important to understand the difference between doing school work each day and taking a test at the end of the school year to show how much has been learned. It is conceivable that completing daily class assignments does improve skill proficiency (accuracy and speed) but may not necessarily lead to better achievement test scores. For example, longer-term studies are almost uniformly negative when it comes to academic achievement (Gadow, 1983b). Even though medication improves school behavior, it does not appear to make a big difference in whether or not a person will graduate from high school or college. In the following sections, an attempt is made to help clarify this situation by describing stimulant drug effects on various academic skills.

Reading

Aman (1982) recently analyzed the results of 10 studies that assessed the effect of stimulant drugs on academic achievement in children selected for the presence of a learning problem. In only four of the studies, however, were the samples limited, according to objective selection criteria, to children with reading problems, of which two selected only children with serious reading disorders. Aman found that while 40 of the 196 perceptual-cognitive measures employed in the 10 studies were significantly improved as a consequence of stimulant treatment, only 2 of the 26 reading measures showed such improvement. On the basis of these findings, he concluded that there was no justification for the use of stimulants in the treatment of reading disorders.

Within the last few years, three studies have been published on the use of stimulant medication with *nonhyperactive* learning disabled children (Aman & Werry, 1982; Gittelman-Klein & Klein, 1976; Gittelman et al., 1983). In their earlier study, Gittelman-Klein and Klein (1976) randomly assigned 61 children to either Ritalin (methylphenidate) or placebo conditions. All subjects were selected on the basis of being 2 years below reading grade level despite average intelligence, and most were receiving academic remediation in school. The average dose was 55 mg, which means that approximately one half of the children received at least 25 mg of Ritalin twice a day. At the end of 4 weeks, the only statistically significant drug effect was for the Wide Range Achievement Test (WRAT) arithmetic score (6-month superiority of medicated over the placebo group). At the end of 12 weeks, however, arithmetic differences were trivial (2 months), but the WRAT reading score difference approached statistical significance ($p = .06$). (Because the WRAT appears to be highly insensitive to drug effects, this finding is noteworthy.) WRAT spelling scores were unaffected by medication. At the end of 12 weeks, teacher global ratings of reading and arithmetic performance did not discriminate between the two treatment groups. On the basis of these and other findings, Gittelman-Klein and Klein concluded that Ritalin was not an effective agent for the remediation of reading deficits in nonhyperactive learning disabled children. They also noted, however, that medication effects may be manifested only in the presence of a specialized academic intervention.

To test this hypothesis, Gittelmen et al. (1983) conducted a second study in which nonhyperactive reading retarded children were randomly assigned to one of three groups: (a) reading remediation (phonics program) and placebo, (b) academic tutoring (without reading instruction) and placebo, and (c) reading remediation and Ritalin. The average dose was 1.19 mg/kg per day, which means that approximately one half of the children received 0.6 mg/kg or more of Ritalin twice a day. The duration of the intervention was 18 weeks. The results indicated that while medication did enhance cognitive task performance, it did not facilitate academic achievement (as measured by the WRAT and Gray Oral Reading Test). Some additional reading achievement measures, however, did show drug effects or trends favoring the medication-treated group, suggesting that the effect of Ritalin on reading instruction was not a strong one. Interestingly, several of the phonics-based tests did show drug effects. Quite unexpectedly, medication did markedly enhance other areas of academic skill performance, namely arithmetic and social studies, which were obviously not part of the reading program. However, a retest of these academic skills 8 months after the termination of treatment failed to show residual drug effects. In other words, the gains in achievement appeared to fade over time after medication was stopped.

Aman and Werry (1982) administered Ritalin, Valium (diazepam), and placebo for 1 week each to 15 children diagnosed as being severely reading retarded (but with normal IQ). Medication was not found to improve cognitive functions presumed to be associated with reading disability.

Although the studies of nonhyperactive learning disabled children *appear* to be discouraging, other investigations with hyperactive children are more hopeful. For example, in one study of 29 elementary school children (most of whom were hyperactive), it was found that Ritalin did increase reading performance (Pelham et al., 1985). All children received various dosages of medication (0.15 mg/kg, 0.3 mg/kg, 0.6 mg/kg) for 1 week each and placebo for 2 weeks. Reading was assessed by counting the number of questions attempted and answered correctly in daily workbook assignments. The results indicated that as the amount of medication increased, the number of questions attempted decreased, but more were answered correctly. This produced an average improvement of 18% between placebo and the highest dose in the *proportion* of questions answered correctly.

Rapport et al. (1982) used an analytical research design to study the effects of Ritalin and response cost on the academic performance of two hyperactive boys. The response cost procedure consisted of an apparatus that was operated by the classroom teacher, which awarded points for doing school work and subtracted points for fooling around. The data for one of the subjects (Mitch) are presented in Figure 3–4. The baseline indicates the child's performance before treatment began. As is clear from the lower panel, the youngster completed more and more problems in his phonics workbook as the dosage increased from 5 mg (0.2 mg/kg) to 15 mg (0.6 mg/kg) administered in the morning. This finding has been replicated in a larger study (Rapport et al., 1985), which is discussed in Chapter 2. When the subject was given 20 mg (0.9 mg/kg), however, academic work dropped dramatically, suggesting that this was too much medication for this particular child. Interestingly, in the upper panel it can be seen that the amount of time Mitch spent on-task (at his desk doing his work) did *not* decrease on the higher dose. In other words, while he appeared to be working at an ever-increasing rate on his school work, the highest dose of medication really was not helping him that much. In fact, he was doing about the same as if he were not taking medication at all. It is also clear from Figure 3–4 that

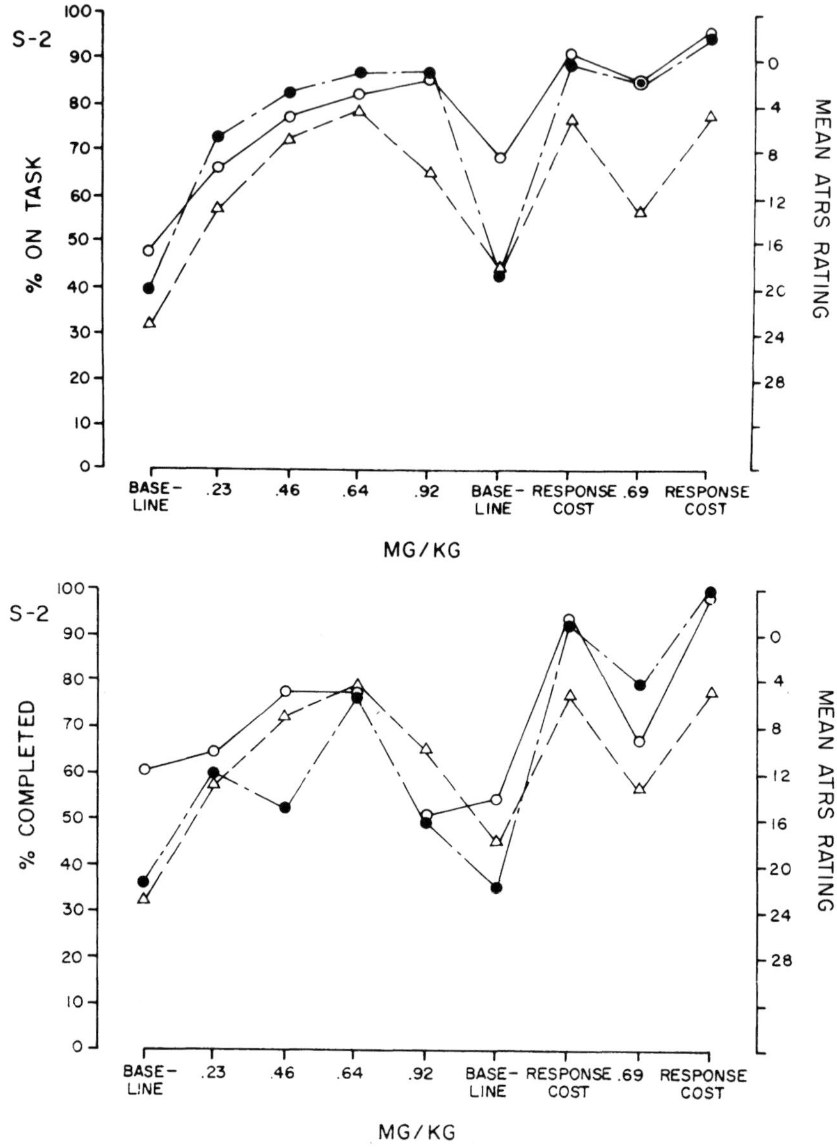

Figure 3–4. The mean percentage of intervals of daily on-task behavior (Upper Panel) across academic areas (math, ●, and phonics, ○), classroom behavior (△, ATRS), and experimental conditions. Mean percentage of daily problems completed presented in Lower Panel. Note: From "Attention Deficit Disorder with Hyperactivity: Critical Treatment Parameters and Their Application in Applied Outcome Research" by M. D. Rapport, in *Progress in Behavior Modification* (Vol. 14, pp. 284–285), by M. Hersen, R. Eisler, and P. Miller (Eds.), 1983, Orlando, FL: Academic Press. Copyright 1983 by Academic Press. Adapted by permission.

response cost was also a very effective procedure for the management of this child.

It is difficult to summarize the findings from research on reading and stimulant medication. On the one hand, medication does not appear to alter the amount of learning, at least as it is measured by standardized achievement tests in short-term studies. This appears to be the case for both nonhyperactive learning disabled children (Gittelman-Klein & Klein, 1976; Gittelman et al., 1983) and hyperactive children (Barkley & Cunningham, 1978). Moreover, it does not correct the underlying problem that is causing the reading disability (Aman & Werry, 1982). On the other hand, there is equally compelling evidence that stimulants do increase the amount of reading-related workbook assignments in underachieving hyperactive children (Pelham et al., 1980, 1985; Rapport et al., 1982, 1985). One would predict that if medication helped students to pay attention and complete more school work, their reading levels would improve. At the present time, however, it is difficult to say with certainty whether this is true or false.

Arithmetic

As noted, Bradley (1937) was the first person to comment that stimulant drugs increased the completion of classroom arithmetic assignments, a finding he later confirmed in a formal study (Bradley & Bowen, 1940). Nevertheless, of the 14 short-term studies in Barkley and Cunningham's (1978) review that employed measures of arithmetic achievement, significant drug effects were reported in only two instances (Bradley & Bowen, 1940; Conners et al., 1969). Although this sounds quite discouraging, there are several recent investigations that suggest a more optimistic outlook.

Pelham, for example, conducted two studies, one with Ritalin (Pelham et al., 1985) and a second with Cylert (pemoline) (Pelham et al., 1980), which showed that stimulant medication does have a powerful effect on classroom arithmetic assignments. These activities consisted of arithmetic calculation problems (e.g., subtraction, multiplication) that the children knew how to do but required more practice to achieve complete mastery. Some have described this reaction as a greater tolerance for overlearning (Ackerman & Dykman, 1982). In other words, the children appear to be less resistant to doing drill activities. In Pelham et al.'s Ritalin study, hyperactive children completed approximately 30% more math problems on the lower dose without a loss of accuracy. Interestingly, increasing the dosage of Ritalin from 0.3 mg/kg to 0.6 mg/kg did not lead to a better academic response. Even bigger gains were reported in the

Cylert study. The findings from both investigations are presented in Figure 3–5.

Several additional studies have also shown that stimulant medication increases arithmetic productivity. Rapport et al. (1982) found that Ritalin markedly increased arithmetic workbook assignments from 25% to 40%. Rapport et al.'s (1985) more recent study also supports this finding. The data for Mitch (see Figure 3–4), however, also appear to show that at higher dosages of medication (0.92 mg/kg), performance decreases again, at least for this particular child.

The Gittelman et al. (1983) study, which was described in the previous (reading) section, found significant Ritalin effects on the arithmetic subtests of the Stanford Achievement Test in nonhyperactive learning disabled children. They reported a 0.8-year difference between drug and placebo groups. In fact, on some arithmetic mea-

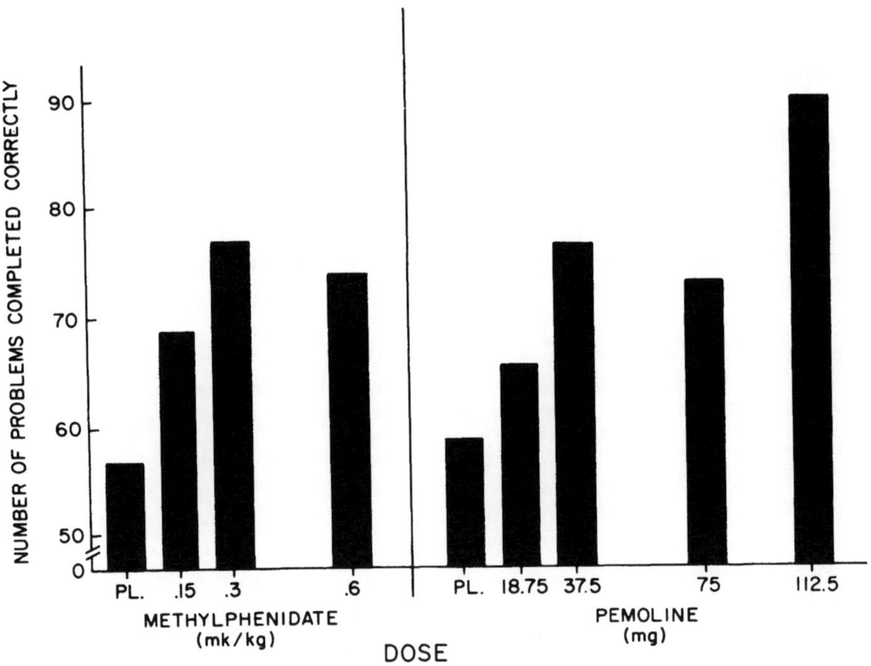

Figure 3–5. Number of arithmetic problems completed correctly in 15-minute, supervised, special classroom periods as a function of methylphenidate [Ritalin] and pemoline [Cylert] doses. Note: From "The Effects of Psychostimulant Drugs on Learning and Academic Achievement in Children with Attention Deficit Disorders and Learning Disabilities" by W. E. Pelham, in *Psychological and Educational Perspectives on Learning Disabilities* by J. K. Torgesen and B. Wong (Eds.), 1985, Orlando, FL: Academic Press. Copyright 1985 by Academic Press. Reprinted by permission.

sures, the Ritalin and reading instruction group scored at grade level even though arithmetic skill development was *not* part of the intervention program.

The findings from studies on stimulant medication and arithmetic productivity are fairly consistent. Drug therapy appears to increase work output without sacrificing accuracy. As with reading, however, there are only a few reports of improved performance on standardized achievement tests (Conners et al., 1969; Gittelman et al., 1983). Nothing is known about the effects of stimulants on children who have a specific arithmetic disability and no other behavior or learning disorder.

Spelling

There were 11 short-term drug studies in Barkley and Cunningham's (1978) review that employed either measures of spelling achievement ($n = 10$) or productivity ($n = 1$), and significant drug effects were demonstrated in only two instances (Conners et al., 1972; Weiss et al., 1971). Pelham et al. (1985) reported a modest Ritalin effect on the proportion of words correct on weekly spelling tests. Weekly spelling assignments consisted of words that the hyperactive children could not spell correctly. In a similar study, however, Cylert failed to enhance spelling performance (Pelham et al., 1980). Another investigation (Stephens et al., 1984) of Ritalin (0.3 mg/kg), Cylert (1.9 mg/kg), and placebo revealed that stimulant drugs produced a 25% reduction in spelling errors (nonsense words) compared with placebo. In addition, Dykman et al. (1980) reported spelling achievement test gains for hyperactive learning disabled children and hyperactive children with both Ritalin and Cylert.

In view of the conflicting results from studies that have examined stimulant drugs and spelling, it is not possible to draw definite conclusions about this topic at present. It is not clear exactly why some tasks are more drug sensitive than others, and only further research can clarify the inconsistencies.

Handwriting

A number of investigators have reported that stimulant drugs can enhance handwriting ability in hyperactive children (Levy, 1973; Schain & Reynard, 1975; Taylor, 1979; Whalen et al., 1981) and adolescents (Yellin et al, 1982). Moreover, there are a number of published handwriting samples (Levy, 1973; Schain & Reynard, 1975; Taylor, 1979) that compellingly demonstrate the magnitude of this effect. In general, these findings have been serendipitous in that poor handwriting would not be expected to prompt medical referral, nor is it a clinical indication for treatment. The only published study that selected children (diagnosed as having MBD) on the basis of poor handwriting was conducted by Lerer et al. (1977). The 50 children who participated in this study received both Ritalin and placebo. They found that handwriting improved with Ritalin in 52% of the cases, compared with only one child receiving placebo. In general, handwriting deteriorated subsequently to drug withdrawal, but improvement was maintained for months in those children who remained on medication.

To give some idea on how powerful the drug effect can be in some children, Figure 3–6 shows the results of two spelling tests for a fourth-grade girl who was involved in a research project. For the test dated January 20, the child was receiving Ritalin, and her handwriting is clear and legible. However, while she was on placebo (February 7) writing skills rapidly deteriorated after the third word.

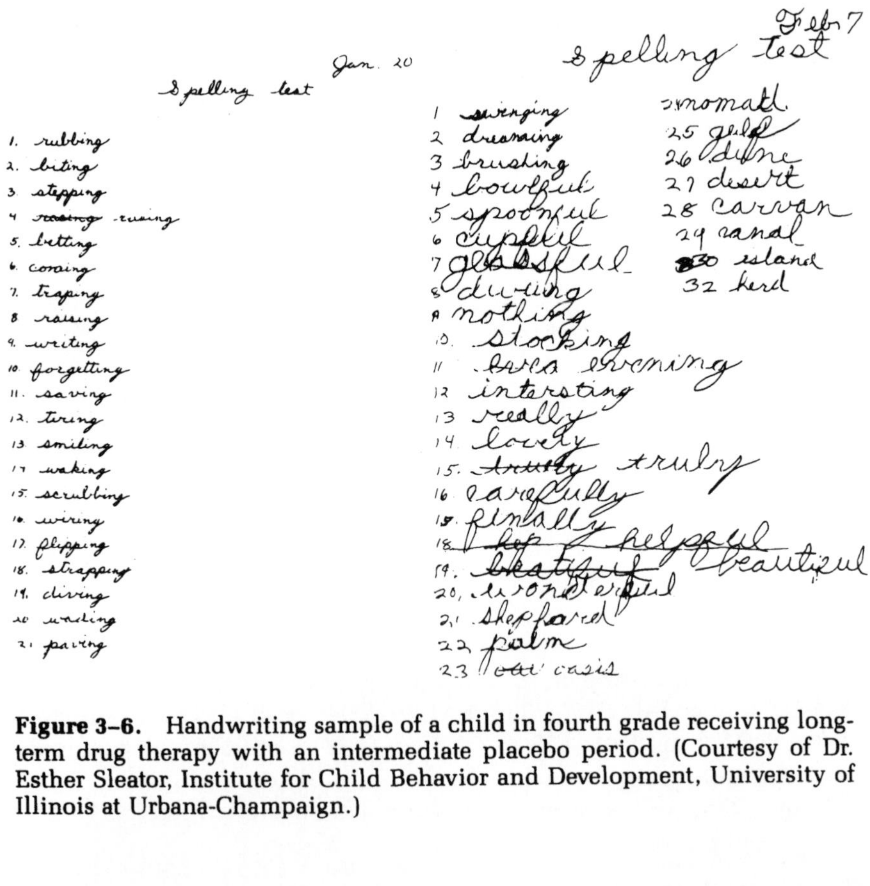

Figure 3–6. Handwriting sample of a child in fourth grade receiving long-term drug therapy with an intermediate placebo period. (Courtesy of Dr. Esther Sleator, Institute for Child Behavior and Development, University of Illinois at Urbana-Champaign.)

Throughout the remainder of the test, the quality of her handwriting varies greatly. In fact, it is easy to visualize her concentration level rising and falling throughout the test.

Although these findings seem exciting, neatness is only one small component of what people generally refer to as written communication skills. The latter includes spelling, sentence structure, grammar, the ability to express and organize ideas, and so forth. It is important not to underestimate neatness and legibility, but we must also realize that little is known about the effect of stimulant drugs on more serious forms of written communication disorders.

Speech, Language, and Communication Disorders

Although it is true that relatively little pharmacotherapy research has been conducted on speech, language, and communication disorders in hyperactive children (Barkley et al., 1983), a careful reading of the stimulant drug literature will reveal a surprising number of case studies or anecdotes about how these drugs affect the speech or language of specific children. Moskowitz (1941), for example, reported on the effects of Benzedrine in 23 mentally retarded adolescents and young adults (IQ: 43 to 75) who were being treated on an outpatient basis by a psychiatric clinic. Although only a few cases showed ''striking improvement,'' the reaction of one youth is noteworthy:

> His speech was virtually unintelligible. . . . Before benzedrine therapy, education and training had been of no avail. There was complete apathy and disinterest in the immediate environment. . . . After administration of 30 mgms. (milligrams) benzedrine daily, speech correction became possible . . . . The patient was able to recognize his failure in speech articulation and would even become angry at his difficulty with 'that lazy old tongue'. . . . When benzedrine (was discontinued) the patient became noticeably more inert and apathetic. (pp. 541–542).

Moskowitz went on to comment that medication appeared to induce spontaneous speech and enhance responsiveness to instruction. It must be emphasized, however, that only a few patients responded in this fashion.

Bender and Cottington (1942) described a case of elective mutism that appeared to respond to Benzedrine. Elective mutism is a disorder in which the individual is fully capable of speech but refuses to talk in some (e.g., school) or all settings.

> Case 2. - A negro boy of twelve was admitted because of a sudden onset of complete mutism . . . . No improvement occurred in response to the therapeutic routines on the ward. He responded to

> benzedrine by beginning to speak in answer to direct questions. . . . In this boy, the effect of benzedrine appeared to be to initiate better social adaptation and to allow freer expression of aggression. (p. 117)

Bender and Cottington went on to describe several other cases (children with developmental aphasia or organic brain damage) for whom stimulant medication had no beneficial effect.

Ginn and Hohman (1953) described the treatment of a 4-year-old hyperactive boy with 7.5 mg of Dexedrine (dextroamphetamine) in the morning. The boy "jabbered only a few words" and stuttered. Medication presumably made him talk more slowly.

The first controlled study of stimulant drugs for speech disorders was conducted by Fish and Bowling (1962), who administered either Dexedrine (15 mg) or placebo to 106 mentally retarded people, primarily adults, with speech defects. Only the stutterers appeared to improve with medication, and therapeutic improvement was limited to only a few cases.

In spite of these early studies, which suggest that stimulant medication may facilitate speech and language therapy in some individuals and possibly improve some speech disorders, there really is not much research on speech and language disorders per se. Most of the additional research on the effects of drugs on verbal behavior pertains to hyperactive children, and the nature of their speech and language problems, if present, is generally not specified.

Creager and VanRiper (1967) administered Ritalin (20 mg twice a day) and placebo to 30 children with "cerebral dysfunction." The children were referred to a psychiatric clinic for a variety of reasons, including "hyperactivity, scholastic difficulty, unmanageable behavior, withdrawal, short attention span, and maturational delay" (p. 624). In the study, the children were asked a few questions and talked about a series of pictures. An analysis of their verbal behavior indicated that medication caused the children to talk more, which the authors believed was important for children undergoing speech therapy because the child must talk if therapy is going to work. Similarly, Ludlow et al. (1979) found that Dexedrine increased verbal productivity and language complexity in hyperactive boys.

The observed effects of stimulant drugs on verbal behavior are determined to a considerable degree by the characteristics of the task and setting, which is obvious from the findings from two additional studies. In one of these, Barkley et al. (1983) administered Ritalin and placebo to hyperactive children who did not exhibit deficits in language complexity, and found that medication reduced the number of vocalizations in both free and structured settings with no concurrent change in complexity. Whalen et al. (1978) also found that Ritalin significantly reduced task-irrelevant speech and verbal productivity to a more normal level.

The studies of hyperactive children suggest that stimulant medication appears to decrease verbal output in situations that call for less talking (participating in a cooperative group activity) and increases output when it is appropriate (describing a picture to an adult). Stimulants also appear to channel speech in such a way as to make it more goal directed and less extraneous or off-task. We must, of course, bear in mind that these generalizations pertain to group effects. In individual cases, stimulant medication can make children excessively talkative or excessively withdrawn (very little speech). When this happens, their reactions are generally considered to be side effects, which typically abate with dosage reduction and are, of course, completely reversible upon drug withdrawal.

Collectively, while these studies provide us with information about stimulants and hyperactive children, they tell us relatively little about the usefulness of stimulant medication for the treatment of communication disorders. Nevertheless, Cantwell and Baker's studies on speech and language impaired children clearly show that such children exhibit a variety of psychiatric disorders, most notably hyperactivity (Baker & Cantwell, 1985; Cantwell & Baker, 1985). Therefore, the management of behavior disorders does have direct bearing on speech and language therapy, and possibly on language development, in learning disability programs.

Other Drugs

Stimulant drugs are by no means the only psychotropic agents that have been studied with regard to their effect on academic achievement. In his excellent review of drugs, learning, and cognition, Mike Aman (1978) shows that there are many studies of how psychotropic drugs affect performance on cognitive tasks and, to a much lesser extent, academic achievement. Unfortunately, much of the earlier research in this area is not particularly good because the studies are poorly designed. This is important because some scientists have reported a fairly powerful placebo effect with some learning disabled children (e.g., Chase et al., 1984). In a certain sense, the problem is a serious one and has prompted John Werry (1981) to note that we really do not have very much information on how the various psychotropic drugs affect academic achievement, which is particularly true for learning disabled children. While there is an occasional well-designed study with neuroleptics, such as Thorazine (chlorpromazine) (Freed et al., 1959), with antianxiety agents such as Valium (diazepam) (e.g., Aman & Werry, 1982), or with antidepressants such as Tofranil (imipramine) (Rapoport et al., 1974), most of what we know is about stimulants. It is therefore accurate to say that there are no other psychotropic drugs being seriously considered as treatments for academic deficits at the present time.

There is another drug, however, whose generic name is piracetam, that is generating a considerable amount of interest. It belongs to a group of compounds called *nootropics*. "Noo" refers to mind and "tropein" means toward. In other words, these drugs have selective cognitive effects. Piracetam is a derivative of the neurotransmitter GABA (gamma-aminobutyric acid). Substances such as GABA appear to increase the ability of nerve cells to process information. While piracetam has been around for 20 years and is approved for use in approximately 86 countries of the world (sold as Nootropyl in some places), it is *not* presently approved by the Food and Drug Administration for use in the United States. It is, however, currently the subject of an intense multiclinic study (DiIanni et al., in press). Research on adult volunteers (e.g., Dimond & Brouwers, 1976) suggested that piracetam increased verbal learning and improved performance on short-term memory tasks. Other researchers found drug effects on tasks that purportedly measured functioning in the left hemisphere of the brain (e.g., Mindus et al., 1976; Squitieri et al., 1975), which is significant because many scientists link the left hemisphere with reading disorders. Based on these and other findings, it seemed logical to study the effects of piracetam in nonhyperactive reading disabled children.

Briefly, the results from several of the child studies indicate that piracetam (a) increases the speed with which children read and write and decreases spelling errors (Chase et al., 1984), (b) improves the ability to read words presented one at a time but not paragraph reading (Helfgott et al., 1984), (c) improves the ability to remember and name pictures of objects (Rudel & Helfgott, 1984), (d) enhances the brain's ability to process verbal stimuli in the left hemisphere (Conners et al., 1984), and produces remarkably few side effects. Although this area of research is most exciting, the size of the treatment effect appears to be modest, and much remains to be learned about this drug, such as its interactive effects with specialized reading instruction.

There is not much to report on treatment practices because this is still a relatively new agent for reading disorders. The dosage levels of piracetam currently employed range from 3,300 to 4,800 mg per day. This is typically divided into two doses, one administered in the morning and a second later in the day.

In addition to piracetam, there are other drugs, vitamins, and foods that are touted as treatments for learning disabilities or reading disorders. In general, their research credentials are scandalous, and subsequently they are not even mentioned here so as not to draw attention to them.

ALTERNATIVE THERAPIES

It is somewhat misleading to talk about alternatives to medication when there is no legally recognized drug for the treatment of learning disabilities in the first place. This is not as straightforward as it sounds, however, because academic underachievement can be associated with another disorder, such as hyperactivity, that is responsive to drug therapy. As we have already seen, stimulant medication does increase academic output in some hyperactive children. Nevertheless, its effect on reading performance in children with reading disability (who are not hyperactive) appears to be limited, but this is controversial (see Pelham, 1985). The notion of alternative treatments is complicated by the fact that there are scores of theories and hypotheses regarding the cause of academic failure, which in turn have prompted the development of an equally mind-boggling array of therapies. Although many of these are nothing more than snake oil remedies, many parents fall victim to the influence of a charismatic clinician. Even parents who should know better are snared into using worthless treatments and obtaining meaningless diagnostic evaluations in their desperate attempt to seek help for their child. Unfortunately, our professional societies often fail us when it comes to monitoring the behavior of therapists who peddle questionable treatments for learning disabled children.

In addition to the problems created by well-meaning but incompetent clinicians and scientific dilettantism, there is the added problem of clinically irrelevant symptomatic improvement. The latter pertains to an alleviation of symptoms associated with the disorder that have little bearing on the primary reason for treatment. For example, say that drug A improves attention span and that a particular nonhyperactive learning disabled child is inattentive, daydreams, and does not follow directions. Drug A could improve all of these symptoms and in so doing produce a more typical student; but if it failed to significantly enhance academic learning as measured by some test of skill acquisition, what good would it be? Caregivers must be wary, therefore, of treatments designed to correct the cause of learning disability in an age where proven causes do not exist.

MEDICATION VERSUS EDUCATION

The beliefs that special education techniques are far superior to pharmacotherapy for the amelioration of academic deficits in learning disabled students, and that medication adds little to the effectiveness of a proven education program, are deeply entrenched in the education establishment. However, until very recently there was not much research on this topic. Educators knew, of course, that unlike educational interventions, medication taught the child nothing. Nevertheless, at the same time that drug therapy for hyperactivity was becoming popular, educators were becoming aware of the fact that teaching strategies designed to reverse or accommodate to presumed etiological (causal) mechanisms (e.g., perceptual-motor and cognitive deficits) were not particularly effective in facilitating academic achievement in learning disabled children either (Arter & Jenkins, 1979; Vellutino et al., 1977; Ysseldyke & Salvia, 1974). Ironically, this was also a serious blow to drug therapy because its strong suit has always been a clear demonstration of treatment effects upon measures of perceptual-motor skills and cognitive abilities such as sustained attention.

Unlike school personnel, many physicians have generally believed that medication does enhance school achievement in hyperactive children who experience school failure. This is based, in part, on research reports, some of which have already been discussed, and actual clinical experience with treated children and their teachers and families. This situation of differing professional opinion ultimately led to a heated debate as to whether medication really played a meaningful role in the treatment of hyperactive children. While it is true that much of the controversy focused on the social behavior of these children, it spilled over into the academic area because many hyperactive children were either underachievers or learning disabled. The debate ultimately settled on the issue of whether or not stimulant medication made children more responsive to instruction, thereby enhancing the effectiveness of education. There are at least three parts to this issue. One is the effect of medication on children who are receiving the standard educational program. The second pertains to the relative efficacy issue—that is, how does medication compare with special academic interventions (i.e., which is superior). The third aspect of this issue is whether or not medication increases the effectiveness of academic interventions that are provided in addition to, or as substitutes for, regular classroom efforts. Because the first part of this issue has already been addressed, this section focuses on the relative efficacy and the treatment enhancement questions.

In an attempt to better understand the relationship between stimulant drug therapy and behavioral interventions designed to improve academic performance, Gadow (1985) examined 16 studies that addressed this topic. Each of these studies, as well as their general findings, is presented in Table 3–1. Most of the studies were conducted with hyperactive children, and only one investigation examined nonhyperactive learning disabled youngsters (Gittelman et al., 1983). In general, the academic deficits of the hyperactive samples were poorly documented. A number of different academic skills were targeted for intervention, but most researchers appeared to study whatever reading or arithmetic skills the children were engaged in at the time. Perhaps the most important distinguishing characteristic of all the academically oriented interventions was whether or not the primary objective of treatment was to increase the motivation to learn, to teach an academic skill, or both.

The behavioral interventions employed in these studies were very diverse (see Table 3–1). Process-oriented treatments, for example, included training perceptual motor skills, impulse control, self-instruction, and metacognitive skills for academic tasks. Two studies employed specialized reading interventions; one was phonics based (Gittelman et al., 1983), and the other was a combined phonics-sight word approach (Winsberg et al., 1983). The behavior therapy approaches included token reinforcement, training of parent, teacher, or both in contingency management, response cost, and a combination of token reinforcement and response cost. Not surprisingly, most of the behavioral interventions in these studies were specifically targeted for academic behaviors; however, there were some exceptions (Abikoff & Gittelman, 1985; Conrad et al., 1971; Firestone et al., 1981).

Which treatment modality is superior? There were nine studies in which medication was directly compared with a behavioral intervention designed to help academic performance. In two cases they were equally effective or equally ineffective; the behavioral intervention was superior in four studies; and medication was demonstrated to be more efficacious in the remaining three investigations (all of which failed to show a significant behavioral intervention effect). Taken together, these comparisons suggest that *effective* behavioral interventions are superior to medication in enhancing academic performance.

Does a behavioral intervention enhance medication? When behavioral intervention plus medication was compared with medication alone, the behavioral intervention was found to be superior in some studies. In the remaining studies, neither was superior. Although this would appear to be somewhat at odds with the pre-

Table 3–1. Studies of Stimulant Medication Versus Behavioral Interventions Versus Combination Therapies

Authors	Behavioral Intervention	Academic Measures	Results[a]
Conrad et al. (1971)	Prescriptive tutoring with perceptual-motor training; 2 sessions per week	WRAT arithmetic and reading subtests	PL = PL + BI = M = M + BI
Ayllon et al. (1975)	Token reinforcement for correct responses; 30 minutes per day	Reading comprehension questions and arithmetic calculations; percent correct	BI >M = NT
Wulbert & Dries (1977)	Token reinforcement for correct responses; 2 sessions per week	Reading comprehension questions; percent correct	BI + PL = BI + M > M = PL
Wolraich et al. (1978)	Token reinforcement for correct responses; 4 afternoons per week	Paragraph copying and reading workbook questions; percent correct	*BI + PL = BI + M > M = PL
Rapport et al. (1980)	Response cost	Writing spelling words, reading comprehension questions, and copying sentences; percent of assignment completed and percent correct	Assignment completion: BI + M = BI > M = NT Assignment accuracy: BI + M = BI = M = NT
Firestone et al. (1981)	Parent and teacher training in behavior modification; 9 parent and 2 teacher sessions	Metropolitan Achievement Test, Gates-MacGinitie Reading Test (GMGRT)	Vocabulary subtest of GMGRT: BI + M = M > BI + PL
Rapport et al. (1982)	Response cost for on-task behavior; 1 hour per day	Phonics and math workbook assignments; percent completed and percent correct	M > NT; BI > NT; BI > M
Pelham et al. (1979)	Parent and teacher training in behavior modification; average of 10 parent and 10 teacher sessions	WRAT	BI + M = BI + PL

Gittelman et al. (1983) and Gittelman & Feingold (1983)	Individualized tutoring in phonics decoding and encoding skills plus systematic reinforcement; 3 sessions per week	WRAT, Gray Oral Reading Test, Stanford Achievement Test, Daniels-Diak Phonetic Reading Test, teacher ratings of academic performance	Reading: BI + PL > BPL; BI + M = BI + PL Stanford arithmetic & social studies: BI + M > BI + PL
Schell et al. (1982)	Token reinforcement and prompting attending behavior; Exp. I 15 sessions, Exp II 10 sessions	Sight word identification; percent correct and number of words learned to criterion	BI + M > BI + PL = M; BI > NT; M > PL
Pelham et al. (1985)	Token reinforcement for accuracy and productivity; 25 sessions	Arithmetic production and accuracy, reading and spelling accuracy	Arithmetic and reading: BI + M = M > BI + + PL = PL Spelling: BI + M = M = BI + PL = PL
Atkins et al. (1983)	Parent and teacher training in behavior modification plus daily report card (BI_1), playgroups (BI_2), and response cost (BI_3)	Academic accuracy (four academic subjects)	English, arithmetic: BI_3 > BI_1 + BI_2 + M > BI_1 + BI_2 = NT
Brown et al. (1985)	Multifaceted cognitive training program based on work of Miechenbaum and Goodman (1971), Douglas et al. (1976), and Cohen et al. (1981) with parent involvement; 22 sessions	WRAT reading and arithmetic subtests, Durrell Analysis of Reading Difficulty (listening comprehension subtest), Detroit Test of Learning Aptitude (three attention subtests)	Durrell: BI + M = M > BI = NT Others: BI + M = M = BI = NT
Abikoff & Gittelman (1985)	Cognitive training program that focused on self-instruction on nonacademic psychoeducational tasks and social problem solving with parent involvement; 2 sessions per week	Gray Oral Reading Test, WRAT spelling, reading, and arithmetic subtests, Stanford Achievement Test (reading and arithmetic subtests), teacher ratings of academic performance	BI + M = M + BPL = M

Table 3–1. Studies of Stimulant Medication Versus Behavioral Interventions Versus Combination Therapies (Continued)

Authors	Behavioral Intervention	Academic Measures	Results[a]
Abikoff (1983)	Cognitive training program that emphasized instructional and planning strategies with academic tasks; 2 sessions per week	WRAT (reading, spelling, arithmetic), Stanford Achievement Test (reading comprehension, math application, math computation), Academic Skills Test (adaptation of Metropolitan Achievement Test)	BI + M (pretest <post-test); M (pretest = post-test)
Winsberg, Kupietz, & Richardson (1983)	Individualized tutoring in phonics skills and sight word recognition with parent involvement; 1 session per week	Gates-MacGinitie Reading† Test, Decoding Skills Test, Peabody Individual Achievement Test, instructional process measures (error rate and response strength)	†BI + M = BI + PL

[a]M = medication, BI = behavioral intervention, PL = pharmacological placebo, BPL = behavioral placebo, NT = no treatment.

*Whether or not these conclusions can be drawn from Wolraich et al.'s (1978) study is controversial. Pelham and Murphy (1985) have noted that the two baseline periods appear to have been analyzed as different levels of the behavioral intervention, which would yield the reported findings uninterpretable.

†Reported here are the preliminary findings from a study that is two-thirds complete. It should be noted that there is a marked trend in the data indicating that BI + 0.7 mg/kg M > BI + PL, which may be substantiated when the number of subjects in each cell is complete.

vious observation, in all instances where the behavioral intervention did not facilitate pharmacotherapy, the behavioral intervention was not found to be effective.

Does medication improve the effectiveness of a behavioral intervention that is designed to improve school learning? The combination treatment (medication plus behavioral intervention) was found to be more effective in approximately one half of the studies designed to test this question. Unfortunately, most either failed to demonstrate that the behavioral intervention was indeed effective, or they contained only a few subjects.

Collectively, the research indicates that certain academically oriented behavioral interventions are clearly superior to stimulant medication in facilitating academic performance in hyperactive, learning disabled, and hyperactive learning disabled children. Moreover, although stimulant drugs enhance a variety of learning-related behaviors (e.g., attention span) and have been shown to increase academic productivity, they do not appear to markedly facilitate academically oriented behavioral interventions unless the latter are ineffective. These findings were fairly consistent across a number of studies that varied greatly, which suggests that if a clinically significant combination treatment effect does exist, it is not particularly robust.

It must be reemphasized that the behavioral interventions in the studies listed in Table 3–1 are most diverse. Because representations of each type of treatment are limited, so too are replications. Therefore, conclusions about efficacy must be tentative. With this qualification in mind, relative efficacy studies suggest the following:

1. Cognitive training programs are more effective when they are clearly focused on academic task performance.

2. Of the two general approaches to behavior modification, teaching caregivers how to use this strategy is much less effective than direct contingency management. With direct contingency management, the therapist actually delivers the treatment or directly supervises the caregiver while they implement the treatment.

3. Punishment (for example, response cost, which incorporates both positive and negative consequences) appears to be an important element in behavioral approaches for hyperactive children (see also Rosen et al., 1984).

4. Stimulant drug therapy and contingency management *may* affect behavior in a similar way. They both appear to improve task motivation, which may explain the limited interactive effects when both are administered at effective levels.

5. Behaviorally oriented approaches that employ multiple techniques with different mechanisms of action, such as special academic curriculums designed for skill acquisition that also use effective contingency management, are generally superior to contingency management alone and are probably little influenced by the addition of medication. Unfortunately, the latter are generally available only in some special education settings and are surprisingly understudied with learning disabled students (see, for example, Gittelman & Feingold, 1983).

IS MEDICATION APPROPRIATE?

There is no easy answer to this question. Stimulant drugs do increase academic productivity in hyperactive (and, in all probability, learning disabled) children. Moreover, treated children are aware of this change in their academic behavior (see Gadow, 1983b), which *may* lead to less stress in their lives. As Bradley (1957) noted, "medication is at best a crutch, but if in the long run it enables the child to experience success and a sense of being loved and appreciated, it is well justified" (p. 1051). It seems plausible that a dramatic improvement in productivity and proficiency may even be more clinically meaningful than a modest increase in standardized achievement test performance. In addition, one of the commonly associated reasons for treatment in the first place is that the child does not complete his or her schoolwork and subsequently does not make satisfactory academic progress. It seems reasonable to conclude, therefore, that if medication makes a child more responsive to educational instruction, then it is clinically useful. After all, the education literature is replete with scientific studies that document how various strategies designed to increase task motivation improve academic productivity. Nevertheless, careful consideration must be given both to the seriousness of academic underachievement and the magnitude of the treatment effect and the safety of the drug.

If one were to seriously consider the clinical implications of learning disabilities, the clear focus is on reading. The other areas are simply not that essential to maintenance in a typical employment setting. Chandler (1978), for example, commented that with regard to arithmetic a fourth-grade skill level in numeration, computation, measurement, and simple problem solving was all that was really necessary. With the advent of the hand-held calculator, basic mathematical competencies can be achieved by almost anyone. As for written communication and its component skill, spelling, very few jobs in our society require writing ability. The typewriter all but eliminates the necessity for good penmanship. This leaves oral communication. While no one would challenge the social obstacles created by a severe inability to understand spoken language or express oneself, the adult outcome of children with such problems has really not been studied that much. Snyder (1979, 1983) even makes a compelling case for the questionable necessity of reading skills in most areas of employment; when necessary, there is usually some way to compensate. The real problem with learning disabilities is that they are handicaps with regard to obtaining most traditional post-secondary education (e.g., college, trade school). The tragedy is that most jobs require very little academic ability; however, in order to get them, one must run the gauntlet of traditional academic instruction. It must be emphasized that followup studies of learning disabled children generally show a favorable adult outcome (Horn et al., 1983). Although the same could be said for clinically diagnosed and treated cases of hyperactivity (see Chapter 2), there is some disagreement on this point.

For a drug to be truly justifiable for the treatment of a learning disability, it would have to be (a) remarkably safe and (b) highly effective for learning disabled students, but (c) relatively ineffective for regular classroom students. You may well wonder about the significance of the last criterion. Well, one would seriously doubt that such an agent would be used solely by learning disabled students. Many average youngsters, with the full support of ambitious parents, would also take this drug. One need only consider the situation of Olympic athletic competition to appreciate the implications of such a drug. Unfortunately, if enough students used it, the entire academic achievement curve would shift to the right, and the learning disabled child could still conceivably remain at the bottom of the scholastic heap.

DRUG-INDUCED LEARNING IMPAIRMENT

One topic that has received only moderate attention in the medical literature is drug-induced learning impairment. Technically, if drug treatment reduced a child's academic performance to a level significantly lower than what would be predicted on the basis of his or her unmedicated ability level, the student could conceivably be considered learning disabled. However, scientists and educators rarely, if ever, talk in terms of drug-induced learning disabilities. Generally, if a particular medication has an adverse affect on mood, thought processes, or behavior, the adverse reaction is referred to as *behavioral toxicity*. Regardless, it seemed appropriate to present a brief summary of adverse drug reactions that could lead to an impairment of academic performance. Unfortunately, it is very difficult to locate studies that actually employed academic tasks or tests, and this is part of a much broader problem in drug research (see Gadow & Swanson, 1985). What research is available generally consists of laboratory studies of child performance on cognitive tasks. Inferences are generally made that if medication impairs the child's ability to do the task, it probably interferes with classroom learning as well. In this section, three groups of drugs are briefly reviewed: stimulants, neuroleptics, and antiepileptics. For more detailed discussions of behavioral toxicity, the reader is referred to Chapter 2 and Chapter 4 for stimulants and neuroleptics, respectively. Antiepileptic drugs are reviewed in the companion volume, *Epilepsy, Emotional Disturbance, and Adolescent Disorders*.

Stimulants

Swanson et al. (1978) reported that 25% to 30% of the hyperactive children in their study made more errors on a paired-associate learning task when receiving Ritalin (i.e., were nonresponders) than while receiving a placebo, regardless of the dosage. In addition, when children who were favorable responders to a smaller dose (e.g., 10 mg) were given a larger dose (e.g., 15 mg), the number of errors increased to the level of the nonresponders (on medication). In other words, they experienced drug-induced cognitive deficit on the larger dose of Ritalin. Similarly, Sprague and Sleator's (1977) data suggest that a high therapeutic dose (1.0 mg/kg) of Ritalin may impair performance on their STM task. These and other findings indicate that at certain dosages stimulants may produce an atypical fixation of attention on a narrow band of task stimuli, which may lead to cognitive perseveration, stereotyped behavior, and decreased levels of social interaction and exploratory behavior (Robbins & Sahakian, 1979).

Studies showing an adverse effect on academic performance are few. This is not to say, however, that such a reaction is not possible. Often, when the signs of behavioral toxicity appear in children who are participating in a drug study, either the physician or the parent requests a dosage reduction or change of medication. Because adverse responders are usually dropped from a study before the investigator has time to examine academic performance, evidence of scholastic deterioration is lacking. Nevertheless, two stimulant drug studies do suggest that these drugs *may* suppress academic productivity at higher doses in certain children (Rapport et al., 1982; Sulzbacher, 1972).

Neuroleptics (Major Tranquilizers)

Two phenothiazines, Mellaril (thioridazine) and Thorazine, are the most commonly prescribed neuroleptics for exceptional children. Recently, Winsberg and Yepes (1978) reviewed the literature on the effects of major tranquilizers in children and concluded that although some studies suggest that these drugs depress performance on laboratory measures of attention and cognitive function, the data with regard to academic achievement and learning were inconclusive. Nevertheless, many scientists (see Aman, 1983) believe that impairment of academic performance is highly probable depending on the dose of medication and the nature of the child. Given the fact that these drugs can produce marked sedation and confusional states in children, it is unrealistic to think that daily work output would not be affected.

Antiepileptic Drugs

The behavioral effects of antiepileptic drugs have been the topic of several literature reviews (e.g., Reynolds, 1983; Stores, 1978). One of the most consistent findings is that higher therapeutic doses of Dilantin (phenytoin), phenobarbital, and Mysoline (primidone) can impair sustained attention on vigilance and short-term memory tasks.

Drowsiness, a frequent side effect of phenobarbital and Mysoline, is self-limiting and usually dissipates within 2 weeks following the onset of treatment. If the drowsiness persists, however, the physician may prescribe a stimulant drug (Livingston, 1978). The findings from two large surveys of special education programs suggest that drug-induced drowsiness may be a pervasive problem (Gadow, 1982). It is not known whether there is a relationship between a drowsy appearance (some students do fall asleep in class) and academic underachievement. Nevertheless, it certainly seems reasonable to hypothesize that a drowsy student is less responsive to instruction than an alert pupil.

Another side effect of phenobarbital is a behavior disorder characterized by irritability, aggressiveness, and hyperactivity. Livingston (1978) estimates that from 15 to 20% of all children treated with this drug are so affected. These side effects are not dose related, but rather demonstrate a specific sensitivity to the drug. Frequently the behavior disorder is so severe that it is a bigger problem than the seizures. Drug-induced behavior disorder would, of course, be an impediment to learning.

SUGGESTED READINGS

Aman, M. G. (1978). Drugs, learning, and the psychotherapies. In J. S. Werry (Ed.), *Pediatric psychopharmacology: The use of behavior modifying drugs in children* (pp. 79–108). New York: Bruner/Mazel. (C, S)

Barkley, R. A., & Cunningham, C. E. (1978). Do stimulant drugs improve the academic performance of hyperkinetic children? *Clinical Pediatrics, 17*, 85–92. (C, S)

Gadow, K. D. (1983). Effects of stimulant drugs on academic performance in hyperactive and learning disabled children. *Journal of Learning Disabilities, 16*, 290–299. (S)

Gadow, K. D. (1983). Pharmacotherapy for learning disabilities. *Learning Disabilities, 2*, 127–140. (S)

Gadow, K. D. (1985). Relative efficacy of pharmacological, behavioral, and combination treatments for enhancing academic performance. *Clinical Psychology Review, 5*, 513–533. (C, S)

Gadow, K. D., & Swanson, H. L. (1985). Assessing drug effects on academic performance. *Psychopharmacology Bulletin, 21*, 877–886. (C, S)

Pelham, W. E. (1985). The effects of psychostimulant drugs on learning and academic achievement in children with attention deficit disorders and learning disabilities. In J. K. Torgesen & B. Wong (Eds.), *Psychological and educational perspectives on learning disabilities*. Orlando, FL: Academic Press. (C, S)

Pelham, W. E., & Murphy, H. A. (1985). Behavioral and pharmacological treatment of attention deficit and conduct disorders. In M. Hersen (Ed.), *Pharmacological and behavioral treatment: An integrative approach*. New York: Wiley. (C, S)

Sprague, R. L., & Berger, B. D. (1980). Drug effects on learning performance: Relevance of animal research to pediatric psychopharmacology. In R. M. Knights & D. J. Bakker (Eds.), *Rehabilitation, treatment and management of learning disorders*. Baltimore: University Park Press. (C, S)

REFERENCES

Abikoff, H. (1983, August). *Academic cognitive training and stimulants in hyperactivity: A pilot study*. Paper presented at the meeting of the American Psychological Association, Anaheim, CA

Abikoff, H., & Gittelman, R. (1985). Hyperactive children treated with stimulants. *Archives of General Psychiatry, 42*, 953–961.

Ackerman, P. T., & Dykman, R. A. (1982). Automatic and effortful information-processing deficits in children with learning and attention disorders. *Topics in Learning & Learning Disabilities, 2*, 12–22.

Aman, M. G. (1978). Drugs, learning, and the psychotherapies. In J. S. Werry (Ed.), *Pediatric psychopharmacology: The use of behavior modifying drugs in children* (pp. 79–108). New York: Brunner/Mazel.

Aman, M. G. (1982). Psychotropic drugs in the treatment of reading disorders. In R. N. Malatesha & P. G. Aaron (Eds.), *Reading disorders: Varieties and treatments* (pp. 453–471). Orlando, FL: Academic Press.

Aman, M. G. (1984). Drugs and learning in mentally retarded persons. In G. D. Burrows & J. S. Werry (Eds.), *Advances in human psychopharmacology* (Vol. 3, pp. 121–163). Greenwich, CT: JAI Press.

Aman, M. G., & Werry, J. S. (1982). Methylphenidate and diazepam in severe reading retardation. *Journal of the American Academy of Child Psychiatry, 1*, 31–37.

Arter, J. A., & Jenkins, J. R. (1979). Differential diagnosis–prescriptive teaching: A critical appraisal. *Review of Educational Research, 49*, 517–555.

Atkins, M., White, K., Adams, P., Case, D., & Pelham, W. E. (1983). *Intensive, long-term behavioral and pharmacological treatment of a hyperactive, aggressive child.* Unpublished manuscript, Department of Psychology, Florida State University, Tallahassee.

Ayllon, T., Layman, D., & Kandel, H. J. (1975). A behavioral-educational alternative to drug control of hyperactive children. *Journal of Applied Behavior Analysis, 8*, 137–146.

Baker, L., & Cantwell, D. P. (1985). Psychiatric and learning disorders in children with speech and language disorders: A critical review. In K. D. Gadow (Ed.), *Advances in learning and behavioral disabilities* (Vol. 4, pp. 1–27). Greenwich, CT: JAI Press.

Barkley, R. A. (1981). *Hyperactive children: A handbook for diagnosis and treatment.* New York: Guilford.

Barkley, R. A., & Cunningham, C. E. (1978). Do stimulant drugs improve the academic performance of hyperkinetic children? *Clinical Pediatrics, 17*, 85–92.

Barkley, R. A., Cunningham, C. E., & Karlsson, J. (1983). The speech of hyperactive children and their mothers: Comparison with normal children and stimulant drug effects. *Journal of Learning Disabilities, 16*, 105–110.

Bender, L., & Cottington, F. (1942). The use of amphetamine sulfate (Benzedrine) in child psychiatry. *American Journal of Psychiatry, 99*, 116–121.

Berk, R. A. (1984). An evaluation of procedures for computing an ability-achievement discrepancy score. *Journal of Learning Disabilities, 17*, 262–266.

Borland, B. L., & Heckman, H. K. (1976). Hyperactive boys and their brothers: A 25-year follow-up study. *Archives of General Psychiatry, 33*, 669–675.

Bradley, C. (1937). The behavior of children receiving Benzedrine. *American Journal of Psychiatry, 94*, 577–585.

Bradley, C. (1957). Characteristics and management of children with behavior problems associated with organic brain damage. *Pediatric Clinics of North America, 4*, 1049–1060.

Bradley, C., & Bowen, M. (1940). School performance of children receiving amphetamine (Benzedrine) sulfate. *American Journal of Orthopsychiatry, 10*, 782–788.

Bradley, C., & Bowen, M. (1941). Amphetamine (Benzedrine) therapy of children's behavior disorders. *American Journal of Orthopsychiatry, 11*, 92–103.

Bradley, C., & Green, E. (1940). Psychometric performances of children receiving amphetamine (Benzedrine) sulfate. *American Journal of Psychiatry, 97*, 388–394.

Brown, R. T., Wynne, M. E., & Medenis, R. (1985). Methylphenidate and cognitive therapy: A comparison of treatment approaches with hyperactive boys. *Journal of Abnormal Child Psychology, 13*, 69–87.

Cantwell, D. P., & Baker, L. (1985). Psychiatric and learning disorders in children with speech and language disorders: A descriptive analysis. In K. D. Gadow (Ed.), *Advances in learning and behavioral disabilities* (Vol. 4, pp. 29–47). Greenwich, CT: JAI Press.

Cantwell, D. P., & Carlson, G. A. (1978). Stimulants. In J. S. Werry (Ed.), *Pediatric psychopharmacology: The use of behavior modifying drugs in children* (pp. 171–207). New York: Brunner/Mazel.

Cantwell, D. P., & Satterfield, J. H. (1978). The prevalence of academic underachievement in hyperactive children. *Journal of Pediatric Psychology, 3*, 168–171.

Chandler, H. N. (1978). Confusion compounded: A teacher tries to use research results to teach math. *Journal of Learning Disabilities, 11*, 361–369.

Chase, C. H., Schmitt, R. L., Russell, G., & Tallal, P. (1984). A new chemotherapeutic investigation: Piracetam effects on dyslexia. *Annals of Dyslexia, 34*, 29–48.

Clements, S. D., & Peters, J. E. (1962). Minimal brain dysfunction in the school-age child. *Archives of General Psychiatry, 6*, 185–197.

Comly, H. H. (1971). Cerebral stimulants for children with learning disorders. *Journal of Learning Disabilities, 9*, 484–490.

Cone, T. E., & Wilson, L. R. (1981). Quantifying a severe discrepancy: A critical analysis. *Learning Disability Quarterly, 4*, 359–371.

Conners, C. K. (1972). Symposium: Behavior modification by drugs. II. Psychological effects of stimulant drugs in children with minimal brain dysfunction. *Pediatrics, 49*, 702–708.

Conners, C. K., Blouin, A. G., Winglee, M., Lougee, L., O'Donnell, D., & Smith, A. (1984). Piracetam and event-related potentials in dyslexic children. *Psychopharmacology Bulletin, 20*, 667–673.

Conners, C. K., Eisenberg, L., & Barcai, A. (1967). Effect of dextroamphetamine on children: Studies on subjects with learning disabilities and school behavior problems. *Archives of General Psychiatry, 17*, 478–485.

Conners, C., Rothschild, G., Eisenberg, L., Stone, L., & Robinson, E. (1969). Dextroamphetamine in children with learning disorders. *Archives of General Psychiatry, 21*, 182–190.

Conners, C. K., Taylor, E., Meo, G., Kurz, M. A., & Fournier, M. (1972). Magnesium pemoline and dextroamphetamine: A controlled study in children with minimal brain dysfunction. *Psychopharmacologia, 26*, 321–336.

Conrad, W. G, Dworkin, E. S., Shai, A., & Tobiessen, J. E. (1971). Effects of amphetamine therapy and prescriptive tutoring on the behavior and achievement of lower class hyperactive children. *Journal of Learning Disabilities, 4*, 45–53.

Creager, R. O., & VanRiper, C. (1967). The effect of methylphenidate on the verbal productivity of children with cerebral dysfunction. *Journal of Speech and Hearing Research, 10*, 623–628.

DiIanni, M., Wilsher, C. R., Blank, M. S., Conners, C. K., Chase, C. H., Funkenstein, H. H., Helfgott, E. Holmes, J. M., Lougee, L, Maletta, G. J., Milewski, J., Pirozzolo, F. J., Rudel, R. G., & Tallal, P. (in press). The effects of Piracetam in children with dyslexia. *Journal of Clinical Psychopharmacology.*

Dimond, S. J., & Brouwers, E. Y. M. (1976). Improvement of human memory through the use of drugs. *Psychopharmacology, 49,* 307–309.

Dykman, R. A., Ackerman, P. T., & McCray, D. S. (1980). Effects of methylphenidate on selective and sustained attention in hyperactive, reading-disabled, and presumably attention-disordered boys. *Journal of Nervous and Mental Disease, 168,* 745–752.

Firestone, P., Kelly, M. J., Goodman, J. T., & Davey, J. (1981). Differential effects of parent training and stimulant medication with hyperactives. *Journal of the American Academy of Child Psychiatry, 20,* 135–147.

Fish, C. H., & Bowling, E. (1962). Effect of amphetamine on speech defects in the mentally retarded. *California Medicine, 94,* 109–111.

Forer, R. K., & Keogh, B. K. (1971). Time understanding of learning disabled boys. *Exceptional Children, 37,* 741–743.

Freed, M., Abrams, J., & Peifer, C. (1959). Reading disability: A new therapeutic approach and its implications. *Journal of Clinical and Experimental Psychopathology and Quarterly Review of Psychiatry and Neurology, 20,* 251–259.

Gadow, K. D. (1982). School involvement in the treatment of seizure disorders: *Epilepsia, 23,* 215–224.

Gadow, K. D. (1983a). Effects of stimulant drugs on academic performance in hyperactive and learning disabled children. *Journal of Learning Disabilities, 16,* 290–299.

Gadow, K. D. (1983b). Pharmacotherapy for learning disabilities. *Learning Disabilities, 2,* 127–140.

Gadow, K. D. (1985). Relative efficacy of pharmacological, behavioral, and combination treatments for enhancing academic performance. *Clinical Psychology Review, 5,* 513–533.

Gadow, K. D., & Swanson, H. L. (1985). Assessing drug effects on academic performance. *Psychopharmacology Bulletin, 21,* 877–886.

Ginn, S. A., & Hohman, L. B. (1953). The use of dextroamphetamine in severe behavior problems of children. *Southern Medical Journal, 46,* 1124–1127.

Gittelman, R., & Feingold, I. (1983). Children with reading disorders—I. Efficacy of reading remediation. *Journal of Child Psychology and Psychiatry, 24,* 167–191.

Gittelman, R., Klein, D. F., & Feingold, I. (1983). Children with reading disorders—II. Effects of methylphenidate in combination with reading remediation. *Journal of Child Psychology and Psychiatry, 24,* 193–212.

Gittelmen-Klein, R., & Klein, D. F. (1976). Methylphenidate effects in learning disabilities. *Archives of General Psychiatry, 33,* 655–664.

Helfgott, E., Rudel, R. G., & Krieger, J. (1984). Effect of piracetam on the single word and prose reading of dyslexic children. *Psychopharmacology Bulletin, 20,* 688–690.

Horn, W. F., O'Donnell, J. P., & Vitulano, L. A. (1983). Long-term follow-up studies of learning disabled persons. *Journal of Learning Disabilities, 16,* 542–555.

Kirk, S. A. (1962). *Educating exceptional children.* Boston: Houghton Mifflin.

Lambert, N., & Sandoval, J. (1980). The prevalence of learning disabilities in a sample of children considered hyperactive. *Journal of Abnormal Child Psychology, 8,* 33–50.

Lerer, R. J., Lerer, M. P., & Artner, J. (1977). The effects of methylphenidate on the handwriting of children with minimal brain dysfunction. *Journal of Pediatrics, 91,* 127–132.

Levy, H. B. (1973). *Square pegs, round holes: The learning-disabled child in the classroom and the home.* Boston: Little, Brown.

Livingston, S. (1978). Medical treatment of epilepsy: Part II. *Southern Medical Journal, 71,* 432–447.

Ludlow, C., Rapoport, J., Brown, G., & Mikkelson, E. (1979). The differential effects of dextroamphetamine on the language and communicative skills of hyperactive and normal children. In R. Knights & D. Bakker (Eds.), *Rehabilitation, treatment, and management of learning disorders.* Baltimore: University Park Press.

Mann, L., Davis, C. H., Boyer, C. W., Metz, C. M., & Wolford, B. (1983). LD or not LD, that was the question: A retrospective analysis of child service demonstration centers' compliance with the federal definition of learning disabilities. *Journal of Learning Disabilities, 16,* 14–17.

Mayron, L. W. (1978). Ecological factors in learning disabilities. *Journal of Learning Disabilities, 11,* 495–505.

Minde, K., Lewin, D., Weiss, G., Lavigueur, H., Douglas, V., & Sykes, E. (1971). The hyperactive child in elementary school: A 5 year, controlled followup. *Exceptional children, 38,* 215–221.

Mindus, P., Cronholm, B., Levander, S. E., & Schalling, D. (1976). Piracetam induced improvement of mental performance: A controlled study on normally aging individuals. *Acta Psychiatrica Scandinavica, 54,* 150–160.

Molitch, M., & Sullivan, J. P. (1937). Effect of benzedrine sulfate on children taking New Stanford Achievement Test. *American Journal of Orthopsychiatry, 7,* 519–522.

Moskowitz, H. (1941). Benzedrine therapy for the mentally handicapped. *American Journal of Mental Deficiency, 45,* 540–543.

Pelham, W. E. (1985). The effects of psychostimulant drugs on learning and academic achievement in children with attention deficit disorders and learning disabilities. In J. K. Torgesen & B. Wong (Eds.), Psycholog*ical and educational perspectives on learning disabilities.* Orlando, FL: Academic Press.

Pelham, W. E., Bender, M. E., Caddell, J., Booth, S., & Moorer, S. H. (1985). Methylphenidate and children with attention deficit disorder: Dose effects on classroom academic and social behavior. *Archives of General Psychiatry, 42,* 948–952.

Pelham, W. E., & Murphy, H. A. (1985). Behavioral and pharmacological treatment of attention deficit and conduct disorders. In M. Hersen (Ed.), *Pharmacological and behavioral treatment: An integrative approach.* New York: Wiley.

Pelham, W. E., Schnedler, R. W., Miller, J., Ronnei, M., Paluchowski, C., Budrow, M., Marks, D., Nilsson, D., & Bender, M. (1979, September). *The combination of behavior therapy and psychostimulant medication in the treatment of hyperactive children: A therapy outcome study.* Paper presented at the meeting of the American Psychological Association, Montreal.

Pelham, W. E., Swanson, J., Bender, M., & Wilson, J. (1980, September). *Effects of pemoline on hyperactivity: Laboratory and classroom measures*. Paper presented at the annual meeting of the American Psychological Association, Montreal.

Prinzmetal, M., & Bloomberg, W. (1935). The use of Benzedrine for the treatment of narcolepsy. *Journal of the American Medical Association, 105*, 2051–2054.

Rapoport, J. L., Quinn, P. O., Bradbard, G., Riddle, K. D., & Brooks, E. (1974). Imipramine and methylphenidate treatments of hyperactive boys. *Archives of General Psychiatry, 30*, 789–793.

Rapport, M. D., Murphy, A., & Bailey, J. S. (1980). The effects of a response cost treatment tactic on hyperactive children. *Journal of School Psychology, 18*, 98–111.

Rapport, M. D., Murphy, H. A., & Bailey, J. S. (1982). Ritalin vs. response cost in the control of hyperactive children: A within-subject comparison. *Journal of Applied Behavior Analysis, 15*, 205–216.

Rapport, M. D., Stoner, G., DuPaul, G. J., Birmingham, B. K., & Tucker, S. (1985). Methylphenidate in hyperactive children: Differential effects of dose on academic, learning, and social behavior. *Journal of Abnormal Child Psychology, 13*, 227–244.

Reynolds, E. H. (1983). Mental effects of antiepileptic medication: A review. *Epilepsia, 24* (Suppl. 2), S85–S95.

Robbins, T. W., & Sahakian, B. J. (1979). "Paradoxical" effects of psychomotor stimulant drugs in hyperactive children from the standpoint of behavioral pharmacology. *Neuropharmacology, 18*, 931–950.

Rosen, L. A., O'Leary, S. G., Joyce, S. A., Conway, G., & Pfiffner, L. J. (1984). The importance of prudent negative consequences for maintaining the appropriate behavior of hyperactive students. *Journal of Abnormal Child Psychology, 12*, 581–604.

Rudel, R. G., & Helfgott, E. (1984). Effect of piracetam on verbal memory of dyslexic boys. *Journal of the American Academy of Child Psychiatry, 23*, 695–699.

Safer, D. J., & Krager, J. M. (1984). Trends in medication therapy for hyperactivity: National and international perspectives. In K. D. Gadow (Ed.), *Advances in learning and behavioral disabilities* (Vol. 3, pp. 125–149). Greenwitch, CT: JAI Press.

Schain, R. J., & Reynard, C. L. (1975). Observations on effects of central stimulant drug (methylphenidate) in children with hyperactive behavior. *Pediatrics, 55*, 709–716.

Schell, R. M., Bender, M. E., Pelham, W. E., & Andre, J. (1982, November). *The use of a multi-element design in the assessment of task structure, reinforcement and methylphenidate on the learning of a five-year-old, language delayed child with attention deficit disorder.* Paper presented at the meeting of the Association for the Advancement of Behavior Therapy, Los Angeles.

Smith, D. D., *Teaching the learning disabled*. Englewood Cliffs, NJ: Prentice-Hall, 1981.

Snyder, R. D. (1979). The right not to read. *Pediatrics, 63*, 791–794.

Snyder, R. D. (1983). Coping strategies for inefficient readers. *Journal of Learning Disabilities, 5*, 261–263.

Sprague, R. L., & Berger, B. D. (1980). Drug effects on learning performance: Relevance of animal research to pediatric psychopharmacology.

In R. M. Knights & D. J. Bakker (Eds.), *Rehabilitation, treatment and management of learning disorders.* Baltimore: University Park Press.

Sprague, R. L., & Sleator, E. K. (1977). Methylphenidate in hyperactive children: Differences in dose effects on learning and social behavior. *Science, 198,* 1274–1276.

Squitieri, G, Cervone, A., & Agnoi, A. (1975). *A study on short-term memory in man: Interactions with nooanaleptic and nootropic drugs.* Paper presented at Third International College of Congress on Psychosomatic Medicine, Rome, Italy.

Stephens, R. S., Pelham, W. E., & Skinner, R. (1984). The state-dependent and main effects of methylphenidate and pemoline on paired-associates learning and spelling in hyperactive children. *Journal of Consulting and Clinical Psychology, 523,* 104–113.

Stores, G. (1978). Antiepileptics (anticonvulsants). In J. S. Werry (Ed.), *Pediatric psychopharmacology: The use of behavior modifying drugs in children* (pp. 274–315). New York: Brunner/Mazel.

Sulzbacher, S. I. (1972). Behavior analysis of drug effects in the classroom. In G. Semb (Ed.), *Behavior analysis and education* (pp. 37–52). University of Kansas.

Swanson, J., Kinsbourne, M., Roberts, W., & Zucker, K. (1978). Time-response analysis of the effect of stimulant medication on the learning ability of children referred for hyperactivity. *Pediatrics, 61,* 21–29.

Taylor, E. (1979). The use of drugs in hyperkinetic states: Clinical issues. *Neuropharmacology, 18,* 951–958.

U. S. Office of Education (1977). Assistance to states for education of handicapped children: Procedures for evaluating specific learning disabilities. *Federal Register, 42,* 65082–65085.

Vellutino, F. R., Steger, B. M., Moyer, S. C., Harding, C. J., & Niles, J. A. (1977). Has the perceptual deficit hypothesis led us astray? *Journal of Learning Disabilities, 10,* 375–385.

Weiss, G., Minde, K., Douglas, V., Werry, J., & Sykes, D. (1971). Comparison of the effects of chlorpromazine, dextroamphetamine and methylphenidate on the behavior and intellectual functioning of hyperactive children. *Canadian Medical Association Journal, 104,* 20–25.

Werry, J. (1981). Drugs and learning. *Journal of Child Psychology and Psychiatry, 22,* 283–290.

Whalen, C., Collins, B., Henker, B., Alkus, S., Adams, D., & Stapp, J. (1978). Behavior observations of hyperactive children and methylphenidate effects in systematically structured classroom environments: Now you see them, now you don't. *Journal of Pediatric Psychology, 3,* 177–187.

Whalen, C. K., Henker, B., & Finck, D. (1981). Medication effects in the classroom: Three naturalistic indicators. *Canadian Journal of Psychiatry, 26,* 385–392.

Wiederholt, J. L. (1974). Historical perspectives on the education of the learning disabled. In L. Mann & D. A. Sabatino (Eds.), *The second review of special education* (pp. 103–152). Philadelphia: JSE Press.

Wiig, E. H., & Semel, E. M. (1976). *Language disabilities in children and adolescents.* Columbus, OH: Charles E. Merrill.

Winsberg, B., Kupietz, S., & Richardson, E. (1983). *NIMH Grant Proposal.* Unpublished manuscript, Child Development Center, Nassau County Medical Center, East Meadow, NY.

Winsberg, B. G., & Yepes, L. E. (1978). Antipsychotics. In J. S. Werry (Ed.), *Pediatric psychopharmacology: The use of behavior modifying drugs in children* (pp. 234–273). New York: Brunner/Mazel.

Wolraich, M., Drummond, T., Salomon, M. K., O'Brien, M. L., & Sivage, C. (1978). Effects of methylphenidate alone and in combination with behavior modification procedures on the behavior and academic performance of hyperactive children. *Journal of Abnormal Child Psychology, 6*, 149–161.

Wulbert, M., & Dries, R. (1977). The relative efficacy of methylphenidate (Ritalin) and behavior-modification techniques in the treatment of a hyperactive child. *Journal of Applied Behavior Analysis, 10*, 21–31.

Yellin, A. M., Hopwood, J. H., & Greenberg, L. M. (1982). Adults and adolescents with attention deficit disorder: Clinical and behavioral responses to psychostimulants. *Journal of Clinical Psychopharmacology, 2*, 133–136.

Ysseldyke, J. E., & Salvia, J. (1974). Diagnostic-prescriptive teaching: Two models. *Exceptional Children, 41*, 181–185.

Chapter **4**

Mental Retardation

Drug treatment for behavior disorders in mentally retarded children, adolescents, and adults is considered a separate topic in this book for several reasons. First, many of the maladies for which psychotropic drugs are prescribed are prevalent in mentally retarded populations. This is particularly true for more severely and profoundly impaired individuals. Second, it is often unclear whether some disorders associated with mental retardation are the same, in terms of both etiology and response to treatment, as apparently similar disorders (e.g., hyperactivity) in nonretarded individuals (Fish, 1971). Third, some drug treated disorders, such as stereotypic behavior, are commonly associated with mental retardation. And fourth, the way in which social agencies and the general public respond to mentally retarded people may interact in complex ways with decisions about drug treatment. For example, the recent emphasis on deinstitutionalization is bringing many severely and profoundly retarded persons into the mainstream of everyday life through community placements. The feasibility of such placements for some individuals with severe behavior problems *may* depend upon effective pharmacotherapy.

It should be noted that psychotropic drugs are not prescribed for mental retardation per se. The objective of drug treatment is not to "cure" or change biochemical processes in such a fashion that a mentally retarded child can perform like his or her nonretarded peers. Although medication may enhance responsiveness to learning and cognitive performance, the typical reason for prescribing medication is the control of behavior disorders, notably hyperactivity, aggressivity, self-injurious behavior, and stereotypic motor movements.

Surveys show that both stimulants and neuroleptics are frequently prescribed for behavior disorders in mentally retarded children and adolescents. These studies have also found that one of the most common reasons for drug use is hyperactivity. Because hyperactivity is a symptom associated with at least several different handicapping conditions, it would be inappropriate to infer that stimulants are the "drugs of first choice" in treating all hyperactive mentally retarded children (Fish, 1971). Nevertheless, it is clear that stimulants are used frequently for the treatment of hyperactivity, behavior problems, and aggressivity in mentally retarded children in public schools (Epstein et al., 1985; Gadow & Kalachnik,1981). In residential settings, however, stimulants are rarely prescribed for behavior disorders, and neuroleptics account for almost all psychotropic drug prescriptions.

In view of this situation, this chapter addresses both stimulant (see also Chapter 2) and neuroleptic drug use. No attempt is made to survey the literature about drug therapy for mentally retarded individuals, as many excellent review articles are already available (e.g., Aman, 1984; Aman & Singh, 1983; Freeman, 1966, 1970a, 1970b; Lipman et al., 1978; Sprague & Werry, 1971). Last, it is instructive to note that the study of psychopharmacotherapy in mentally retarded people is a science of institutions (see Gadow, 1985). Very little effort has been made to study psychotropic drug use with children and adolescents in public school programs.

Before discussing the clinical literature in this area, the reader should understand that the use of psychotropic drugs for the treatment of various disorders in mentally retarded people is a controversial topic. Moreover, it has *always* been a matter of controversy. In a truly insightful commentary on this issue, Theodore Greiner stated in 1958 that "in the years to come, the retarded may claim an all-time record, of having the greatest variety and largest tonnage of chemical agents shoveled into them" (p. 346). Unfortunately, his prophecy became reality. He went on to admonish scientists who conducted shoddy research by saying, "If your aim is helping the retarded, I urge you to avoid the casual clinical trial of drugs. Make them good trials, or don't make them at all" (p. 347). Greiner also identified what has remained one of the most troubling features of pharmacotherapy for this population and for children in general:

> Sensible adult patients will usually balk when a drug is causing symptoms, but the very young and the very old are forced to take drugs, can't complain or stop on toxic symptoms, may not even connect them with the drug. The mentally deficient of any size or age cannot protect themselves either, and they also merit special care to avoid toxic doses. (p. 349)

DISORDERS ASSOCIATED WITH MENTAL RETARDATION

The prevalence of behavior problems is much higher among mentally retarded children as compared with their nonretarded agemates. A study of 9 to 11 year old British children on the Isle of Wight showed that this relationship holds up whether the source of information is behavioral ratings obtained from parents or teachers or psychiatric examinations (Rutter, 1971; Rutter et al., 1970).

Payne et al. (1969) conducted what must certainly be one of the most comprehensive surveys of mentally retarded persons in residential facilities. Twenty-two institutions in the western United States were asked to provide detailed data on a total of 24,257 residents in 1968. Ward personnel completed behavioral ratings using a four-point scale: never, seldom, occasionally, and frequently. Of primary interest were behaviors considered maladaptive (i.e., those that interfered with institutional programming). The most common behaviors rated "frequently" were hyperactivity, aggressivity, and running. Other "frequent" behaviors were self-destructiveness, requiring restraints, destroying clothing, and attacking other residents. Of the residents, 21% were characterized as "occasionally" hyperactive or aggressive or both.

Eyman and Call (1977) studied the prevalence of maladaptive behavior in mentally retarded individuals living in residential facilities, community settings, or their own homes. Using a behavior rating scale, social workers in community settings and direct care personnel in institutions evaluated 6,870 mentally retarded children and adults. Clients were divided into three groups according to level of retardation: profound, severe, and mild-moderate. Group comparisons revealed a greater frequency of behavior problems in profoundly retarded than in mildly-moderately retarded persons. The prevalence of behavior disorders was also much higher in institutions than in community settings. Three behavior problems were quite common, with some variation across age and level of retardation: stereotypies, hyperactivity, and aggressivity. The latter was subdivided into violence toward others, violence toward oneself or self-injurious behavior, and the destruction of property.

Approximately half of the individuals under 13 years of age in institutions had *stereotypies* (repetitive, often bizarre motor activity). In general, the figures were lower for those in community placements and for older, moderately retarded residents. Examples of such behavior are rhythmic rocking, head weaving, mouthing, hand or arm flapping, and rubbing parts of the body (see Baumeister & Forehand, 1973).

PREVALENCE AND PATTERN OF DRUG TREATMENT

Largely as a result of lawsuits concerning the mistreatment of mentally retarded people in institutions, we now have a fairly substantial amount of information about how pharmacotherapy is managed in real-world situations. While these data were generally not collected in response to a court order, the lawsuits drew so much attention to this area that a number of scientists became interested in documenting the extent of alleged wrongdoing. Drug treatment practices are described here for three different settings: institutions, community placements, and public schools.

Institutions

Lipman (1970) conducted one of the first questionnaire surveys on psychotropic drug use in state and private institutions for mentally retarded people and found that the extent of drug use was considerable; 51% of the residents had received psychotropic agents at some time. Two major tranquilizers, Mellaril (thioridazine) and Thorazine (chlorpromazine), accounted for over half of all reported drugs, and they were the preferred agents in 91% of the institutions. Some of the reported maximum dosages were quite high: 3,000 mg per day for Thorazine and 1,800 mg per day for Mellaril (cf. Table 4–4). Even more disturbing was the chronic nature of drug use; 25% of the drug-treated residents had received medication for 4 or more years.

Sprague (1977a; Cohen & Sprague, 1977) reported data about the extent and pattern of psychotropic drug therapy from the records of mentally retarded residents in two midwestern facilities, one old and one new. The older institution housed 1,639 residents in buildings with day rooms and open wards. Residents ranged from moderately to profoundly retarded, with a mean age of 27.4 years. The new (small) facility housed 286 residents who lived in group homes, each designed for eight people. The entire facility was modeled after community living, and from outward appearances, it looked much like a suburban housing division. The residents were moderately to profoundly retarded with a mean age of 29.4 years. Despite differences in the philosophy and type of care represented by these two facilities, the prevalence of drug treatment was quite similar: 50% in the older large institution and 51% in the new community-styled facility. Over half the residents on medication in both facilities were receiving two or more psychotropic and/or antiepileptic drugs. The most frequently reported psychotropic drugs were Mellaril and Thorazine.

Some of the most extensive studies of institutions have been conducted by Brad Hill at the University of Minnesota (Hill et al., 1983, 1986). In 1977, he and his colleagues identified 55,438 mentally retarded individuals in public residential facilities (institutions) under the age of 22 years in the United States. Staff interviews concerning a randomly selected sample of children and adolescents revealed the following drug treatment prevalence rates: total psychotropics (31%), neuroleptics (20%), and stimulants (0.7%) (Hill, 1984). Over three fourths of the subjects in the institutional sample were severely or profoundly retarded (IQ < 36). The primary reason for drug use was "overactive behavior."

On an international level, psychotropic drugs are commonly prescribed for institutionalized mentally retarded people in many countries of the world. Figure 4–1 shows treatment prevalence rates for Canada (Tu, 1979), England (Kirman, 1975), New Zealand (Pulman et al., 1979; Sewell & Werry, 1976), and the United States (Cohen & Sprague, 1977; Hill et al., 1983). While the rates reported in these and other studies are quite high, this does not necessarily have to be the case. Briggs et al. (1984), for example, reviewed the results of six programs to reduce or regulate institutional drug use, which indicated that treatment rates can be lowered to the 20 to 30% level.

Although there is an emerging picture of the extent and pattern of drug treatment for mentally retarded individuals in residential facilities, very little has been reported about the exact reasons for which these drugs are prescribed. Klebanoff et al. (1973) made one attempt to determine why these drugs are prescribed by surveying staff physicians working in state institutions in Massachusetts. They reported that Mellaril and Thorazine were prescribed primarily for the control of agitated and/or aggressive behavior and of psychotic states. However, drug use for the control of agitation or aggression was reported twice as often as for psychosis.

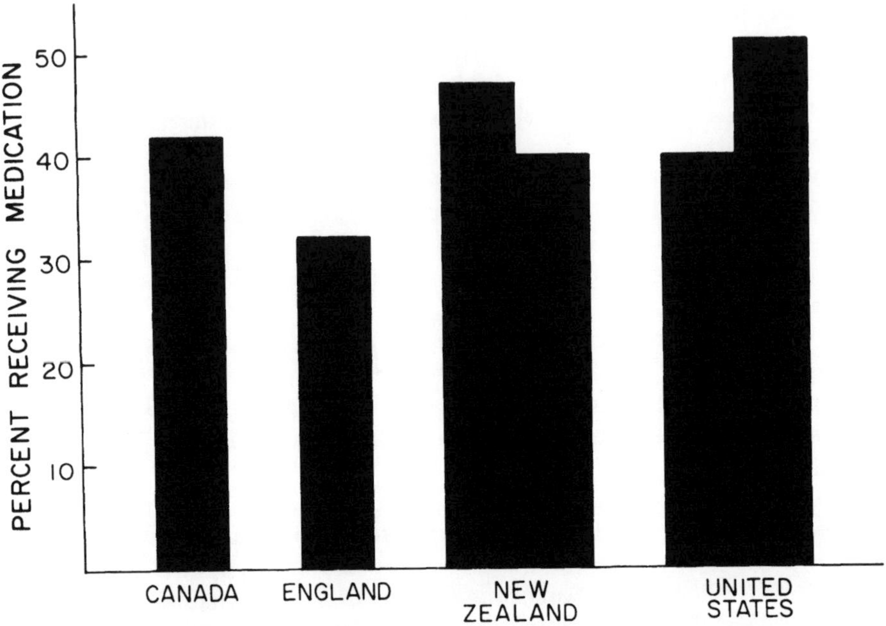

Figure 4–1. Prevalence of psychotropic drug use in institutions for the mentally retarded as reported in six surveys

In another study of the reasons for drug use, Sewell and Werry (1976) surveyed resident records in a facility in New Zealand. They found that Thorazine and Mellaril were the most frequently prescribed drugs. The target symptoms for which they were prescribed (in rank order of frequency) were hyperactivity, noisiness, aggressiveness, destructiveness, self-mutilation, and perverseness. Similarly, Briggs et al. (1984) found that physical aggression, self-injurious behavior, verbal aggression, and damaging property were among the most common reasons for prescribing psychotropic drugs.

Community Placements

The most extensive studies of psychotropic drug use in specially licensed community residential facilities (e.g., foster homes, group homes) have been conducted by Hill and his associates (1983, in press). In 1977, they identified 35,751 mentally retarded children and adolescents in community residential placements (Fig. 4–2). Staff interviews concerning a randomly selected sample indicated the following: total psychotropics (19%), neuroleptics (13%), and

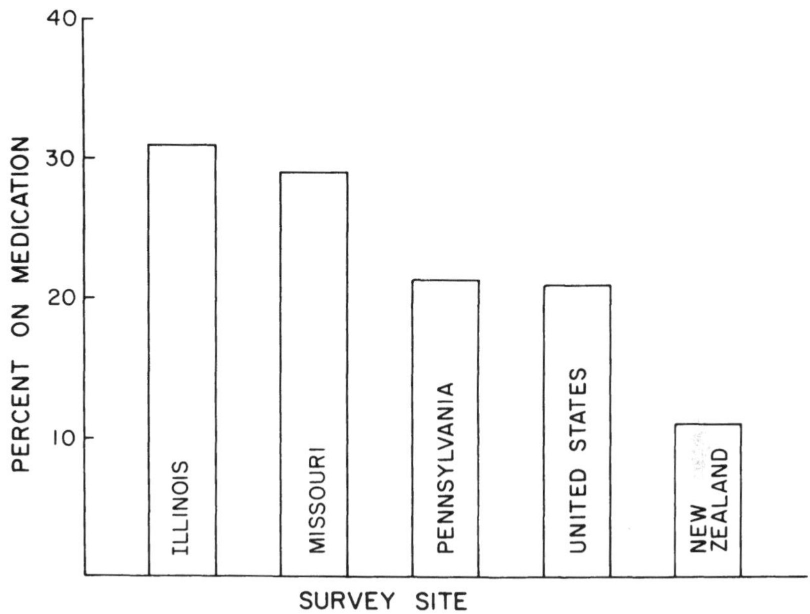

Figure 4–2. Prevalence of neuroleptic drug use for mentally retarded people in community placements as reported in five surveys.

(Hill, 1984). Approximately half of the youngsters in the community sample were moderately to severely retarded. Psychotropic drugs were prescribed primarily for "overactive behavior."

Several surveys of community placements have now been conducted, and an accurate description of drug use is emerging. In Figure 4–2, the prevalence of *neuroleptic* drug use is presented from studies conducted in Illinois (Martin & Agran, 1985), Missouri (Intagliata & Rinck, 1985), Pennsylvania (Radinsky, 1984), United States (Hill et al., 1983), and Auckland, New Zealand (Aman et al., 1985). The data from Illinois and New Zealand pertain only to adults (Aman et al., 1985; Martin & Agran, 1985). Stimulant drug use was uncommon, even for individuals under 21 years of age.

Public Schools

Because two laws (Public Law 89-313 and Public Law 94-142) require states to report to the federal government the number of children between the ages of 3 and 21 years who are receiving special education services, it is possible to obtain fairly accurate figures for school-labeled mentally retarded students in the United States. Pub-

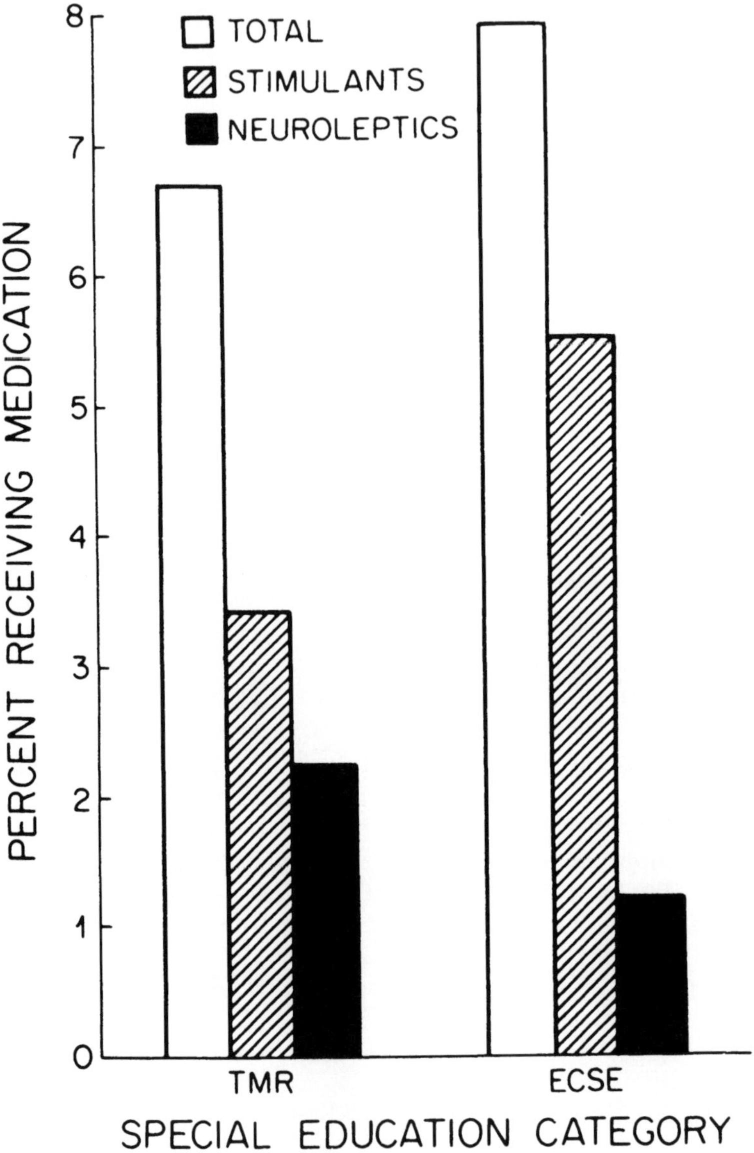

Figure 4–3. Percentage of children in classes for the trainable mentally retarded (TMR) and in early childhood special education (ECSE) receiving medication. *Note:* From "Prevalence and Efficacy of Stimulant Drug Use with Mentally Retarded Children and Youth" by K. D. Gadow, 1985, *Psychopharmacology Bulletin, 21*, p. 293.

lic Law 94-142 pertains to children receiving special education and other services primarily in public school classes, whereas Public Law 89-313 refers to children in state-operated and/or state-supported schools that receive federal funds. Table 4–1 lists the number of children reported as being mentally retarded or multiply handicapped in December 1983 (U.S. Department of Education, 1985). In general, severely and profoundly mentally retarded (SPMR) children are represented by the "multiply handicapped" category and, to a certain extent, the Public Law 89-313 figures, whereas the Public Law 94-142 figures pertain primarily to educable mentally retarded (EMR) and trainable mentally retarded (TMR) students. Although these data are not without their limitations (see Gadow, 1985), they are the best available estimates of school-labeled mentally retarded children and adolescents.

Trainable Mentally Retarded Students. In general, programs for TMR pupils serve children and adolescents who score between 30/35 and 50/55 on standardized IQ tests. What is known about the pattern and prevalence of drug use among children in these programs comes from one statewide study conducted in Illinois (Gadow & Kalachnik, 1981), and one city-wide survey conducted in New Zealand (Aman et al., 1985).

The results of the Illinois study showed that 4.9% were taking medication for behavior disorders, and an *additional* 1.8% of the sample were administered drugs for both behavior problems and seizures. Psychotropic drugs were also prescribed for other disorders, the most common being cerebral palsy, anxiety, and enuresis. The New Zealand figure was somewhat lower. There, it was found that 3.4% of the "special school" children and adolescents were receiving psychotropic medication.

Stimulants and neuroleptics were the most commonly prescribed drugs for the management of behavior disorders in the Illinois study (see Figure 4–3). Stimulants accounted for 45% of the *total* number of psychotropic drugs, and neuroleptics accounted for 37%. Approximately two thirds of the youngsters in the neuroleptic-treated sample were 14 years of age or older. The two most frequently administered drugs were Ritalin (methylphenidate) and Mellaril. However, almost two dozen different drugs were reportedly used for the management of behavior disorders (see Table 4–2).

In New Zealand, stimulants were rarely prescribed to special school mentally retarded children. Approximately 2% received neuroleptics; Mellaril and Haldol (haloperidol) were the most popular.

Table 4–1. Number of Children Receiving Special Education and Related Services in the United States[a]

Category	Public Law 94-142	Public Law 89-313[b]
Mentally retarded		
3–5 years	19,052	
6–17 years	557,909	
18–21 years	76,121	
Total	653,082	97,452
Multiply handicapped		
3–5 years	12,500	
6–17 years	33,083	
18–21 years	5,123	
Total	50,706	16,808

Note: Children counted under Public Law 89-313 are excluded from the count under Public Law 94-142.

[a]Children reported as of December 1, 1983.

[b]Public Law 89-313 does not provide a breakdown by age. Totals refer to children between 3 and 21 years old.

The most common reasons for drug treatment in the Illinois sample were hyperactivity, behavior problems, and aggressivity. Other reasons for prescribing medication were psychotic behavior and attentional deficits. When asked to list specific behavioral changes as a result of drug therapy, teachers most often reported less motor restlessness (hyperactivity), improved attention to tasks, fewer behavior problems, and greater manageability.

Compared with the prevalence of psychotropic drug treatment in residential facilities and community placements, pharmacotherapy for TMR children and adolescents is much less frequent. Also, when medication is prescribed for behavior management, the TMR child in school is more apt to receive a stimulant, whereas the institutionalized child will probably be given a neuroleptic.

From both teacher questionnaires and interviews with parents of TMR children on medication, some generalizations can be made about the pattern of treatment (Gadow, 1981; Gadow & Kalachnik, 1981). First, only a small percentage of children are actually placed on medication during the school year. The incidence (number of new cases) of drug treatment for behavior disorders was 6.3 cases per 1,000. This is a far cry from some popular scenarios that depict teachers and doctors in a conspiracy to enslave mentally retarded children in chemical straitjackets. Second, drug treatment often is begun early and is maintained, sometimes intermittently, for long periods of time. Although differences among age groups in the prev-

Table 4–2. Drugs Prescribed for the Management of Behavior Disorders

Generic Name	Trade Name[a]	BD[b]	SD-BD[c]
Stimulants		(90)	(30)
Methylphenidate	Ritalin	68	21
Pemoline	Cylert	11	5
Dextroamphetamine	Dexedrine	9	2
Other	Other	2	2
Major tranquilizers		(68)	(15)
Thioridazine	Mellaril	40	6
Chlorpromazine	Thorazine	12	6
Haloperidol	Haldol	6	1
Trifluoperazine	Stelazine	5	1
Other	Other	5	1
Minor tranquilizers		(12)	(9)
Diazepam	Valium	7	3
Hydroxyzine	Atarax, Vistaril	3	6
Chlordiazepoxide	Librium	2	0
Miscellaneous		(31)	(9)
Imipramine	Tofranil	9	2
Phenobarbital	Luminal	6	1
Other	Other	12	4
Unknown	Unknown	4	2
Total[d]		201	63

[a]Only the trade name under which the drug was originally marketed in the United States is cited.

[b]Behavior disorder (n = 161).

[c]Behavior and seizure disorder (n = 60).

[d]Totals are inflated because 34 BD and 3 SD-BD students received more than one psychotropic drug during the school year.

Note: From "Prevalence and Pattern of Drug Treatment for Behavior and Seizure Disorders of TMR Students" by K. D. Gadow and J. Kalachnik, 1981, *American Journal of Mental Deficiency*, 85, p. 591. Copyright 1981 by the American Association on Mental Deficiency. Reprinted by permission.

alence of drug treatment for behavior disorders were not significant, the trend was for increased use during the 9 to 14 year old age range (see Table 4–3). Finally, multiple drug regimens were relatively infrequent: only 13% of the behavior disordered children were on more than one medication. Additional drugs were usually prescribed to control the side effects produced by neuroleptics or to help induce sleep at night. Of the few psychotropic drug combinations reported, the two most frequent were Ritalin–Mellaril and Tofranil–Mellaril.

Educable Mentally Retarded Students. In general, children and adolescents who are referred to as educable mentally retarded (EMR) score between 50/55 and 75/80 on standardized IQ tests.

Table 4–3. Treatment Prevalence Rates by Age

Age (Years)	*n*	BD[a]	SD[b]	SD-BD
3–5	193	1.0	14.0	2.1
6–8	487	4.3	10.7	1.6
9–11	507	6.7	10.8	2.6
12–14	642	6.9	9.3	2.3
15–17	670	4.0	10.6	1.5
18–21	603	5.0	10.4	1.7

[a]Behavior disorder.
[b]Seizure disorder.

Note: From "Prevalence and Pattern of Drug Treatment for Behavior and Seizure Disorders of TMR Students" by K. D. Gadow and J. Kalachnik, 1981, *American Journal of Mental Deficiency, 85*, p. 591. Copyright 1981 by the American Association on Mental Deficiency. Reprinted by permission.

Although recent efforts in mainstreaming have focused on EMR children, many remain in segregated programs for at least part of the school day (Borginsky, 1974; Epstein et al., 1985).

Information about psychotropic drug use for behavior disorders in EMR students is limited to one pilot study by Epstein et al. (1985). They collected drug treatment data for 294 children enrolled in EMR programs (i.e., resource rooms, self-contained classes) in northern Illinois and found that 13.3% were receiving medication for behavior disorders, a rate comparable to that for emotionally disturbed students. The treatment prevalence rate for 6 to 11 year olds (28%) was much higher than the figure for 12 to 18 year olds (11.3%). The stimulants were clearly the most commonly administered psychotropic drugs for this group of children. Given the small sample size and its restricted geographic range, generalizations about and estimates derived from these data must, of course, be qualified. It is unfortunate that we know so little about the use of psychotropic medication with EMR youngsters because they are by far the largest subgroup of mentally retarded children in our schools.

STIMULANT DRUGS

Unquestionably, some of the most commonly prescribed psychotropic drugs for mentally retarded children and youth are the stimulants. Moreover, what limited data are available suggest that they are highly effective in the treatment of hyperactivity in mildly to moderately retarded individuals (Gadow, 1985). At first blush, these statements appear far-fetched, given the widespread use of neuroleptics in institutions throughout the world and the popularly held belief (at least in some professional groups) that these drugs are *not* effective for the treatment of behavior disorders in mentally retarded people. Because stimulants are widely used with mentally retarded children and youth, it was decided that a separate section devoted to these agents was not only desirable, but also necessary from the standpoint of clarifying some common misconceptions.

It is a generally unappreciated fact that mentally retarded children were often included in early stimulant drug studies. This was true for all the primary stimulant drugs: Benzedrine (amphetamine sulfate) (Molitch & Eccles, 1937; Molitch & Sullivan, 1937), Dexedrine (dextroamphetamine) (Laufer et al., 1957; Ounsted, 1955), and even Ritalin (Zimmerman & Burgemeister, 1958). These early investigators found that mentally retarded subjects improved in much the same way as their nonretarded peers. In spite of this early interest in mentally retarded people, we really know very little about the effect of these drugs on mildly to moderately retarded children. There are many reasons for this, but the most important was the adoption of mental retardation as an exclusion criterion in drug studies with hyperactive children, as one of several measures designed to decrease sample heterogeneity. While this was understandable and in a certain sense commendable, it has created a glaring gap in our clinical knowledge.

Hyperactivity

It bears repeating that the term *hyperactivity* is used both as a symptom and as a diagnostic construct. This distinction is particularly important in the mental retardation area because, as Fish (1971) has pointed out, not all children who exhibit motor restlessness are behaviorally comparable, nor are stimulants always the drugs of choice (see Chapter 2).

Hyperactive and nonhyperactive EMR children appear to respond to stimulant medication much the same way as nonretarded children (Alexandris & Lundell, 1968; Blacklidge & Ekblad, 1971; Blue et al., 1960; Molitch & Eccles, 1937; Molitch & Sullivan, 1937; Varley & Trupin, 1982). The results of these studies support this conclusion with regard to a variety of dependent measures including caregiver ratings and psychological tests. The only contradictory findings for hyperactive EMR children were reported by Christensen (1975), who compared behavior therapy plus Ritalin with behavior therapy plus placebo. Given the fact that it has long been recognized that the presence of ongoing psychological interventions can obscure drug effects (Greenblatt et al., 1959), this finding is not surprising, and Christensen reached a similar conclusion. Although the EMR studies are few in number, their results are certainly comparable to those from mainstream hyperactivity research.

The TMR studies include several with hyperactive children (Christensen, 1975; Davis, 1971; McConnell et al., 1964); unfortunately, they really do not clarify the situation. The Christensen (1975) study, as noted, did not contain drug alone or placebo alone conditions; the Davis (1971) study selected subjects on the basis of stereotypies; and the McConnell et al. (1964) study used very low dosages. Some support for the efficacy of stimulant drugs for hyperactive TMR students can be found in Gadow's (1982b, 1983a) survey of TMR classes in public schools. Both parent and teacher ratings indicated that Ritalin was effective for hyperactivity in some cases. These surveys, however, were not designed to be well-controlled clinical trials, so their findings should only be used as an indication for the need to do research in this area.

As for SPMR individuals who exhibit overactivity, hyperactivity, or conduct problems, the findings are mixed in the sense that improvement in specific individuals is reported (e.g., Spencer, 1970; Triantafillou, 1972), but group findings are overwhelmingly negative (e.g., Aman & Singh, 1982; Anton & Greer, 1969; Spencer, 1970). This is *not* to suggest that drug effects are not present because several investigators have reported increased heart rate, anorexia, exacerbation of symptoms, weight loss, and so forth. Collectively, these studies fail to support the indiscriminant use of these agents in this subpopulation of mentally retarded individuals.

Stereotypic Behavior

Several studies have focused on stereotypies, either in subject selection, dependent measures, or both (Aman & Singh, 1982; Berkson, 1965; Davis, 1971; Davis et al., 1969). The data indicate that stimulants are by no means effective for the treatment of stereotypies, nor do they appear to aggravate the disorder, at least in SPMR individuals.

Drug-Induced Drowsiness

There are at least two studies of stimulants being used to counteract neuroleptic and antiepileptic drug-induced drowsiness in mentally retarded individuals (Carter, 1956; Levy et al., 1957). In both cases, the drugs were found to be highly effective.

Speech Disorders

A commonly reported, though not necessarily common, side effect of stimulant medication is increased talkativeness. In one uncontrolled study of a large number of mentally retarded children and adults with speech and language disorders, Fish and Bowling (1962) identified several subjects who appeared to respond favorably by showing greater task motivation and fluent language output. Moskowitz (1941) also reported increased responsiveness to speech therapy in a few individuals.

Hyperactive-Epileptic Children

Many mentally retarded children with seizure disorders are also hyperactive or exhibit conduct problems. While stimulant drugs are generally recommended for such cases (e.g., Livingston, 1972; Millichap, 1969), the actual number of studies on this group of children is limited. In one such investigation, Ounsted (1955) found that while Dexedrine was very effective for some children, many others responded by becoming withdrawn, depressed, and weepy. While this reaction is commonly reported in the literature, it is generally considered an indication of excessive medication. Although mentally retarded, epileptic children *may* be less responsive to these agents, treatment prevalence studies (Gadow, 1981; Gadow & Kalachnik, 1981) suggest that many take them with apparent success. Livingston (1978) noted that stimulants are also an effective treatment for barbiturate-induced hyperactivity in epileptic children, but there does not appear to be any research on this practice.

NEUROLEPTICS: GENERAL TOPICS

The first report of the use of a neuroleptic (Thorazine) in the treatment of adult psychiatric disorders appeared in 1952. A year later, the first article about the use of Thorazine (known as Largactil in Europe and Canada) with children was published (Heuyer et al., 1953). Since then, dozens of neuroleptics have been developed and marketed. A listing of many of these agents appears in Appendix A. Although it would seem that ample time has elapsed to collect a considerable amount of research information about the effects of these agents in children, relatively few studies have actually been conducted (see Aman, 1984; Aman & Singh, 1983; DiMascio et al., 1970; Sprague & Werry, 1974). Much of what has been done contains serious methodological flaws and lacks systematic documentation of side effects.

This section describes neuroleptic drug effects in adults. Although this may sound at odds with the primary focus of this text, there are really three good reasons for so doing. First, the distinction between late adolescence and adulthood is probably not an important one in terms of drug response. Second, the highest rates of neuroleptic use with mentally retarded people are found in these two age groups. Third, in institutional settings, treatment-related issues are similar for all residents, regardless of age. It is also worthy of note that in contrast to pediatric research, there is a voluminous literature about the use of neuroleptics in the treatment of adult psychiatric disorders.

Neuroleptics are used extensively with mentally retarded people, particularly in residential facilities. Although it would be inappropriate to consider all the behavior disorders of mentally retarded persons as comparable to psychiatric disorders in nonretarded people, there are many similarities between the bizarre behavior of some mentally retarded persons and psychotic individuals. It is also the case that some mentally retarded people in institutions and community placements exhibit identifiable psychiatric disorders (see, for example, Eaton & Menolascino, 1982). One of the objectives of pharmacotherapy for psychotic patients is the suppression of maladaptive behavior (i.e., behavior that is injurious to self and others, is socially unacceptable, and interferes with therapeutic progress). It is reasonable to assume that drug therapy for severe behavior disorders in mentally retarded children, adolescents, and adults is similarly motivated. However, the high rate of psychotropic drug use in residential facilities has prompted a number of researchers, clinicians, and educators to question whether or not the resident's wellbeing is always the overriding concern (Sprague, 1978, 1982).

The neuroleptics consist primarily of three subgroups of drugs: *phenothiazines* (e.g., Mellaril, Thorazine, Stelazine), *butyrophenones* (e.g., Haldol), and *thioxanthenes* (e.g., Taractan, Navane). The phenothiazines are the most widely used neuroleptics and, for this reason, they are the primary focus of the following discussion. There are two more categories of neuroleptics (see Appendix A), but at present they are used infrequently with mentally retarded individuals. Although there are some marked differences in the prevalence of certain adverse drug reactions, all the neuroleptics have similar effects on behavior disorders. They have proved to be effective in the suppression of some symptoms associated with certain psychiatric disorders such as schizophrenia, character disorders, manic states, and agitated depression (Klein et al., 1980). These drugs can have a pronounced effect on disordered thought, hyperactive behavior, combativeness, and uncooperativeness. Patients who suffer dramatic changes in mood in a relatively short period of time are also aided by these agents due to their mood-regulating effects. Other therapeutic benefits for schizophrenic patients include making them less withdrawn and more responsive and suppressing hallucinations and delusions. Because many severely and profoundly mentally retarded individuals exhibit behaviors similar to those of people diagnosed as having certain types of psychiatric disorders, it is not unusual that a medical approach to the treatment of mental retardation should draw heavily upon psychiatry.

The general behavioral effects of the phenothiazines in psychiatric patients are "suppression of spontaneous movements and complex behavior . . . a striking lack of initiative, disinterest in the environment, little display of emotion, and limited range of affect" (Baldessarini, 1980, p. 397). To an observer, adults receiving phenothiazines are not upset by situations or events that would normally arouse them, perceiving the world with a detached serenity. Although fully capable of thinking clearly and conversing, they appear indifferent to feelings and express thoughts without emotion. Spontaneous motor activity can be greatly reduced. People taking phenothiazines perform less well on tasks that require sustained attention, and there is a general impairment in cognitive performance and learning at higher dosages (Hartlage, 1965). Initially, Mellaril and Thorazine produce a considerable degree of sedation (drowsiness, lethargy) for which the patient usually develops a tolerance within several days to a few weeks, often without a reduction in dosage.

Side Effects

In addition to their ability to alter mood, thought processes, and behavior, phenothiazines affect a number of bodily functions (Baldessarini, 1980; Klein et al., 1980). They produce a variety of autonomic nervous system reactions that include blurred vision, dry mouth, nausea, decreased sweating and salivation, nasal stuffiness, dizziness, constipation, and inhibition of ejaculation (but may not interfere with erection). The latter is particularly true of Mellaril. Another common autonomic nervous system side effect is *orthostatic hypotension*, which refers to lowered blood pressure upon standing erect. The person experiencing such a reaction may feel faint, dizzy, or weak, especially when getting up in the morning. It usually appears during the first week of treatment but is seldom a problem because tolerance for this reaction develops rather quickly.

The endocrine system can also be affected by treatment with the phenothiazines. Drug-induced changes in the release of growth hormones may account for frequent reports of increased appetite and weight gain.

Jaundice is observed in fewer than 2 to 4% of the patients treated with Thorazine. Current estimates, however, put the prevalence of this reaction at less than 1% (Klein et al., 1980). This is generally mild and commonly occurs between the second and fourth week of treatment. If jaundice occurs, treatment is usually terminated and another drug is substituted.

Skin reactions are fairly common, with *urticaria* or *dermatitis* reported in about 5% of those treated with phenothiazines. This usually occurs within the first to fifth week of treatment, clearing up when medication is discontinued. Most skin rashes are *self-limiting* (disappear with time).

Phototoxicity is another type of skin reaction. In some people taking phenothiazines, exposure to the sun for even a few minutes results in a severe sunburn. This can be prevented by simply keeping clothed areas well covered and using a sunscreen on skin exposed to sunlight. Long-term drug use at high dosages can also produce a gray-blue pigmentation in skin areas exposed to the sun.

Neuroleptics, particularly high doses or rapid increases in dosage, can cause tonic-clonic (grand mal) seizures. This can be easily managed by making a slight decrease in dosage.

After reviewing the psychiatric literature, Klein and Davis (1969) classified the frequency of side effects as very frequent (20% or more), frequent (10 to 20%), and occasional (5 to 10%). For Mellaril, the very frequent side effects were nausea, vomiting, drowsiness, dizziness, and dry mouth. Frequent adverse effects were visual disturbance and constipation; occasionally, patients were confused or had urinary disturbances. The very frequent side effects of Thorazine were drowsiness, dry mouth, and weight increase. Frequent effects were depression, visual disturbance, and constipation; occasional effects included confusion, allergic reactions, and endocrine disturbances.

Dose and side effect information for frequently prescribed neuroleptics are presented in Table 4–4. The dosage information is in reference to adult psychiatric disorders, but it is also relevant to adolescents in residential facilities for the mentally retarded (see Table 4–1).

Table 4–4. Selected Neuroleptic Drugs: Adult Doses and Side Effects

Generic Name	Trade Name	Daily Oral Dose (mg) Usual	Daily Oral Dose (mg) Extreme*	Sedative Effects	Extra-pyramidal Effects	Hypotensive Effects
Phenothiazines						
Acetophenazine	Tindal	60–120	20–600	+ +	+ +	+
Chlorpromazine	Thorazine	300–800	25–2000	+ + +	+ +	+ +
Fluphenazine	Prolixin	2.5–20	1–30	+	+ + +	+
Mesoridazine	Serentil	75–300	25–400			
Perphenazine	Trilafon	8–32	4–64	+ +	+ + +	+
Piperacetazine	Quide	20–160	5–200			
Prochlorperazine	Compazine	75–100	15–150	+ +	+ + +	+
Thioridazine	Mellaril	200–600	50–800	+ + +	+	+ +
Trifluoperazine	Stelazine	6–20	2–60	+	+ + +	+
Triflupromazine	Vesprin	100–150	50–300	+ +	+ + +	+ +
Thioxanthenes						
Chlorprothixene	Taractan	50–400	30–600	+ + +	+ +	+ +
Thiothixene	Navane	6–30	6–60	+ to + +	+ +	+ +
Others						
Haloperidol	Haldol	6–20	2–100	+	+ + +	+
Loxapine	Loxitane	6–100	20–250	+	+ +	+
Molindone	Moban	50–225	15–400	+ +	+	0

*Extreme dosage ranges are occasionally exceeded cautiously and only when appropriate measures have failed.

Note: From "Drugs and the Treatment of Psychiatric Disorders" by R. J. Baldessarini, in *The Pharmacological Basis of Therapeutics* (6th ed., pp. 408–411) by A. G. Gilman, L. S. Goodman, and A. Gilman, 1980, New York: Macmillan. Copyright 1980 by Macmillan Publishing Co. Adapted by permission

Extrapyramidal Syndromes

Perhaps the most disquieting and alarming side effects of neuroleptics are the *extrapyramidal syndromes*. These are disorders that involve certain motor areas of the brain called the *extrapyramidal tract*. The various *nuclei* (groups of nerve cells) and nerve fibers that make up this structure control and coordinate motor activities, especially walking, posture, muscle tone, and patterns of movement. Drugs that affect the extrapyramidal tract can cause spasms in skeletal muscles and changes in body posture, facial expression, and movement of the limbs. Four different extrapyramidal syndromes are associated with the use of major tranquilizers: *Parkinsonian syndrome, akathisia, acute dystonic reactions*, and *tardive dyskinesia*. These side effects are most common in treatment with Haldol, Stelazine (trifluoperazine), and Compazine (prochlorperazine) and are least likely to occur with Mellaril (see Table 4–4).

Parkinsonian Syndrome

The Parkinsonian syndrome caused by the neuroleptics appears similar to the symptoms of Parkinson's disease. The syndrome is characterized by a decrease in spontaneous movements. The patient may appear depressed, with a masklike facial expression which parents and other caregivers may refer to as "looking like a zombie." Associated with this is muscle rigidity, changes in posture, and tremor (involuntary shaking, trembling, or quivering). Other features may include drooling, a shuffling walk without free swing of the arms, and "pill-rolling." The latter refers to movements of the hand as if the patient is rolling a pill between his or her fingers. There is disagreement as to the best way of managing this side effect. Some patients may respond to dosage reduction, whereas others may require *anticholinergic* agents, such as Arthane (trihexyphenidyl) or Cogentin (benztropine). For children, oral doses of 1 mg of Artane three times a day or 1 to 2 mg of Cogentin three times a day rapidly alleviate these symptoms (Winsberg et al., 1976).

Akathisia

This reaction is characterized by involuntary motor restlessness. The patient is unable to sit still, is constantly fidgeting, and appears to be agitated. The disorder responds to dosage reduction and in some cases to anticholinergic drugs.

Acute Dystonic Reaction

A third type of extrapyramidal syndrome is acute dystonic reaction. Symptoms include one or more of the following: facial grimacing, *oculogyric crisis* (fixed upward gaze), and *torticollis* (a twisting of the neck and an unnatural positioning of the head due to contraction of the neck muscles). The tongue may be protruded or the teeth tightly clenched. In rare cases, the patient may have difficulty swallowing. Although this reaction responds well to treatment, it can be terrifying for both patient and caregivers. Acute dystonic reactions are common with Compazine and Stelazine compared with the other neuroleptics. They are more apt to occur in younger patients and when medication is first initiated. A child having a severe reaction should receive immediate medical attention. The physician may use an intramuscular injection of Benadryl (diphenhydramine) or of anticholinergic agents for immediate relief of symptoms, and later prescribe oral doses of Cogentin or Artane for the continued control of this reaction.

Tardive Dyskinesia

The fourth extrapyramidal syndrome, tardive dyskinesia, typically appears late, often months after drug treatment has been initiated, and may not be evident until medication is discontinued. Tardive dyskinesia is characterized by rhythmic, repetitive stereotyped movements that appear to be involuntary but can usually be inhibited. Some of the major features are sucking and smacking movements of the lips and side-to-side shifts of the chin, giving the appearance of a cow "chewing its cud." The tongue may dart in and out in a "fly catching" fashion. Other symptoms include a sudden flying of the arms, up-and-down movements of the toes, in-and-out movements of the fingers or "piano playing," and jerky body movements. (See Kalachnik, 1985, for a detailed description of the syndrome.) Tardive dyskinesia is more common among patients who receive large dosages of neuroleptic medication over extended periods. Prevalence figures for this adverse reaction range as high as 15 to 30% among psychiatric patients. There is no one best method for treating tardive dyskinesia (Kobayashi, 1977). When the disorder appears while the person is on medication, treatment should be stopped, if possible, or another agent selected if drug therapy is necessary. For individuals who develop the disorder after treatment has been terminated, a variety of drugs that have helped some people are available. Some patients are benefited by resuming the drug that caused the tardive dyskinesia. The disorder can persist indefinitely after medication is terminated, but for at least half of the patients, there is gradual improvement over time after medication has been stopped. Some very preliminary data suggest that gradual neuroleptic drug withdrawal in mentally retarded people produces fewer dyskinesias than abrupt drug withdrawal (Schroeder & Gualtieri, 1985).

Several large studies of drug treatment with psychotic, emotionally disturbed, and mentally retarded children have clearly documented tardive dyskinesia in children (McAndrew et al., 1972; Paulson et al., 1975; Polizos et al., 1973). Involuntary movements of the lips, tongue, and jaw are much less common among children than adults. *Choreiform* (ceaseless, rapid, jerky, and involuntary) movements of the arms, legs, and head were the most frequently reported symptoms in children with tardive dyskinesia. For many children, the syndrome did not become apparent until medication was terminated. Off medication, some children improved over time and others became worse. Resuming drug treatment alleviated symptoms in many children who remained unchanged or became worse when drug treatment was stopped. McAndrew et al. (1972) reported that tardive dyskinesia was more common among children who received higher dosages for longer periods of time than among children on short-term regimens at lower dosages.

Children Versus Adults

There are some general differences between children and adults in the prevalence of extrapyramidal reactions (Winsberg & Yepes, 1978). The Parkinsonian syndrome is most common among older adult patients and is not often observed in children. When it does occur in children, the reaction is usually mild. Acute dystonic reactions are found more often in children, and appear within 24 to 72 hours after the onset of treatment. The most common extrapyramidal syndrome in adults is akathisia, which is typically seen in middle-aged women. It is also reported in children, but the prevalence rate is difficult to determine. Tardive dyskinesia seems to occur with similar frequency in both children and adults, especially at higher doses. In one study of schizophrenic children receiving neuroleptics at doses comparable to those recommended for adults, 48% exhibited neurological symptoms similar to tardive dyskinesia upon withdrawal of medication (Engelhardt et al., 1975).

NEUROLEPTICS: TREATMENT APPLICATIONS

There has been very little research on the use of neuroleptics with mentally retarded children, adolescents, and adults since the late 1950s and early 1960s when these drugs were first becoming widely used. These early studies were often, but not always, poorly done, at least according to contemporary standards. Subsequently, much of what has been written about the use of these agents with prepubertal children has been extrapolated from research and clinical experience with adolescents and adults. In addition, many of the truly well-designed studies have been conducted with nonretarded children (e.g., Gittelman-Klein et al., 1976; Sprague et al., 1970; Werry & Aman, 1975).

Hyperactivity

Although it is generally assumed that neuroleptics are effective for hyperactivity in mentally retarded people regardless of the level of intellectual ability (see Aman & Singh, 1980, 1983), the research in this area generally is not particularly compelling. Nevertheless, well-designed studies do show a drug effect on hyperactivity (e.g., Singh & Aman, 1981). Studies of intellectually normal hyperactive children (e.g., Gittelman-Klein et al., 1976) have shown that Mellaril does lead to behavioral improvement in some hyperactivity symptoms, particularly in the area of conduct problems.

Stereotypies

Sterotypic behaviors are of concern to caregivers because they interfere with educational and habilitative efforts. Moreover, they can also be an impediment to normalization, in that bizarre behaviors are generally perceived in a negative way by others. There is now substantial evidence that Mellaril reduces levels of stereotypic behavior in mentally retarded people (e.g., Davis, 1971; Davis et al., 1969; Singh & Aman, 1981; Zimmerman & Heistad, 1982). Whether drug-induced reductions in stereotypic behaviors do in fact lead to performance gains in other areas is unknown. It is noteworthy that Singh and Aman (1981) found that a low dose (2.5 mg/kg) of Mellaril was just as effective as higher therapeutic doses in controlling stereotypies.

Self-Injurious Behavior (SIB)

Studies of mentally retarded people in institutions (e.g., Schroeder et al., 1978) suggest that approximately 10% exhibit self-injurious behavior (generally referred to as SIB). The extent of this problem is often underappreciated. Schroeder et al. (1986), for example, estimated that as many as 34,000 severely and profoundly mentally retarded persons exhibit serious SIB, which may result in tissue damage, permanent impairment, and even death. Despite the seriousness of this disorder and our heartfelt reactions to it, there are few well-conducted studies that have examined the effectiveness of neuroleptics, even though these drugs are generally considered to be therapeutic (see Aman & Singh, 1980, 1983; Singh & Millichamp, 1985). Both phenothiazines (see Aman & Singh, 1983) and butyrophenones such as Haldol (Burk & Menolascino, 1968) have been reported to reduce SIB. A variety of behavioral techniques can also be used to suppress SIB (see Romanczyk, 1986), and one survey study found that while the majority of mentally retarded individuals with severe SIB were on neuroleptic medication, all were receiving behavior modification. Durand (1982) showed that Haldol in combination with mild punishment was more effective than either treatment used alone in reducing SIB in a profoundly retarded adolescent.

Psychiatric Disorders

There is no reason to assume that mentally retarded people are not susceptible to the same psychiatric disorders that afflict nonretarded people. In fact, the medical literature describes successful neuroleptic treatment for a wide variety of psychiatric problems, ranging from assault trauma (Varley, 1984) to schizophrenia (Menolascino et al., 1985) and Tourette syndrome (Golden & Greenhill, 1981) in mentally retarded people. It should be noted, however, that there may be differences between mentally retarded and nonmentally retarded psychotic persons with regard to specific aspects of treatment. Menolascino et al. (1985), for example, found that mentally retarded schizophrenic patients required *less* medication.

Side Effects in Children

Side effects of neuroleptics in children are similar to those reported for adults. Sedative effects (drowsiness, lethargy, apathy) are quite common with Thorazine, but children usually develop a tolerance for this reaction within several days to a few weeks. Dosage reduction may be necessary in some cases. It is noteworthy that irritability and excitability are also possible. Skin reactions are infrequent. Also reported are diarrhea, upset stomach, dry mouth, blurred vision, constipation, urinary retention, and abdominal pain (Winsberg & Yepes, 1978). A number of studies report increased appetite, weight gains, or both, during drug treatment.

Side effects are believed to be less frequent with Mellaril than with Thorazine. Adverse drug reactions commonly associated with Mellaril are drowsiness, lethargy, irritability, hyperactivity, ataxia, and dizziness. Increased appetite and weight gain are also not unusual. Because Mellaril has been reported to have a favorable effect on seizure reduction, this drug can be used with some confidence for the treatment of behavior disorders in epileptic children (Kamm & Mandel, 1967).

Katz et al. (1975) stated that in their experience with nonretarded hyperactive children the side effects of Mellaril were frequent and severe. Drowsiness was the most common adverse reaction that was difficult to manage. If the dose was reduced, the drowsiness was less severe, but the therapeutic response was weaker. Many children developed enuresis and had to be taken off medication. Increased appetite was also common, as was puffiness around the eyes and mild dry mouth. Stomachache, nausea, and vomiting necessitated dosage reduction in a number of children. Other side effects included nosebleed, mild tremor, and orthostatic hypotension. Some children who reacted well to Mellaril later developed changes in temperament. They became irritable, moody, and belligerent, and medication eventually had to be stopped.

Extrapyramidal syndromes are frequently reported in studies using Haldol to control behavior disorders in children. Clinicians manage these side effects by administering an anticholinergic agent either at the beginning of drug treatment (a practice that is controversial), after symptoms appear, or after the discontinuation of treatment. Although Haldol is usually not associated with sedative effects (see Table 4–4), drowsiness was sometimes reported in studies with children. Other side effects include nausea, ataxia, slurred speech, and weight gain.

Perhaps the most controversial side effect of neuroleptics is cognitive and academic impairment. This is controversial because the studies in this area are not particularly well designed (see Aman, 1984). There are, nevertheless, good examples of research with neuroleptics in nonretarded (e.g., Sprague et al., 1970; Werry & Aman, 1975) and mentally retarded (e.g., Wysocki et al., 1981) individuals which strongly suggest that mental impairment is a definite *possibility.* It is important, therefore, to monitor adaptive behavior during dosage adjustment to assess the extent to which desirable behaviors may be adversely affected.

Treatment Practices

There has been relatively little research (compared with stimulants) on the clinical utility of various treatment practices involving neuroleptic drugs for prepubertal children. Much of what has been written are either discussions of clinical experience or descriptions of treatment procedures employed in specific studies.

Dosage and Schedule

There is a considerable range in reported dosages across studies with children. The dose for Thorazine and Mellaril ranges from 10 to 1,000 mg per day, with an average daily dose of 75 to 200 mg. Some clinicians prescribe one large dose at night to avoid daytime drowsiness, whereas others divide the total amount into two or three doses during the day (Katz et al., 1975; Winsberg et al., 1976). Most hyperactive children require no more than 50 mg to 100 mg three times per day. Relative to body weight, the average dose is 3 to 6 mg/kg per day. The effective dose of Haldol ranges from 2 to 5 mg per day, which is divided into three daily doses. It is noteworthy that significant improvements in cognitive performance have been reported with doses of Haldol as low as 0.025 mg/kg in nonretarded hyperactive boys (Werry & Aman, 1975). Daily doses for Stelazine range from 2 mg to 50 mg per day, with an average of 6 to 15 mg per day. In most studies, medication is given in divided doses, usually three times per day.

Duration

At this point it would be desirable to provide information about the duration and termination of drug treatment for behavior disorders associated with mental retardation. Unfortunately, there are almost no data available on this topic and virtually no well-controlled followup studies. TMR children who are treated for behavior disorders often are placed on medication when younger and are treated for a number of years. In fact, the median duration of treatment for children still on medication was approximately 4 years in one study (Gadow, 1981).

OTHER DRUGS

Surveys of mentally retarded children and adolescents (regardless of setting) reveal that all kinds of drugs are prescribed for the management of behavior disorders. Nevertheless, the many reviewers (e.g., Aman & Field, 1985; Aman & Singh, 1983) of the mental retardation literature have found little evidence for the utility of antiepileptic drugs or antianxiety agents for the treatment of behavior disorders in general. The tricyclic antidepressants have not been shown to have widespread use for depression in mentally retarded people (see Gualtieri & Hawk, 1982), and a recent study found that imipramine actually caused a worsening of behavior in "depressed" profoundly retarded people (Aman et al., in press). One drug, however, has received a considerable amount of attention in recent years and may prove to be useful for the treatment of both mood disorders and aggressivity in mentally retarded people. This drug is lithium carbonate and is sold as a generic and under a variety of trade names (e.g., Eskalith, Lithane, Lithonate).

Lithium has been reported to be effective for the treatment of aggressive-oppositional behavior and overactivity (e.g., Dostal & Zvolsky, 1970; Goetz et al., 1977), self-injurious behavior (Cooper & Fowlie, 1973; Micev & Lynch, 1974), and affective disorders (Naylor et al., 1974; Rivinus & Harmatz, 1979) in mentally retarded people. In prepubertal children reported dosages range from 50 to 2,000 mg per day (Gualtieri et al., 1983), and dosages close to adult levels may be necessary to achieve therapeutic blood levels. It is recommended that therapy be carefully monitored (e.g., blood level analyses at appropriate intervals). Early signs of toxicity include loss of appetite (*anorexia*), upset stomach, nausea, thirst, and hand tremor. Last, while the scientific literature suggests that lithium may help some individuals, it is not always effective and may even aggravate the child's problems.

Another relatively new drug for the treatment of aggression and explosive aggressive outbursts is Inderal (propranolol), a beta-adrenergic blocking agent, or "beta-blocker." This drug is used primarily for the treatment of *hypertension* (high blood pressure), *angina* (intense chest pains), and *cardiac arrhythmias* (irregularities in heart beat). A growing number of studies (see Gualtieri et al., 1983) indicate that Inderal may be effective in the treatment of a variety of psychiatric disorders. However, it is not yet approved by the FDA for use in the treatment of these disorders in the United States. Reports of Inderal's effectiveness for childhood behavior disorders have focused on children with some form of organic brain damage or brain dysfunction (e.g., Williams et al., 1982). The average dose for children and adolescents is 160 mg per day (the optimal range is 50 to 960 mg per day). When Inderal is used with the right children and dosage is gradually increased, side effects are not a major problem. A key point here is use with the "right" children. Inderal should be employed in cases where conventional pharmacological and behavioral treatments have failed. The use of this drug is contraindicated for children and youth with a history of cardiac or respiratory disease, who have hypoglycemia, or who are taking MAOIs (Gualtieri et al., 1983).

Yet another drug that has very recently drawn considerable interest is Narcan (naloxone), an opiate antagonist that is used to treat respiratory depression due to narcotic overdose. Two reports indicate that Narcan can suppress SIB (Davidson et al., 1983; Sandman et al., 1983). Narcan can be administered intravenously, intramuscularly, or subcutaneously. In the adult study (Sandman et al., 1983), three intramuscular doses were used (0.1, 0.2, and 0.4 mg), and in the child study (Davidson et al., 1983), two intramuscular doses (0.15 mg and 0.075 mg) were used.

ISSUES RELATING TO DRUG TREATMENT

Psychotropic drug therapy with mentally retarded people has been the focus of controversy for several reasons. First, after reviewing the research in this area, Sprague and Werry (1971) concluded that much of the data was of questionable value due to serious methodological flaws in most studies. Unfortunately, new research on the use of medication for mentally retarded people is very infrequent. There are many reasons for this, but suffice it to say that Sprague and Werry's observation is, for the most part, still true today. Very little research has been conducted comparing drug therapy with other treatment approaches (for example, behavior modification), and there have been few published accounts about how to improve the way in which pharmacotherapy is used with mentally retarded people. Second, the manner in which these drugs are prescribed and administered (e.g., dosage, duration of treatment, monitoring) raises questions about possible drug misuse (Lipman, 1970; Sprague, 1977b, 1978). Third, recent court cases involving residential facilities for mentally retarded persons have raised serious questions about the competence of caregivers (Sprague, 1977b, 1978, 1982). Some of the major issues in these court cases are the focus on symptom suppression instead of responsiveness to habilitation, overmedication, poor monitoring procedures, and a cavalier approach to record keeping on the use and effects of psychotropic drugs. An excellent review of this material has been prepared by Sprague (1982). Fourth, the exclusion of teachers in public schools and of direct care personnel in residential facilities from meaningful participation in the treatment process is also a major problem (Gadow, 1981, 1982a). Although psychotropic drugs affect the very behaviors that often become objectives in educational and habilitative programming, nonmedical personnel are frequently excluded from diagnostic and drug evaluation procedures. Finally, because neuroleptics can produce serious side effects when used for long periods of time at high dosages and can suppress adaptive behavior, disagreements about the risks versus benefits are unavoidable. Central to this issue is whether or not medication is being used in a manner that is in the best interests of the mentally retarded child.

These problems are, of course, highly interrelated and well known to many who have direct experience with residential facilities, and, to a lesser extent, public school programs. This is not to suggest that exemplary treatment evaluation programs do not exist because they do (e.g., Fielding et al., 1980). The misuse of psychotropic medication is therefore the product of inadequate training, incomplete medical knowledge, inappropriate diagnostic and drug assessment practices, and, in some cases, incompetence and societal irresponsibility. This section addresses three topics of considerable concern to caregivers: litigation, model drug monitoring programs, and tardive dyskinesia.

Litigation

Less-than-adequate drug monitoring procedures and the use of medication as a substitute for habilitation are two major legal issues. They have been attended to in several recent court cases. In *Wyatt v. Stickney*, Judge Frank M. Johnson ruled that the mentally retarded residents at the Partlow State School in Alabama have a right to appropriate treatment (habilitation), which he defined as "the process by which the staff of the institution assists the resident to acquire and maintain those life skills which enable him to cope more effectively with the demands of his own person and of his environment and to raise the level of his physical, mental, and social efficiency" (*Wyatt v. Stickney*, 1972, p. 395). The court developed a set of standards describing what adequate habilitation of the mentally retarded person meant, including a section about drug treatment. Several of the items are particularly noteworthy:

1. "Residents shall have a right to be free from unnecessary or excessive medication. The resident's records shall state the effects of psychoactive medication on the resident. When dosages of such are changed or other psychoactive medications are prescribed, a notation shall be made in the resident's record concerning the effect of the new medication or new dosages and the behavior changes, if any, that occur."
2. "Notation of each individual's medication shall be kept in his medical records. . . . At least weekly the attending physician shall review the drug regimen of each resident under his care. All prescriptions shall be written with termination date, which shall not exceed 30 days."
3. "Medication shall not be used as punishment, for the convenience of staff, as a substitute for a habilitative program, or in quantities that interfere with the resident's habilitation program."

Another case, *New York State ARC v. Rockefeller* (1975), resulted in a consent decree that established standards for drug therapy at the Willowbrook State School. Among the guidelines were these:

1. "Only appropriately trained staff shall be allowed to administer drugs."
2. "Written policies and procedures that govern the safe administration and handling of all drugs shall be developed."
3. "Medication errors and drug reactions shall be recorded and reported immediately to the practitioner who ordered the drug."

One last example presented here is from a consent decree pertaining to Pineland Center in Maine (*Wuori v. Zitnay*), which was issued in 1978 (see Sprague, 1982):

1. "Psychotropic drugs shall be used only as an integrated part of an individualized habilitation plan that is designed to lead to a less restrictive way of treating, and ultimately to the elimination of the behaviors for which the drugs are employed."
2. "Before any new psychotropic medication is prescribed, the attending physician shall ascertain, consider and record in the resident's medical record:

   (a) the reasons for the choice of medication including such matters as careful balancing of expected therapeutic effects and potential adverse effects, the history of the resident's response to the same or similar medication, and why techniques other than medication are not deemed adequate or appropriate treatment for the resident, and

(b) the fact that the physician or nurse has explained in lay terms to the resident and to the resident's correspondent the reasons for the treatment and possible benefits and consequences of the medication."

3. "The physician will ensure that appropriate persons responsible for the resident's habilitation, education, care and other treatment are informed as to the significant potential effects of the medication and record their observations thereof, including effects on the resident's progress in habilitation and education programs and his participation in other activities."

Only a few excerpts have been presented here from an ever-growing number of court cases involving mentally retarded people in residential facilities. A more detailed discussion of these and other cases and their clinical implications is available elsewhere (see Sprague, 1982).

Tardive Dyskinesia

Tardive dyskinesia (TD) has become an important issue in the mental retardation area for several reasons: (a) high neuroleptic drug exposure in terms of prevalence, dosage, and duration of treatment (see Gualtieri et al., 1984), (b) inadequate side effect monitoring systems, and (c) vulnerability to professional incompetence and societal irresponsibility. Add to this the fact that some mentally retarded people receive medication for trivial reasons and many exhibit symptoms similar to TD in their unmedicated state, and you have a situation that invites disaster. For example, there have been several recent court cases involving TD (see Kalachnik, 1985), one of which involved a mentally retarded adolescent (see Sprague, 1982, pp. 402–405). The details of these cases are often shocking, but rather than dwell on the tragedy it is more instructive here to discuss ways in which caregivers can minimize the risks of neuroleptic drug use.

For mentally retarded people in residential facilities who must receive neuroleptic medication, the most prudent course of action for caregivers is the development of a TD monitoring system. Several are described in the literature (e.g., Glazer & Moore, 1981; Whall et al., 1983), but none are more detailed than Kalachnik's program for residential facilities (1985; Kalachnik et al., 1983a, 1984). Several TD assessment scales have been developed to date; two of the more popular are the Abnormal Involuntary Movement Scale (Guy, 1976) and the Dyskinesia Identification System–Coldwater (Sprague et al., 1984a, 1984b). The latter (which is called DIS-CO) appears in Appendix E and item descriptions in Appendix F. An abbreviated version (DISCUS) is presented in Appendix G, the manual for which can be obtained from Sprague et al. (1985). A sample parent letter about side effects formulated by Kalachnik (1985) appears in Appendix H.

Drug Monitoring Programs

The need for effective drug assessment procedures is self-evident to anyone who is concerned about the use of psychotropic and antiepileptic drugs with mentally retarded people. Almost all of the effort in this area concerns residential facilities because it is very difficult to either regulate or monitor drug use with children and adolescents in public schools, for a variety of reasons. Several articles have appeared in recent years that describe procedures to successfully reduce unnecessary psychotropic drug use (e.g., Ellenor & Frisk, 1977; Ferguson et al., 1982; Fielding et al., 1980; Inoue, 1982; LaMendola et al., 1980) and unnecessary neuroleptic multiple drug therapy (Ellenor, 1977). Moreover, this is an international effort, as is evidenced by reports from England (Carter, 1983; James, 1983) and Australia (Horten, 1982). One program (Fielding et al., 1980) is briefly described here to show how much can be done to improve the welfare of these often unfortunate people.

Fielding et al. (1980) formulated a two-phase assessment procedure that greatly reduced psychotropic drug use in an institution for mentally retarded people. During Phase One, residents received their regular medication for 20 days, followed by 30 days of no medication (baseline). The daily number of occurrences of maladaptive behaviors were recorded, and the individual's behavioral intervention was in effect. Unless problem behaviors during baseline were twice as high as during drug therapy, the medication was stopped. The Phase One procedure was repeated a second time for those still receiving treatment. In Phase Two, the *minimum effective dose* was determined for those residents who needed to take neuroleptic medication. The normal dose was decreased by 25%, or the equivalent of 100 mg of Thorazine, whichever was less, for 30 days. If problem behavior did not increase one standard deviation above baseline, the dosage was again reduced and reevaluated. With this two-phase procedure, Fielding et al. were able to take 60% of the treated residents off medication altogether.

In addition to conducting periodic dosage and drug-free period evaluations, consideration must also be given to the development of efficient and cost-effective procedures to assess response to treatment. One example of this is an interdisciplinary medication review form developed by Kalachnik et al. (1983b) that provides a systematic record of both behavioral and pharmacological interventions. With this form, the interdisciplinary treatment team can monitor therapeutic progress and subsequently take steps to avoid the misuse of medication. It is particularly noteworthy that this procedure actually *reduced* the amount of time necessary to monitor neuroleptic drug therapy by structuring interdisciplinary interaction and focusing attention clearly on target behaviors. Moreover, it also led to an increase in the quality and quantity of data available for making treatment-related decisions.

In addition to the need for more effective treatment evaluation procedures, there is a serious shortage of reliable and valid drug assessment instruments. A newly developed measure, the Aberrant Behavior Checklist (see Aman et al., 1985a, 1985b), holds considerable promise in helping fill this void. A testing manual is available. Information regarding this rating scale can be obtained by contacting Dr. Michael Aman, Department of Psychiatry, University of Auckland, New Zealand.

Although much discussion has focused on private and public residential facilities, information collected about TMR children in public schools is equally discouraging (Gadow, 1981). It was found that teachers received very little formal training regarding psychotropic drugs even though they frequently encountered children on medication (Gadow, 1983b). Nor were they provided basic information about the effects of medication on their students' behavior (Gadow, 1982a). Interaction between school, parent, and physician was limited, and there was almost no direct contact between the teacher and the doctor (Gadow, 1982b, 1982c). Inadequate monitoring procedures were the result of poorly developed channels of communication, lack of standardized evaluation instruments, ambiguities in role behavior, and failure to establish drug evaluation procedures (Gadow, 1983a). In general, teachers were excluded from what most experts in pediatric psychopharmacology believe should be an interdisciplinary team effort. One cannot help but draw comparisons between the standards established as a result of federal court cases and the situation that exists in the public schools.

SUGGESTED READINGS

Aman, M. G. (1984). Drugs and learning in mentally retarded persons. In G. D. Burrows & J. S. Werry (Eds.), *Advances in human psychopharmacology* (Vol. 3, pp. 121–163). Greenwich, CT: JAI Press. (C, S)

Aman, M. G., & Singh, N. N. (1983). Pharmacological intervention. In J. L. Matson & J. A. Mulick (Eds.), *Handbook of mental retardation* (pp. 317–337). New York: Pergamon. (C, S)

Gadow, K. D. (1982). School involvement in pharmacotherapy for behavior disorders. *Journal of Special Education, 16,* 385–399. (S)

Gadow, K. D. (1983). Pharmacotherapy for behavior disorders: Typical treatment practices. *Clinical Pediatrics, 22,* 48–53. (C, S)

Kalachnik, J. E. (1985). Applied aspects of tardive dyskinesia monitoring: Over, under, sideways, down; backward, forward, square, and round. In K. D. Gadow (Ed.), *Advances in learning and behavioral disabilities* (Vol. 4, pp. 133–180). Greenwich, CT: JAI Press. (C)

Keogh, D., & Whitman, T. (1983). Mental retardation in children. In M. Herson, V. B. Van Hasselt, & J. L. Matson (Eds.), *Behavior therapy for the developmentally and physically disabled* (pp. 205–246). Orlando, FL: Academic Press. (C, S)

Lipman, R. L., DiMascio, A., Reatig, N., & Kirson, T. (1978). Psychotropic drugs and mentally retarded children. In M. A. Lipton, A. DiMascio, & K. F. Killam (Eds.), *Psychopharmacology: A generation of progress* (pp. 1437–1449). New York: Raven Press. (C)

Matson, J., & McCartney, J. R. (Eds.) (1981). *Handbook of behavior modification with the mentally retarded.* New York: Plenum.

Matson, J. L., & Mulick, J. A. (Eds.). (1983). *Handbook of mental retardation.* New York: Pergamon. (C, S)

Pharmacotherapy and mental retardation workshop. (1985). *Psychopharmacology Bulletin, 21,* 258–333. (C)

Sprague, R. L. (1982). Litigation, legislation, and regulations. In S. E. Breuning & A. D. Poling (Eds.), *Drugs and mental retardation* (pp. 377–414). Springfield, IL: Charles C Thomas. (C, S)

Sprague, R. L., & Werry, J. S. (1971). Methodology of psychopharmacological studies with the retarded. In N. R. Ellis (Ed.), *International review of research in mental retardation* (Vol. 5, pp. 147–219). Orlando, FL: Academic Press. (C)

Whitman, T. L., Scibak, J. W., & Reid, D. H. (1983). *Behavior modification with the severely and profoundly retarded.* Orlando, FL: Academic Press.

REFERENCES

Alexandris, A., & Lundell, F. W. (1968). Effect of thioridazine, amphetamine, and placebo on the hyperkinetic syndrome and cognitive area in mentally deficient children. *Canadian Medical Association Journal, 98,* 92–96.

Aman, M. G. (1984). Drugs and learning in mentally retarded persons. In G. D. Burrows & J. S. Werry (Eds.), *Advances in human psychopharmacology* (Vol. 3, pp. 121–163). Greenwich, CT: JAI Press.

Aman, M. G., & Field, C. J. (1985). Pharmacological management. In N. N. Singh & K. M. Wilton (Eds.), *Mental retardation in New Zealand: Provisions, services and research* (pp. 223–249). Christchurch, NZ: Whitcoulls.

Aman, M. G., Field, C. J., & Bridgman, G. D. (1985). City-wide survey of drug patterns among non-institutionalized retarded persons. *Applied Research in Mental Retardation, 6*, 159–171.

Aman, M. G., & Singh, N. N. (1980). The usefulness of thioridazine for treating childhood disorders—Fact or folklore? *American Journal of Mental Deficiency, 84*, 331–338.

Aman, M. G., & Singh, N. N. (1982). Methylphenidate in severely retarded residents and the clinical significance of stereotypic behavior. *Applied Research in Mental Retardation, 3*, 345–358.

Aman, M. G., & Singh, N. N. (1983). Pharmacological intervention. In J. L. Matson & J. A. Mulick (Eds.), *Handbook of mental retardation* (pp. 317–337). New York: Pergamon.

Aman, M. G., Singh, N. N., Steward, A. W., & Field, C. J. (1985a). The Aberrant Behavior Checklist: A behavior rating scale for the assessment of treatment effects. *American Journal of Mental Deficiency, 89*, 485–491.

Aman, M. G., Singh, N. N., Stewart, A. W., & Field, C. J. (1985b). Psychometric characteristics of the Aberrant Behavior Checklist. *American Journal of Mental Deficiency, 89*, 492–502.

Aman, M. G., & White, A. J. (1986). Measures of drug change in mental retardation. In K. D. Gadow, *Advances in learning and behavioral disabilities* (Vol. 5). Greenwich, CT: JAI Press.

Aman, M. G., White, A. J., Vaithianathan, C., & Field, C. J. (in press). Preliminary study of imipramine in profoundly retarded residents. *Journal of Autism & Developmental Disorders.*

Anton, A. H., & Greer, M. (1969). Dextroamphetamine, catecholamines, and behavior. *Archives of Neurology, 21*, 248–252.

Baldessarini, R. J. (1980). Drugs and the treatment of psychiatric disorders. In A. G. Gilman, L. S. Goodman, & A. Gilman (Eds.), *The pharmacological basis of therapeutics* (6th ed., pp. 391–447). New York: Macmillan.

Baumeister, A. A., & Forehand, R. (1973). Stereotyped acts. In N. R. Ellis (Ed.), *International review of research in mental retardation* (Vol. 6, pp. 55–96). Orlando, FL: Academic Press.

Bennett, H. S., Dunlop, T., & Ziring, P. (1983). Reduction of polypharmacy for epilepsy in an institution for the retarded. *Developmental Medicine and Child Neurology, 25*, 735–737.

Berkson, G. (1965). Stereotyped movements of mental defectives: VI. No effect of amphetamine or a barbiturate. *Perceptual and Motor Skills, 21*, 698.

Blacklidge, V., & Ekblad, R. (1971). The effectiveness of methylphenidate hydrochloride (Ritalin) on learning and behavior in public school educable mentally retarded children. *Pediatrics, 47*, 923–926.

Blue, A. W., Lytton, G. J., & Miller, O. W. (1960). The effect of methylphenidate on intellectually handicapped children (Abstract). *American Psychologist, 15*, 393.

Borginsky, M. E. (1974). *Provision of instruction to handicapped pupils in local public schools. Spring 1970.* Washington, DC: U.S. Office of Education.

Briggs, R., Garrard, S., Hamad, C., & Wills, F. (1984). A model for evaluating psychoactive medication use with mentally retarded persons. In J.

A. Mulick & B. L. Mallory (Eds.), *Transitions in mental retardation (Vol. 1): Advocacy, technology, and science*. Norwood, NJ: Ablex.

Burk, H. W., & Menolascino, F. J. (1968). Haloperidol in emotionally disturbed mentally retarded individuals. *American Journal of Psychiatry, 124*, 1589–1591.

Carter, C. H. (1956). The effects of reserpine and methylphenidate (Ritalin) in mental defectives, spastics, and epileptics. *Psychiatric Research Reports, 4*, 44–48.

Carter, G. (1983). The abrupt withdrawal of antiparkinsonian drugs in mentally handicapped patients. *British Journal of Psychiatry, 142*, 166–168.

Christensen, D. E. (1975). Effects of combining methylphenidate and a classroom token system in modifying hyperactive behavior. *American Journal of Mental Deficiency, 80*, 266–276.

Cohen, M. (1978, May). *Survey of psychotropic drug treatment in residential facilities for the mentally retarded*. Paper presented at the annual meeting of the Council for Exceptional Children, Kansas City.

Cohen, M. N., & Sprague, R. L. (1977, March). *Survey of drug usage in two midwestern institutions for the retarded*. Paper presented at the Gatlinburg Conference on Research in Mental Retardation, Gatlinburg, TN.

Cooper, A. F., & Fowlie, H. C. (1973). Control of gross self-mutilation with lithium carbonate. *British Journal of Psychiatry, 122*, 370–371.

Davidson, P. W., Kleene, B. M., Carroll, M., & Rockowitz, R. J. (1983). Effects of naloxone on self-injurious behavior: A case study. *Applied Research in Mental Retardation, 4*, 1–4.

Davis, K. V. (1971). The effect of drugs on stereotyped and nonstereotyped operant behavior in retardates. *Psychopharmacology, 22*, 195–213.

Davis, K. V., Sprague, R. L., & Werry, J. S. (1969). Stereotyped behavior and activity level in severe retardates: The effect of drugs. *American Journal of Mental Deficiency, 73*, 721–727.

DiMascio, A., Soltys, J. J., & Shader, R. I. (1970). *Psychotropic drug side effects*. Baltimore: Williams & Wilkins.

Dostal, T., & Zvolsky, P. (1970). Antiaggressive effects of lithium salts in severely mentally retarded adolescents. *International Pharmacopsychiatry, 5*, 203–207.

Durand, V. M. (1982). A behavioral/pharmacological intervention for the treatment of severe self-injurious behavior. *Journal of Autism & Developmental Disorders, 12*, 243–251.

Eaton, L. F., & Menolascino, F. J. (1982). Psychiatric disorders of the mentally retarded: Types, problems, and challenges. *American Journal of Psychiatry, 139*, 1297–1303.

Ellenor, G. L. (1977). Reducing irrational antipsychotic polypharmacy prescribing. *Hospital Pharmacy, 12*, 369–376.

Ellenor, G. L., & Frisk, A. (1977). Pharmacist impact on drug use in an institution for the mentally retarded. *American Journal of Hospital Pharmacy, 34*, 604–608.

Englehardt, D. M., Polizos, P., & Waizer, J. (1975). CNS consequences of psychotropic drug withdrawal in autistic children: A follow-up report. *Psychopharmacology Bulletin, 11*, 6–11.

Epstein, M. H., Cullinan, D., & Gadow, K. D. (1985). *Prevalence of psychotropic drug use with learning disabled, emotionally disturbed, and mentally retarded children*. Unpublished manuscript, Northern Illinois

University, Department of Learning Development, and Special Education, DeKalb.

Eyman, R. K., & Call, T. (1977). Maladaptive behavior and community placement of mentally retarded persons. *American Journal of Mental Deficiency, 82*, 137–144.

Ferguson, D. G., Cullari, S., Davidson, N. A., & Breuning, S. E. (1982). Effects of data-based interdisciplinary medication reviews on the prevalence and pattern of neuroleptic drug use with institutionally mentally retarded persons. *Education and Training of the Mentally Retarded, 16*, 103–108.

Fielding, L. T., Murphy, R. J., Reagan, M. W., & Peterson, T. L. (1980). An assessment program to reduce drug use with the mentally retarded. *Hospital & Community Psychiatry, 31*, 771–773.

Fish, B. (1971). The "one child, one drug" myth of stimulants in hyperkinesis. *Archives of General Psychiatry, 25*, 193–203.

Fish, C. H., & Bowling, E. (1962). Effect of amphetamine on speech defects in the mentally retarded. *California Medicine, 94*, 109–111.

Freeman, R. D. (1966). Drug effects on learning in children: A selective review of the past thirty years. *Journal of Special Education, 1*, 17–43.

Freeman, R. D. (1970a). Use of psychoactive drugs for intellectually handicapped children. In N. R. Bernstein (Ed.), *Diminished people: Problems and care of the mentally retarded* (pp. 277–304). Boston: Little, Brown.

Freeman, R. D. (1970b). Psychopharmacology and the retarded child. In F. Menolascino (Ed.), *Psychiatric approaches to mental retardation*. New York: Basic Books.

Gadow, K. D. (1981). Drug therapy for hyperactivity: Treatment procedures in natural settings. In K. D. Gadow & J. Loney (Eds.), *Psychosocial aspects of drug treatment for hyperactivity* (pp. 13–76). Boulder, CO: Westview Press.

Gadow, K. D. (1982a). Problems with students on medication. *Exceptional Children, 49*, 20–27.

Gadow, K. D. (1982b). School involvement in pharmacotherapy for behavior disorders. *Journal of Special Education, 16*, 385–399.

Gadow, K. D. (1982c). School involvement in the treatment of seizure disorders. *Epilepsia, 23*, 215–224.

Gadow, K. D. (1983a). Pharmacotherapy for behavior disorders: Typical treatment practices. *Clinical Pediatrics, 22*, 48–53.

Gadow, K. D. (1983b). Educating teachers about pharmacotherapy. *Education and Training of the Mentally Retarded, 18*, 69–73.

Gadow, K. D. (1985). Prevalence and efficacy of stimulant drug use with mentally retarded children and youth. *Psychopharmacology Bulletin, 21*, 291–303.

Gadow, K. D., & Kalachnik, J. (1981). Prevalence and pattern of drug treatment for behavior and seizure disorders of TMR students. *American Journal of Mental Deficiency, 85*, 588–595.

Gittelman-Klein, R., Klein, D. F., Katz, S., Saraf, K., & Pollack, E. (1976). Comparative effects of methylphenidate and thioridazine in hyperkinetic children. *Archives of General Psychiatry, 33*, 1217–1231.

Glazer, W., & Moore, D. C. (1981). A tardive dyskinesia clinic in a mental health center. *Hospital & Community Psychiatry, 32*, 572–574.

Goetz, U., Grunberg, F., & Berkowitz, B. (1977). Lithium carbonate in the management of hyperactive aggressive behavior of the mentally retarded. *Comprehensive Psychiatry, 18,* 599–606.

Golden, G. S., & Greenhill, L. (1981). Tourette syndrome in mentally retarded children. *Mental Retardation,* 17–19.

Greenblatt, M., Levinson, D. J., & Shapiro, A. K. (1959). Placebo effect, social milieu, and the evaluation of psychiatric therapies. *Journal of Chronic Diseases, 9,* 327–333.

Greiner, T. (1958). Problems of methodology in research with drugs. *American Journal of Mental Deficiency, 64,* 346–352.

Gualtieri, C. T., Golden, R. N., & Fahs, J. J. (1983). New developments in pediatric psychopharmacology. *Developmental and Behavioral Pediatrics, 4,* 202–209.

Gualtieri, C. T., & Hawk, B. (1982). Antidepressant and antimanic drugs. In S. E. Breuning & A. D. Poling (Eds.), *Drugs and mental retardation* (pp. 215–234). Springfield, IL: Charles C Thomas.

Gualtieri, C. T., Quade, D., Hicks, R. E., Mayo, J. P., & Schroeder, S. R. (1984). Tardive dyskinesia and other clinical consequences of neuroleptic treatment in children and adolescents. *American Journal of Psychiatry, 141,* 20–23.

Guy, W. (Ed.). (1976). *ECDEU assessment manual for psychopharmacology.* Washington, DC: U.S. Government Printing Office.

Hartlage, L. C. (1965). Effects of chlorpromazine on learning. *Psychological Bulletin, 64,* 235–245.

Heuyer, G., Gerard, G., & Galibert, J. (1953). Traitement de l'excitation psychometrics chez l'enfant pare (le 4560 r.p.). *Archives Francaises de Pediatrie, 9,* 691.

Hill, B. K., Balow, E. A., & Bruininks, R. H. (1983). *A national study of prescribed drugs in institutions and community residential facilities for mentally retarded people* (Brief No. 20). Minneapolis: University of Minnesota, Department of Educational Psychology.

Hill, B. K., Lakin, K. C., & Bruininks, R. H. (1986). Trends in residential services for mentally retarded people: 1977–1982. *Journal for the Association for Persons with Severe Handicaps.*

Horten, I. (1982). A new caring model reduces need for drug therapy for intellectually handicapped persons. *Australia & New Zealand Journal of Developmental Disabilities, 8,* 219–225.

Inoue, F. (1982). A clinical pharmacy service to reduce psychotropic medication use in an institution for mentally handicapped persons. *Mental Retardation, 20,* 70–74.

Intagliata, J., & Rinck, C. (1985). Psychoactive drug use in public and community residential facilities for mentally retarded persons. *Psychopharmacology Bulletin, 21,* 268–278.

James, D. H. (1983). Monitoring drugs in hospitals for the mentally handicapped. *British Journal of Psychiatry, 142,* 163–165.

Kalachnik, J. E. (1985). Applied aspects of tardive dyskinesia monitoring: Over, under, sideways, down; backward, forward, square, and round. In K. D. Gadow (Ed.), *Advances in learning and behavioral disabilities* (Vol. 4, pp. 133–180). Greenwich, CT: JAI Press.

Kalachnik, J. E., Larum, J. G., & Swanson, A. (1983a). A tardive dyskinesia monitoring policy for applied facilities. *Psychopharmacology Bulletin, 19,* 277–282.

Kalachnik, J. E., Miller, R. F., Jamison, A. G., & Harder, S. R. (1983b). Results of a system to monitor effects of psychotropic medication in an applied setting. *Psychopharmacology Bulletin, 19,* 12–15.

Kalachnik, J. E., Young, R. C., & Offerman, D. (1984). A tardive dyskinesia evaluation and diagnosis form for applied facilities. *Psychopharmacology Bulletin, 20,* 303-308.

Kamm, I., & Mandel, A. (1967). Thioridazine in the treatment of behavior disorders in epileptics. *Diseases in the Nervous System, 28,* 46–48.

Katz, S., Saraf, K., Gittelman-Klein, R., & Klein, D. F. (1975). Clinical pharmacological management of hyperkinetic children. *International Journal of Mental Health, 4,* 157–181.

Kirman, B. (1975). Drug therapy in mental handicap. *British Journal of Psychiatry, 127,* 545–549.

Klebanoff, L. B., DiMascio, A., & Lowe, L. M. (1973). *Report on a survey of the use of psychopharmacological agents in Massachusetts state residential facilities for the mentally retarded.* Unpublished manuscript.

Klein, D. F., & Davis, J. M. (1969). *Diagnosis and drug treatment of psychiatric disorders.* Baltimore: Williams & Wilkins.

Klein, D. F., Gittelman, R., Quitkin, F., & Rifkin, A. (1980). *Diagnosis and drug treatment of psychiatric disorders: Adults and children* (2nd ed.). Baltimore: Williams & Wilkins.

Kobayashi, R. (1977). Drug therapy of tardive dyskinesia. *New England Journal of Medicine, 296,* 257–260.

LaMendola, W., Zaharia, E., & Carver, M. (1980). Reducing psychotropic drug use in an institution for the retarded. *Hospital & Community Psychiatry, 31,* 271–272.

Laufer, M. W., Denhoff, E., & Riverside, R. I. (1957). Hyperactive behavior syndrome in children. *Journal of Pediatrics, 50,* 463–474.

Levy, J. M., Jones, B. E., & Croley, H. T. (1957). Effects of methylphenidate (Ritalin) on drug-induced drowsiness in mentally retarded patients. *American Journal of Mental Deficiency, 62,* 284–287.

Lipman, R. S., DiMascio, A., Reatig, N., & Kirson, T. (1978). Psychotropic drugs and mentally retarded children. In M. A. Lipton, A. DiMascio, & K. F. Killam (Eds.), *Psychopharmacology: A generation of progress* (pp. 1437–1449). New York: Raven Press.

Lipman, R. S. (1970). The use of psychopharmacological agents in residential facilities for the retarded. In F. J. Menolascino (Ed.), *Psychiatric approaches to mental retardation* (pp. 387–398). New York: Basic Books.

Livingston, S. (1972). *Comprehensive management of epilepsy in infancy, childhood and adolescence.* Springfield, IL: Charles C Thomas.

Livingston, S. (1978). Medical treatment of epilepsy: Part II. *Southern Medical Journal, 71,* 432–447.

Martin, J. E., & Agran, M. (1985). Psychotropic and anticonvulsant drug use by mentally retarded adults across community residential and vocational placements. *Applied Research in Mental Retardation, 6,* 33–49.

McAndrew, J. B., Case, Q., & Treffert, D. A. (1972). Effects of prolonged phenothiazine intake on psychotic and other hospitalized children. *Journal of Autism and Childhood Schizophrenia, 2,* 75-91.

McConnell, T. R., Cromwell, R. L., Bialer, I., & Son, C. D. (1964). Studies in activity level: VII. Effects of amphetamine drug administration on the activity level of retarded children. *American Journal of Mental Deficiency, 68*, 647–651.

Menolascino, F. J., Ruedrich, S. L., Golden, C. J., & Wilson, T. E. (1985). Diagnosis and pharmacotherapy of schizophrenia in the retarded. *Psychopharmacology Bulletin, 21*, 316–322.

Micev, V., & Lynch, D. M. (1974). Effect of lithium on disturbed severely mentally retarded patients. *British Journal of Psychiatry, 125*, 110.

Millichap, J. G. (1969). Management of hyperkinetic behavior in children with epilepsy. *Modern Treatment, 6*, 1233–1246.

Molitch, M., & Eccles, J. P. (1937). Effect of benzedrine sulfate on the intelligence scores of children. *American Journal of Psychiatry, 94*, 587–590.

Molitch, M., & Sullivan, J. P. (1937). Effect of benzedrine sulfate on children taking New Stanford Achievement Test. *American Journal of Orthopsychiatry, 7*, 519–522.

Moskowitz, H. (1941). Benzedrine therapy for the mentally handicapped. *American Journal of Mental Deficiency, 45*, 540–543.

Naylor, G. J., Donald, J. M., LePoidevin, D., & Reid, A. H. (1974). A double-blind trial of long-term lithium therapy in mental defectives. *British Journal of Psychiatry, 124*, 52–57.

New York State Association for Retarded Children, Inc. v. Nelson Rockefeller, No. 72 356, 72 357 (E.D. New York, 1975).

O'Neill, B. P., Ladon, B., Harris, L. M., Riley, H. L., & Dreifuss, F. E. (1977). A comprehensive, interdisciplinary approach to the care of the institutionalized person with epilepsy. *Epilepsia, 18*, 243–250.

Ounsted, C. (1955). The hyperkinetic syndrome in epileptic children. *Lancet, 2*, 303–311.

Paulson, G. W., Rizvi, C. A., & Crane, G. E. (1975). Tardive dyskinesia as a possible sequel of long-term therapy with phenothiazines. *Clinical Pediatrics, 14*, 953–955.

Payne, D., Johnson, R. C., & Abelson, R. B. (1969). *Comprehensive description of institutionalized retardates in Western United States*. Boulder, CO: Western Interstate Commission for Higher Education.

Polizos, P., Engelhardt, D. M., Hoffman, S. P., & Waizer, J. (1973). Neurological consequences of psychotic drug withdrawal in schizophrenic children. *Journal of Autism and Childhood Schizophrenia, 3*, 247–253.

Pulman, R. M., Pook, R. B., & Singh, N. N. (1979). Prevalence of drug therapy for institutionalized mentally retarded children. *Australian Journal of Mental Retardation, 5*, 212–214.

Radinsky, A. M. (1984). *A descriptive study of psychotropic and antiepileptic medication use with mentally retarded persons in three residential environments*. Unpublished doctoral dissertation, University of Pittsburgh.

Rivinus, T. M., & Harmatz, J. S. (1979). Diagnosis and lithium treatment of affective disorder in the retarded: Five case studies. *American Journal of Psychiatry, 136*, 551–554.

Romanczyk, R. G. (1986). Self-injurious behavior: Conceptualization, assessment, and treatment. In K. D. Gadow (Ed.), *Advances in learning and behavioral disabilities* (Vol. 5). Greenwich, CT: JAI Press.

Rutter, M. L. (1971). Psychiatry. In J. Wortis (Ed.), *Mental retardation: An annual review* (Vol 3, pp. 186–221). Orlando, FL: Grune & Stratton.

Rutter, M., Tizard, J., & Whitmore, K. (Eds.). (1970). *Education, health, and behavior*. London: Longmans.

Sandman, C. A., Datta, P. C., Barron, J., Hoehler, F. K., Williams, C., & Swanson, J. M. (1983). Naloxone attenuates self-abusive behavior in developmentally disabled clients. *Applied Research in Mental Retardation, 4*, 5–11.

Schroeder, S. R., Bickel, W. K., & Richmond, G. (1986). Primary and secondary prevention of self-injurious behaviors: A life-long problem. In K. D. Gadow (Ed.), *Advances in learning and behavioral disabilities* (Vol. 5). Greenwich, CT: JAI Press.

Schroeder, S. R., & Gualtieri, C. T. (1985). Behavioral interactions induced by chronic neuroleptic therapy in persons with mental retardation. *Psychopharmacology Bulletin, 21*, 310–315.

Schroeder, S. R., Schroeder, C. S., Smith, B., & Dalldorf, J. (1978). Prevalence of self-injurious behaviors in a large state facility for the retarded: A three-year follow-up study. *Journal of Autism and Childhood Schizophrenia, 8*, 261–269.

Sewell, J., & Werry, J. S. (1976). Some studies in an institution for the mentally retarded. *New Zealand Medical Journal, 84*, 317–319.

Singh, N. N., & Aman, M. G. (1981). Effects of thioridazine dosage on the behavior of severely mentally retarded persons. *American Journal of Mental Deficiency, 85*, 580–587.

Singh, N. N., & Millichamp, C. J. (1985). Pharmacological treatment of self-injurious behavior in mentally retarded persons. *Journal of Autism and Developmental Disorders, 15*, 257–267.

Spencer, D. A. (1970). Ronyl (pemoline) in overactive mentally subnormal children. *British Journal of Psychiatry, 117*, 239–240.

Sprague, R. L. (1977a). Overview of psychopharmacology for the retarded in the United States. In P. Mittler (Ed.), *Research to practice in mental retardation* (Vol. 3, pp. 199–202). Baltimore: University Park Press.

Sprague, R. L. (1977b). Psychopharmacotherapy in children. In M. F. McMillan & S. Henao (Eds.), *Child psychiatry: Treatment and research* (pp. 130–149). New York: Brunner/Mazel.

Sprague, R. L. (1978). Principles of clinic drug trials. In J. S. Werry (Ed.), *Pediatric psychopharmacology: The use of behavior modifying drugs in children* (pp. 109–135). New York: Brunner/Mazel.

Sprague, R. L. (1982). Litigation, legislation, and regulations. In S. E. Breuning & A. D. Poling (Eds.), *Drugs and mental retardation* (pp. 377–414). Springfield, IL: Charles C Thomas.

Sprague, R. L., Barnes, K. R., & Werry, J. S. (1970). Methylphenidate and thioridazine: Learning, reaction time, activity, and classroom behavior in emotionally disturbed children. *American Journal of Orthopsychiatry, 40*, 615–628.

Sprague, R. L., Kalachnik, J. E., Breuning, S. E., Davis, V. J., Ullmann, R. K., Cullari, S., Davidson, N. A., Ferguson, D. G., Anderson, B., & Hoffer, B. S. (1984a). The Dyskinesia Identification System-Coldwater (DIS-Co): A tardive dyskinesia rating scale for the developmentally disabled. *Psychopharmacology Bulletin, 20*, 328–338.

Sprague, R. L., Kalachnik, J. E., & White, D. M. (1985). *Dyskinesia Identification System: Condensed User Scale (DISCUS)*. University of Illinois, Institute for Child Behavior and Development, 51 Gerty Drive, Champaign, IL 61820.

Sprague, R. L., & Werry, J. S. (1971). Methodology of psychopharmacological studies with the retarded. In N. R. Ellis (Ed.), *International review of research in mental retardation* (Vol. 5, pp. 147–219). Orlando, FL: Academic Press.

Sprague, R. L., & Werry, J. S. (1974). Psychotropic drugs and handicapped children. In L. Mann & D. A. Sabatino (Eds.), *The second review of special education* (pp. 1–50). Philadelphia: JSE Press.

Sprague, R. L., White, D. M., Ullmann, R., & Kalachnik, J. E. (1984b). Methods for selecting items in a tardive dyskinesia rating scale. *Psychopharmacology Bulletin, 20*, 339–345.

Triantafillou, M. (1972). Pemoline in overactive mentally handicapped children. *British Journal of Psychiatry, 121*, 577.

Tu, J. B. (1979). A survey of psychotropic medication in mental retardation facilities. *Journal of Clinical Psychiatry, 40*, 125–128.

U.S. Department of Education. (1985). *Seventh Annual Report to Congress on the Implementation of P.L. 94-142: The Education for All Handicapped Childrens Act*. Washington, DC: Author.

Varley, C. K. (1984). Schizophreniform psychoses in mentally retarded adolescent girls following sexual assault. *American Journal of Psychiatry, 141*, 593–595.

Varley, C. K., & Trupin, E. W. (1982). Double-blind administration of methylphenidate to mentally retarded children with Attention Deficit Disorder: A preliminary study. *American Journal of Mental Deficiency, 86*, 560–566.

Werry, J. S., & Aman, M. G. (1975). Methylphenidate and haloperidol in children. *Archives of General Psychiatry, 32*, 790–795.

Whall, A. L., Engle, V., Edwards, A., Bobel, L., & Haberland, C. (1983). Development of a screening program for tardive dyskinesia: Feasibility issues. *Nursing Research, 32*, 151–156.

Williams, D. T., Mehl, R., & Yudofsky, S. (1982). The effect of propranolol on uncontrolled rage outbursts in children and adolescents with organic brain dysfunction. *Journal of the American Academy of Child Psychiatry, 21*, 129–135.

Winsberg, B. G., & Yepes, L. E. (1978). Antipsychotics. In J. S. Werry (Ed.), *Pediatric psychopharmacology: The use of behavior modifying drugs in children* (pp. 234–273). New York: Brunner/Mazel.

Winsberg, B. G., Yepes, L. E., & Bialer, I. (1976). Pharmacologic management of children with hyperactive/aggressive/inattentive behavior disorders. *Clinical Pediatrics, 15*, 471–477.

Wyatt v. Stickney. 344F. Supp. 387 (1972).

Wysocki, T., Fuqua, W., Davis, V. J., & Breuning, S. E. (1981). Effects of thioridazine (Mellaril) on titrating delayed matching-to-sample performance of mentally retarded adults. *American Journal of Mental Deficiency, 85*, 539–547.

Zimmerman, F. T., & Burgemeister, B. B. (1958). Action of methyl-phenidylacetate (Ritalin) and reserpine in behavior disorders in children and adults. *American Journal of Psychiatry, 115*, 323–328.

Zimmerman, R. L., & Heistad, G. T. (1982). Studies of the long term efficacy of antipsychotic drugs in controlling the behavior of institutionalized retardates. *Journal of the American Academy of Child Psychiatry, 21*, 136–143.

Chapter 5

Early Childhood

The use of psychotropic medication, at least on a long-term basis, with children under 6 years of age is a sensitive topic for most caregivers. We are probably most concerned about the possibility that an immature and rapidly developing body may be at greater risk for adverse drug reactions than either older children or adults. Moreover, it is often difficult to accept the fact that a child so young needs to take medication on a regular basis. It is important to know, however, that in spite of these concerns, psychotropic drugs are often prescribed for young children and that they are generally safe and effective. Because early childhood is recognized as a very special period of development for many reasons, a separate discussion of the use of medication with young children for the treatment of behavior disorders (primarily hyperactivity) is presented here. Before addressing this topic, it is probably useful to have a basic understanding of some of the issues associated with pharmacotherapy during early childhood and a general idea of the kinds of drugs that are most commonly prescribed.

The symptoms of many childhood behavior disorders first appear during the preschool years, but in most cases drug therapy is not initiated until the child goes to school. Nevertheless, there are always some preschool-aged children who are going to be given psychotropic medication. Many hyperactive elementary school children who participated in research studies and were treated with stimulant drugs were found to have been hyperactive at a very early age (e.g., Conners et al., 1972; Schain & Reynard, 1975; Sleator et al., 1982). For example, in one stimulant drug study with 6 to 12 year olds, Conners et al. (1972) found that two thirds of the children had been hyperactive since the age of 2 years. Numerous studies have clearly shown that hyperactivity is a relatively common behavior disorder in preschool-aged children (see Campbell, 1985a, and Ross & Ross, 1982, for reviews), and in many cases, severe problems during early childhood continue into the elementary school years (Campbell, 1985b). Given the prevalence of behavior disorders and their responsiveness to drug therapy, it is fair to say that a relatively large number of young children receive psychotropic medication.

Unquestionably the most significant cultural event to draw attention to the needs of young handicapped children has been the development of public education programs, generally referred to as early childhood special education (ECSE). In the United States, approximately three fourths of all states have some form of legislation that provides for a free public school education for preschool-aged handicapped children. Of course, there have always been a number of private nonprofit organizations such as the Association to Help Retarded Citizens (AHRC), United Cerebral Palsy, and so forth, who have traditionally provided such services. While it is certainly true that not all or even most children who take psychotropic medication are enrolled in some type of ECSE, many of the children who do receive these services are on medication. The importance of this fact lies in an appreciation of the potential interaction of these two therapies. In other words, because early childhood intervention programs can have marked effects on later academic performance and social adjustment (Darlington et al., 1980; Hunt, 1975; see also Odom & Fewell, 1983), medication could have a big impact on the effectiveness of ECSE. If the drug increases the child's responsiveness to instruction, the benefits from education could be even greater than if medication were not administered. Conversely, if pharmacotherapy dulls the child's awareness or interferes with adaptive behavior, the results could be most counterproductive. The sad fact is that for some youngsters, it will be a no-win situation because the underlying disorder is so severe.

This is a serious consideration because large numbers of preschool-aged children are registered for these and related services. Because United States federal law (Public Law 94-142) requires individual states to report on a regular basis the number of children receiving special education, it is now possible to generate national statistics (U.S. Department of Education, 1985) on the number of children enrolled in ECSE programs (see Table 5–1). These data are

Table 5-1. Number of Children Receiving Early Childhood Special Education

Deaf	1,740
Deaf-blind	139
Emotionally disturbed	5,860
Hard of hearing	3,634
Learning disabled	19,214
Mentally retarded	19,052
Multiply handicapped	12,500
Other health impaired	4,015
Orthopedically handicapped	7,031
Speech-language impaired	168,176
Visually impaired	1,736
Total	243,097

Note: The children represented in these figures are from the December 1, 1983, Public Law 94-142 count and do *not* include children under the age of 6 reported in the Public Law 89-313 count.

limited, however, because they exclude many handicapped children who attend private schools, programs funded by nonprofit agencies, Head Start, daycare centers, public institutions, and so forth. As is evident from Table 5-1, many of these youngsters are labeled "speech and language impaired." This label is not, however, very descriptive of their social behavior or cognitive functioning. Many programs have elected to use this term because (a) they use a noncategorical approach and "speech and language impaired" is a fairly benign label, (b) diagnostic constructs in this age group are poorly defined, and (c) there is a reluctance to identify a child as emotionally disturbed or mentally retarded at such a young age unless the disability is particularly severe for fear that it may become a self-fulfilling prophecy.

Perhaps one of the biggest problems in this area from a clinical management perspective is the limited amount of drug research with young children. There are many reasons for this; certainly one of the most compelling in the case of psychotropic medication is that few scientists are really equipped to study this age group. Pharmacotherapy is usually reserved for only severe cases, and unless one had access to a special clinic, it would probably be difficult to locate enough children to study. Moreover, before a scientist can conduct a drug research study, he or she has to go through a special review process where a committee of other scientists (often called an Institutional Review Board or IRB for short) evaluates the research proposal. With a sensitive topic such as psychotropic medication with preschoolers, or even more controversial infants and toddlers, it would be very difficult to obtain approval. This has led to a situation where many physicians use these drugs with young children and occasionally describe their experiences in medical journals, but little or no systematic research is ever conducted.

One consequence of all this has been the creation of *therapeutic orphans*, i.e., children for whom drugs determined to be safe and effective in older children and adults are not recommended because little is known about their use in the pediatric age range (Shirkey, 1972). In other words, the package insert for many psychotropic drugs states that the product is not recommended for children under 12, 6, or 3 years of age. This has resulted in two problems. The most serious is that the quasi-legal status of the package insert possibly prevents or discourages the use of needed and effective therapeutic agents (Klein, 1974; Shirkey, 1971). Also, because many parents, teachers, and other care providers do have access to the *Physicians' Desk Reference*, this warning may prompt unnecessary concern because the package insert really does not provide any information on the nature of the warning, the findings from current research, or treatment practices.

As previously mentioned, the thought of giving medication to a young child for an extended period of time is a sensitive topic for many caregivers. While parents certainly prefer not to use long-term drug therapy, they are often left with few alternatives, and in many instances, the failure to administer medication can have serious consequences. The emotional tone of this situation can be best captured in their own words:

> A number of the parents at one time or another during the interview expressed guilt about giving drugs to their child. Some typical comments were, "I don't want him on medication, but right now it means my sanity or his," or "The doctor says I can increase the dose to 40 mg a day but I don't want to hurt him." The mother of one child receiving a large dose of Ritalin said, "Every time I give him one [pill], I think about it [long-term effects]. It's sort of like taking a butterfly that's wild and free and caging it. If we could live on a farm where he could run it would be different, but I guess in our society he has to learn to conform and accept learning that kind of thing." (Gadow, 1977, pp. 42–43).

PREVALENCE OF MEDICATION USE

It is very difficult to obtain information on the use of medication with young children. Because more are not enrolled in public schools, there is no efficient way to obtain medication data unless one went from door to door, which would be impractical for low prevalence disabilities. Therefore, most of what we do know about drug use with preschool-aged children has been reported in two studies of several thousand children enrolled in ECSE programs in the United States (Gadow, 1975, 1977). Briefly, these programs were noncategorical; that is, they served children with all kinds of handicaps ranging from mild to severe. Most of the youngsters were between 3 and 5 years old. The first study found that 12½% of the children received psychotropic or antiepileptic medication at some time during the school year, while the rate for the second study was 14%. It is possible to make a rough estimate of the total number of children in ECSE programs nationally who are on medication by simply multiplying the total in Table 5–1 by 14%, which is approximately 34,000. This estimate, of course, excludes all the other 3 to 5 year olds who are either at home or in other types of early childhood programs and most children under the age of 3 years.

The most common reasons for which medication was prescribed were as follows: Approximately 6¾% were on medication for a behavior disorder, usually hyperactivity, and about 5½% were being treated for seizures. An additional 1% were taking medication for both a behavior and a seizure disorder. As for the rest of the children on medication, a few were receiving treatment for enuresis, spasticity, sleep problems, and nervousness (anxiety). The ratio of boys to girls in ECSE programs was approximately 2:1, and not surprisingly, pharmacotherapy for behavior disorders was more common for boys than girls (see Figure 5–1).

As noted, the most common behavior disorder for which psychotropic medication is prescribed is hyperactivity. It is incorrect, however, to assume that all children with extremely high activity levels are hyperactive in a diagnostic sense. As was discussed in Chapter 2 (Hyperactivity) and again in Chapter 4 (Mental Retardation), the term *hyperactivity* is used to refer to both a particular disorder and a behavioral characteristic. In other words, while some children are diagnosed as having hyperactivity, other children who show excessive motor restlessness may really suffer from a different type of disorder. The important point is that not all children who appear to be hyperactive respond to the same type of medication. A diagnosis of hyperactivity in young children is more difficult to make than it is in older children because (a) normal levels of the behavioral symptoms of hyperactivity are relatively high to begin with in preschoolers, (b) young children are highly reactive to environmental stressors that may induce these symptoms, (c) there is considerable variability in caregiver perceptions of what is considered normal behavior in young children, (d) there are few normative data for diagnostic instruments in this age group, and (e) if the child

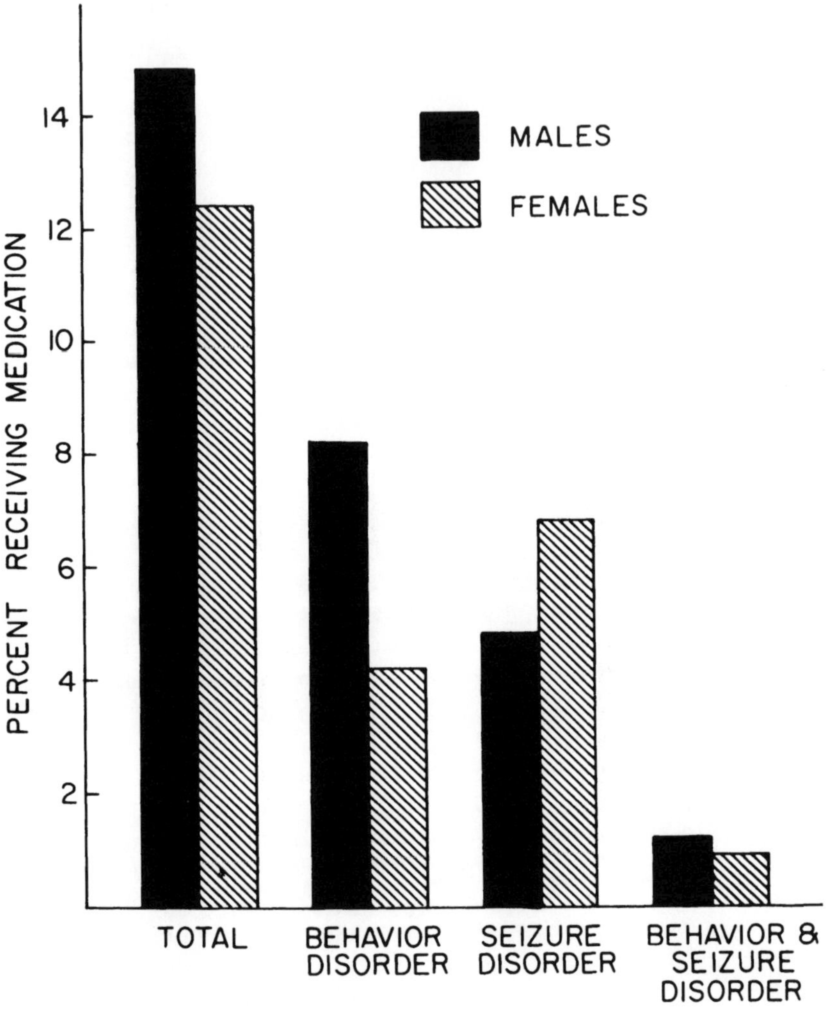

Figure 5–1. Prevalence of drug therapy by sex. *Note:* From *Psychotropic and Antiepileptic Drug Treatment in Early Childhood Special Education* (p. 17) by K. D. Gadow, 1977, Institute for Child Behavior and Development, University of Illinois at Urbana-Champaign. (ERIC Document Reproduction Service No. 162 494)

is not enrolled in some type of school program, it is very difficult to corroborate parental perceptions of deviant behavior (see Campbell, 1985a, for a discussion of these diagnostic difficulties).

As is evident from Table 5–2, a variety of different drugs are prescribed for behavior disorders in young children (Gadow, 1977).

Table 5-2. Drugs Used for the Management of Behavior Disorders

Generic name	Trade name	BD (N = 175)[a]	BD-SD (N = 24)[a]
Stimulants		(130)	(14)
Methylphenidate	Ritalin	112	11
Dextroamphetamine	Dexedrine	11	2
Pemoline	Cylert	5	1
Deanol	Deaner	1	0
Amphetamine	Benzedrine	1	0
Neuroleptics		(23)	(6)
Thioridazine	Mellaril	19	4
Chlorpromazine	Thorazine	2	1
Haloperidol	Haldol	1	0
Piperacetazine	Quide	1	0
Trifluoperazine	Stelazine	0	1
Antianxiety Agents		(9)	(1)
Diazepam	Valium	4	1
Hydroxyzine	Atarax, Vistaril	5	0
Antidepressants		(7)	(3)
Imipramine	Tofranil	6	3
Nortriptyline	Aventyl	1	0
Hypnotics-Sedatives		(7)	(1)
Phenobarbital		5	1
Mephobarbital	Mebaral	1	0
Sodium butabarital	Butisol	1	0
Antiepileptics		(22)	(0)
Phenytoin	Dilantin	20	0
Primidone	Mysoline	2	0
Miscellaneous		(8)	(2)
Diphenhydramine	Benadryl	5	2
Unknown		3	0
Total[b]		206	27

[a]BD = on medication for behavior disorder; BD-SD = on medication for both behavior and seizure disorders.

[b]Totals are inflated because some children received more than one medication during the school year.

Note: From *Psychotropic and Antiepileptic Drug Treatment in Early Childhood Education* (p. 21, 24), by K. D. Gadow, 1977, Institute for Child Behavior and Development, University of Illinois at Urbana-Champaign. (ERIC Document Reproduction Services No. ED 162 494)

Nevertheless, two major drug classes, the stimulants and the neuroleptics, account for most of the medication. The most common reasons for prescribing medication were hyperactivity, behavior problems, and aggressiveness.

Although research on hyperactivity in infants is scant, marked irritability, colic, and poor sleep habits appear to be the most important symptoms (Nichamin, 1972; Weiss, 1975; Werry et al., 1964).

As toddlers and young children, their behavioral peculiarities become more troublesome, and they begin to exhibit the classic symptoms of hyperactivity. When asked about their hyperactive child (Schleifer et al., 1975; Weiss, 1975), parents make comments such as these: "he never walked but ran," "climbed out of his crib," "wore down the crib mattress by jumping up and down," "is always on the go," "cannot stick to anything for more than a few minutes," "does not listen," and "can't play alone." Their activity gets them into a lot of mischief, which includes an increased risk of accidental poisoning (Stewart et al., 1970). Anecdotes about these children often focus on their impulsivity.

> "Nothing helps, neither praise nor punishment: we can spank him, and he will cry for a minute, but then go on to do the very same thing again." A rather striking example of the failure to respond to negative reinforcement was a little boy who burned himself on a hot iron. He was told not to touch the iron ever again and understood the warning; but the very next day this bright four-year-old burned himself again. (Weiss, 1975, p. 217).

In preschool-aged children, the symptoms of hyperactivity can be extremely troublesome for caregivers. One aspect of this behavior that is most challenging are the rapid shifts of involvement from one activity to another in a relatively short period of time. It is difficult to capture in words what it is like to be around such a child, but the following observation may help. Ounsted (1955) described the behavior of a 5-year-old hyperactive boy in a playroom as follows:

> Runs to couch; climbs via chair; puts head on pillow; says: "I'm in bed"; laughs; reaches out to blanket (11 sec.).
>
> Rolls off couch (unhurt); darts to 4 spatulas on floor arranged in a square; picks up each in turn, dropping each immediately; breaks one spatula (8 sec.).
>
> Runs to door; opens; shuts; opens; shuts; opens and peeps out; shuts; turns key; withdraws key; reinserts key; half opens door (10 sec.).
>
> Runs to table; picks up book; leafs rapidly through (no pauses); leafs through again and laughs; tears out page; looks at page; says "it's a Robin Redbreast on a shovel"; starts to put page back into book (12 sec.). (p. 305)

STIMULANTS: EFFICACY OF TREATMENT

Clinicians have described their experiences treating hyperactive infants (Denhoff, 1973; Oettinger, 1973; Nichamin, 1972; Weinberg & Brumback, 1976), toddlers (Denhoff, 1973; Husain et al., 1980; Nichamin, 1972; Renshaw, 1974), and preschoolers (numerous reports) with stimulant medication, and there are four published group studies of medication with hyperactive children under 6 years old (Cohen et al., 1981; Conners, 1975; Schleifer et al., 1975; Zara, 1973). There are also at least two group studies with seriously disturbed children (Campbell et al., 1972; Fish, 1971). Nevertheless, Dexedrine (dextroamphetamine) and Benzedrine (amphetamine sulfate) are not approved for children under 3 years and Ritalin (methylphenidate) and Cylert (pemoline) are not approved by the Food and Drug Administration (FDA) in the United States for children under 6 years of age. This is interesting because approximately 5% of all the children enrolled in ECSE were receiving Ritalin, and several had begun treatment before they were 3 years old (Gadow, 1977). To keep this situation in perspective, it must be realized that preschool-aged children have always participated in stimulant drug research. A careful reading of the literature will reveal the fact that a number of early studies of Benzedrine (Bender & Cottington, 1942), Dexedrine (Ginn & Hohman, 1953; Laufer et al., 1957; Ounsted, 1955); and Ritalin (Zimmerman & Burgemeister, 1958a, 1958b) included at least a few preschool-aged children in their subject samples. Moreover, it is not unusual for physicians to use a newly released medication with young children. For example, when Cylert was first approved it was picked up immediately in an ECSE medication survey. It was generally prescribed to preschoolers who failed to respond to other types of medication (Gadow, 1977).

The whole situation regarding the package insert and therapeutic orphans is unfortunate. As previously noted, parents, teachers, and other lay people gain access to the information in the package insert by consulting the *Physicians' Desk Reference* or some other drug reference book and get a distorted or incomplete view of the situation. Moreover, physicians are not excluded from this process. For example, an advertisement for Mellaril (thioridazine) in the October 17, 1980, issue of *Psychiatric News* reads, "Suitable for use in children aged 2 or over (methylphenidate [Ritalin] not to be used in those under 6; amphetamines [Dexedrine, Benzedrine] not in those under 3)" (p. 13). In other words, the drug company was encouraging the use of neuroleptic drugs with hyperactive preschoolers instead of stimulant medication. It must be emphasized that regardless of the package insert warnings, few scientists or clinicians treating hyperactivity would recommend neuroleptics as the drugs of first choice. It is true, nevertheless, that for some youngsters, neuroleptics will be the most effective.

Stimulant medication appears to affect the behavior of young hyperactive children in much the same way as older children, with three notable exceptions. One, experimental drug studies do not always find the same degree of therapeutic benefit or improvement in as many different areas with the younger children (Conners, 1975; Schleifer et al., 1975). Two, although stimulant drug effects are clearly present, they appear to be "more variable and unpredictable than in similar treatment of older children" (Conners, 1975, p. 74). Three, younger children *may* be particularly sensitive to the effects of overmedication. Schleifer et al. (1975), for example, noted that while mothers perceived their hyperactive preschoolers as improved on medication, they also observed the following:

> Clinical observations indicated that methylphenidate very often had a negative effect on the child's mood and also on his relationship with peers, causing less social behavior and interaction. These almost always appeared and were reported as unwanted side effects of the drug, and included sadness, irritability, excessive hugging and clinging, and increased solitary play, as well as the more usual side effects of poor appetite and difficulty getting to sleep, and were determinate factors in the psychiatrist and the mothers deciding that all but three of the 28 children discontinue medication after the experiment ended. (p. 49)

Interestingly, some of these same children who exhibited social withdrawal after taking medication when younger did not have this reaction to Ritalin when they were older (Weiss, 1980).

Because the effects of stimulant drugs on child behavior are described in detail in Chapter 2 (Hyperactivity), they are not reviewed here. However, a few comments from parents (Gadow, 1977) may provide a more qualitative insight into therapeutic response. For example, one stated, "He's less impulsive, can sit still now; his attention span is increased. He's a happier child now, seems more at peace with himself." Comments about activity level were frequent (e.g., "still active but channels it better" and "slowed down enough to read to"). Parents also reported that their child was more manageable, saying, "It (Ritalin) calms him down to where you can get through to him" or "can reason with him." Also reported were changes in aggressive behavior, "He was mean (before Ritalin treatment) but now I don't have to watch him because he doesn't hurt others" and improvement in sleep cycle, "Without it (Ritalin) he is up at 5:00 am and goes to bed at midnight."

Schedule

Although it has been shown that many hyperactive children can get by on one morning dose of medication (Safer & Allen, 1973; Sleator & von Neumann, 1974; Sprague et al., 1974), it is not unusual for children to take medication two or more times per day. As can be seen in Figure 5–2, most young hyperactive children receive stimulants in divided dosages (Gadow, 1977). In fact, many are even given stimulant medication in the evening to help them go to sleep. This sounds somewhat paradoxical because we expect stimulants to keep us awake and even cause insomnia. Nevertheless, a recent study has confirmed the effectiveness of this practice (Chatoor et al., 1983). Stimulants are not the only drugs, of course, that may be given before bedtime. Others include the antianxiety agents (e.g., Atarax, Vistaril, Valium) and hypnotics such as chloral hydrate. The fact that 42% of the children receiving medication for a behavior disorder required an evening dose suggests that sleep difficulties (i.e., getting the child to go to bed) are a frequent problem in this age group.

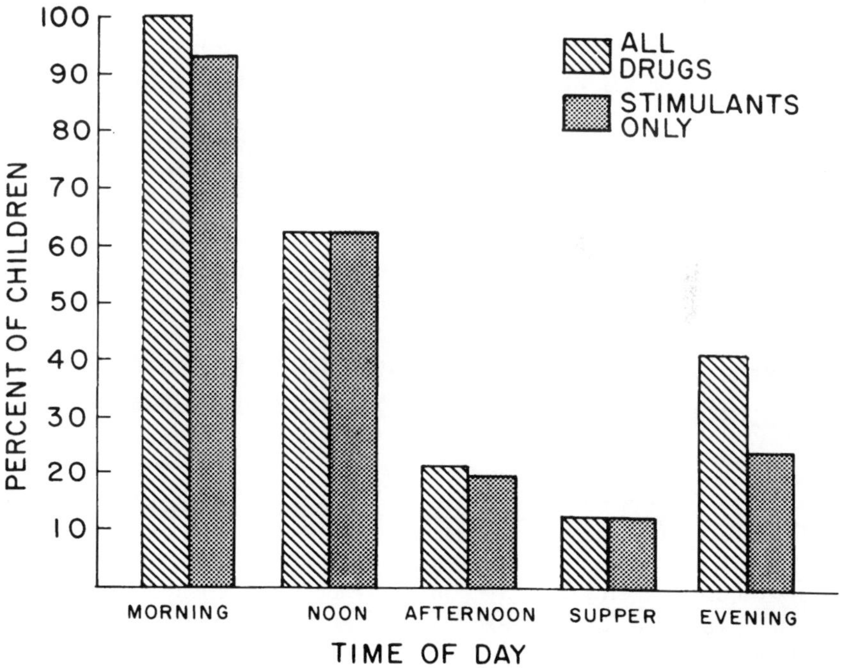

Figure 5–2. Time of day drugs administered to hyperactive children enrolled in ECSE programs. *Note:* From *Psychotropic and Antiepileptic Drug Treatment in Early Childhood Special Education* (pp. 34, 36) by K. D. Gadow, 1977, Institute for Child Behavior and Development, University of Illinois at Urbana-Champaign. (ERIC Document Reproduction Service No. 162 494)

Dosage

The recommended stimulant drug dosages for infants, toddlers, and preschoolers are presented in Table 5–3. These figures are based upon reports from several sources: Ritalin (Cohen et al., 1981; Conners, 1975; Hasser et al., 1978; Schleifer et al., 1975), Dexedrine (Denhoff, 1973; Hasser et al., 1978, Nichamin, 1972; Oetinger, 1973), Cylert (Husain et al., 1980), and Benzedrine (Hasser et al., 1978). Because Dexedrine is available in liquid form, it may be easier to administer to young children. One survey of drug use with 3 to 5 year olds found that the median *daily* dose of Ritalin was 15 mg (range: 5 to 45 mg); the figures for Dexedrine were similar.

STIMULANTS: SIDE EFFECTS

As with older children, the two most common side effects of stimulant drugs in young children are anorexia and insomnia. Many children develop a tolerance for these reactions; others improve with a dosage reduction or a schedule change. Over an extended period of time, drug-induced anorexia could lead to growth suppression (see Chapter 2). While this is not a problem for most children, particularly those receiving lower therapeutic doses, each child must be evaluated and monitored on an individual basis. For example, one mother that we (Gadow, 1977) interviewed stated that her 6 year old son, who was severely hyperactive, had lost 17 to 18 pounds after 5 months of treatment with Ritalin (dosage ranged from 35 to 55 mg per day). This situation was particularly sad because she was clearly distraught over her son's loss of weight and yet trapped by her inability to cope with the stress induced by the severity of his behavior problems.

Another relatively common side effect of stimulants in young children is what is often referred to as a "depressive reaction." Parents (Gadow, 1977) describe their children as "overly quiet," "more quiet than she should have been," "sat in a corner, sucked her thumb, and wouldn't speak at all," "stared in space," and "has a stillness about him that I don't like." As previously noted, Schleifer et al. (1975) reported similar adverse effects.

Conners (1975) stated that the number of complaints of side effects was "remarkably low." In fact, mothers of children receiving placebo reported just as many side effects as the mothers of children taking Ritalin! The list of things the mothers inquired about included insomnia, anorexia, ataxia, nausea, headache, vomiting,

Table 5–3. Reported Dosages (mg) of Stimulants for Infants and Young Children

Drug	Starting Dose	Adjusting Dose	Morning Dose	Daily Dose
Benzedrine				
3 to 5 years	2.5	2.5	2.5	20.0
Dexedrine				
birth to 1 year*			2.0	4.0
1 to 3 years			2.5	5.0
3 to 5 years	2.5	2.5	5	10.0
Ritalin				
1 to 3 years			2.5	5 to 10
3 to 5 years	2.5	5	2.5 to 5	5 to 20

*Reported by Denhoff (1973).

jitteriness, sadness, cramps, thirst, rash, irritability, and nightmares.

Fortunately, because stimulants are short-acting drugs, adverse reactions to a single dose are also limited to a few hours. The following excerpt from a classic paper by Christopher Ounsted (1955) on the use of Dexedrine with hyperactive children clearly shows the time-course of the "depressive reaction":

> One child aged 5 years 6 months, who had been euphoric and was intensely over-active for more than a year, without remission, was given 2-5 mg. of dextro-amphetamine orally at 9-0 A.M. At 10:15 A.M. he sat down and became, abruptly, still. At 10:30 A.M. he began silently to weep and his usual rosiness was replaced by a grey pallor. He remained withdrawn, motionless, and weeping for four hours, and then reverted, over a period of two hours, to his habitual euphoria and energy. . . . (p. 305)

The perceived seriousness of these "depressive" reactions varies with the researcher. Both Schain and Reynard (1975) and Schleifer et al. (1975) see this as an indication to stop treatment, whereas others feel that it is simply a matter of decreasing the dosage for a few days until a tolerance to this side effect develops (Safer & Allen, 1976). Dr. Esther Sleator, research pediatrician at the Institute for Child Behavior and Development, states that she has observed these reactions in older elementary school–aged children on higher doses of Ritalin, and that reducing the dosage not only eliminates this side effect but produces a more desirable therapeutic response from the standpoint of cognitive performance. As one parent of a child in ECSE stated, "It [Ritalin at 65 mg/day] seemed to sedate him a bit. He has a language problem and talks on a 2-year-old level. So we are changing the dosage . . . and with less Ritalin he's a little more hyperactive but talks much better. It's a matter of getting a happy medium.'' Due to the short duration of stimulant drug effects, parents may never observe this reaction (Sprague & Gadow, 1976):

> One parent commented to a survey interviewer: ''The school called and said she was . . . like a zombie. . . She used to have a high vocabulary and was very social. On it [Ritalin] she sat in a corner, sucked her thumb, wouldn't speak at all. I never saw this behavior because she went off to school right after taking it. By the time I picked her up it had worn off enough so that I saw the behavior I was used to. I never caught this at all, but the school did.'' (p. 121)

One unexpected side effect of stimulant medication is lethargy and drowsiness. One parent of an ECSE child, for example, said that after 4 months of treatment her son developed a tolerance to the therapeutic response and that Ritalin ''made him very drowsy, he would just sit in the corner and yawn. When it wore off he was worse than ever, 10 times more active than before. But at first it worked.'' Another mother said the school had called and told her the Ritalin was ''making him dopey in class and sometimes he'd fall asleep.''

Stimulants can also induce psychotic, bizarre, or autistic-like behaviors, including stereotypies (e.g., Mattson & Calverley, 1968). A few parents in the ECSE study (Gadow, 1977) made comments such as ''Ritalin calmed her down but made her nervous in other ways—bit her nails and moving tongue around'' or ''rocks much more with the medicine [Ritalin] than without it.''

NEUROLEPTICS

While it is true that neuroleptic drugs are prescribed for hyperactivity and aggression in preschool-aged children, there is very little well-controlled research *per se* on the management of these disorders in this age group. In fact, the only condition for which there has been any systematic program of neuroleptic drug research is (early) *infantile autism*. The seriousness of this situation can be appreciated more fully by examining Table 5–2 and Figure 4–3 (in the chapter on mental retardation), both of which show that neuroleptics are used with some frequency for children under the age of 6 years. On the basis of available survey data, it can be concluded that at least several thousand preschoolers are currently receiving neuroleptic drugs.

Because neuroleptic medication will be the most effective drugs for decreasing severe hyperactivity, aggression, or noncompliance in *some* children, there is a real need for more information about the use of these agents with this age group. Unfortunately, the reader will simply have to draw inferences from the findings of studies with older children who have a comparable disorder. The research on autistic children may also be helpful, and the medical management of this condition is discussed in the companion volume, *Epilepsy, Emotional Disturbance, and Adolescent Disorders*. It goes without saying, but nevertheless must be emphasized, that in the case of treatments where the clinical data base is limited, adequate drug monitoring procedures become critically important. Unfortunately, there is little evidence of preferential treatment for young children (see Gadow, 1982, 1983).

Among the neuroleptic drugs currently approved by the Food and Drug Administration in the United States for use with children under 6 years of age are Mellaril (thioridazine) and Thorazine (chlorpromazine). Dosages for Mellaril and Thorazine reported in the *Physicians' Desk Reference* (1985) are as follows: For Mellaril, the dose for children between 2 and 12 years ranges from 0.5 mg/kg per day to 3.0 mg/kg per day. For Thorazine, the dosage for child outpatients with a psychiatric disorder is 0.25 mg per *pound*, administered every 4 to 6 hours.

Dosage adjustment is a critical procedure any time one is dealing with a drug whose intended effect is the facilitation of adaptive behavior. For young children receiving special education and other services, neuroleptic medication should be used only when it facilitates cognitive or social development. The following is a description of dosage adjustment procedures for autistic children prepared by Campbell et al. (1984) that is applicable to all preschool-aged children receiving neuroleptic drug therapy:

> Dosage regulation in children requires daily observations performed in a variety of different settings with the close cooperation of the physician, parents, and teachers. Dosage regulation is also difficult because optimal dosage can differ between children of the same approximate size, weight and body surface area. In most instances, dosage regulation can be more easily performed in an inpatient setting. After an adequate period of baseline assessment, drug therapy should begin with the administration of low, often therapeutically ineffective doses. The baseline assessment should include the identification of target symptoms (e.g., aggressiveness, hyperactivity, stereotypies, withdrawal) and careful recording of any involuntary movements (frequency and topography). Dosage increments should be gradual and made on a regular basis no more frequently than twice weekly. The major therapeutic task is to avoid excessive sedation at doses which attenuate target symptoms: Polypharmacy in children is to be avoided.

> The emergence of untoward effects may necessitate dosage reduction. Unlike in adults, affectomotor side effects (e.g., irritability, alterations in level of motor activity) occur commonly with neuroleptic administration to children. On the other hand, parkinsonian side effects appear to be a function of age: the younger the child, the less frequent their occurrence. These side effects in children are best treated by dosage reduction. Antiparkinsonian medication is avoided because there is some evidence that they may reduce serum neuroleptic levels (Rivera-Calimlin et al., 1976) and contribute to worsening of behavioral symptoms and cognition due to central anticholinergic properties. Acute dystonic reactions are less frequent if drug is begun with very lose doses and increases are gradual. However, should they occur, they are usually rapidly responsive to diphenhydramine (Benadryl), either orally or intramuscularly (25 mg). These dystonic reactions result from involuntary contractions of skeletal muscle groups and may be manifest as painful stiffening or arching of the back, neck, or tongue, and oculogyric crisis. (pp. 112–113).

In addition to *acute dystonic reaction,* preschoolers are at risk for the development of other *extrapyramidal* symptoms as well (see also Chapter 4). One long-term treatment study of Haldol (haloperidol) for autistic children found that 22% developed *dyskinesias* (like those associated with *tardive dyskinesia*) either during treatment or when switched to placebo. In a few cases the dyskinesias were manifest as an aggravation of preexisting stereotypies. The dyskinesias appeared any time from 5 weeks to 16 months after the onset of treatment. The dyskinesias stopped with 16 days to 9 months after they first began. In some cases they ceased while the child was on medication, and in others, after they had been switched to placebo or medication was discontinued.

SUGGESTED READINGS

Campbell, M., & Deutsch, S. I. (1985). Neuroleptics in children. In G. D. Burrows, T. Norman, & B. Davies (Eds.), *Drugs in psychiatry (Vol. 3): Antipsychotics* (pp. 213–238). New York: Elsevier Biomedical. (C)

Campbell, S. B. (1985). Hyperactivity in preschoolers: Correlates and prognostic implications. *Clinical Psychology Review,* 5, 405–428.

Conners, C. K. (1975). Controlled trial of methylphenidate in preschool children with minimal brain dysfunction. *International Journal of Mental Health,* 4, 61–74. (C, S)

Gadow, K. D. (1977). *Psychotropic and antiepileptic drug treatment with children in early childhood special education.* Champaign, IL: Institute for Child Behavior and Development, University of Illinois. (ERIC Document Reproduction Service No. ED 162 294) (C, S)

Gadow, K. D. (1982). School involvement in pharmacotherapy for behavior disorders. *Journal of Special Education,* 16, 385–399. (S)

Ounsted, C. (1955). The hyperkinetic syndrome in epileptic children. *Lancet, 2,* 303–311. (C)

Ross, D. M., & Ross, S. A. (1982). *Hyperactivity: Research, theory, and action* (2nd ed.). New York: Wiley. (C, S)

Schleifer, M., Weiss, G., Cohen, N., Elman, M., Cvejic, H., & Kruger, E. (1975). Hyperactivity in preschoolers and the effect of methylphenidate. *American Journal of Orthopsychiatry, 45,* 38–50. (C, S)

REFERENCES

Bender, L., & Cottington, F. (1942). The use of amphetamine sulfate (Benzedrine) in child psychiatry. *American Journal of Psychiatry, 99,* 116–121.

Campbell, M., Anderson, L. T., Deutsch, S. I., & Green, W. H. (1984). Psychopharmacological treatment of children with the syndrome of autism. *Pediatric Annals, 13,* 309–316.

Campbell, M., Fish, B., Shapiro, T., Collins, P., & Koh, C. (1972). Response to triiodothyronine and dextroamphetamine: A study of preschool schizophrenic children. *Journal of Autism and Childhood Schizophrenia, 2,* 343–358.

Campbell, S. B. (1985a). Hyperactivity in preschoolers: Correlates and prognostic implications. *Clinical Psychology Review, 5,* 405–428.

Campbell, S. B., Breaux, A. M., Ewing, L. J., & Szumowski, E. K. (1985b, April). *Family characteristics and child behavior as precursors of externalizing symptomatology at school entry.* Paper presented at the biennial meeting of the Society for Research in Child Development, Toronto.

Chatoor, I., Wells, K. C., Conners, C. K., Seidel, W. T., & Shaw, D. (1983). The effects of nocturnally administered stimulant medication on EEG sleep and behavior in hyperactive children. *Journal of the American Academy of Child Psychiatry, 22,* 337–342.

Cohen, N. J., Sullivan, S., Minde, K., Novak, C., & Helwig, C. (1981). Evaluation of the relative effectiveness of methylphenidate and cognitive behavior modification in the treatment of kindergarten-aged hyperactive children. *Journal of Abnormal Child Psychology, 9,* 43–54.

Conners, C. K. (1975). Controlled trial of methylphenidate in preschool children with minimal brain dysfunction. *International Journal of Mental health, 4,* 61–74.

Conners, C. K., Taylor, E., Meo, G., Kurtz, M. A., & Fournier, M. (1972). Magnesium pemoline and dextroamphetamine: A controlled study in children with minimal brain dysfunction. *Psychopharmacologia, 26,* 321–336.

Darlington, R. B., Royce, J. M., Snipper, A. S., Murray, H. W., & Lazar, I. (1980). Preschool programs and later school competence of children from low-income families. *Science, 208,* 202–204.

Denhoff, E. (1973). The natural history of children with minimal brain dysfunction. *Annals of the New York Academy of Sciences, 205,* 188–205.

Fish, B. (1971). The "one child, one drug" myth of stimulants in hyperkinesis. *Archives of General Psychiatry, 25,* 193–203.

Gadow, K. D. (1975, October). *Pills and preschool: Medication usage with young children in special education.* Paper presented at the Illinois Council for Exceptional Children, Chicago.

Gadow, K. D. (1977). *Psychotropic and antiepileptic drug treatment with children in early childhood special education.* Champaign, IL: Institute for Child Behavior and Development, University of Illinois. (ERIC Document Reproduction Service No. ED 162 294)

Gadow, K. D. (1982). School involvement in pharmacotherapy for behavior disorders. *Journal of Special Education, 16,* 385–399.

Gadow, K. D. (1983). Pharmacotherapy for behavior disorders: Typical treatment practices. *Clinical Pediatrics, 22,* 48–53.

Ginn, S. A., & Hohman, L. B. (1953). The use of dextroamphetamine in severe behavior problems of children. *Southern Medical Journal, 46,* 1124–1127.

Hasser, C. R., Conners, C. K., Denhoff, E., Millichap, J. G., & O'Leary, S. G. (1978). Take a slow approach to hyperkinesis. *Patient Care, 12*(11), 22–73.

Hunt, J. McV. (1975). Reflections on a decade of early education. *Journal of Abnormal Child Psychology, 3,* 275–330.

Husain, A., Chapel, J., & Malek, A. P. (1980). Methylphenidate, neuroleptics and dyskinesia-dystonia. *Canadian Journal of Psychiatry, 25,* 254–258.

Klein, D. F. (1974). What should the package insert be? *Archives of General Psychiatry, 31,* 735–741.

Laufer, M. W., Denhoff, E., & Riverside, R. I. (1957). Hyperactive behavior syndrome in children. *Journal of Pediatrics, 50,* 463–474.

Mattson, R. H., & Calverley, J. R. (1968). Dextroamphetamine-sulfate-induced dyskinesias. *Journal of the American Medical Association, 204,* 400–402.

Nichamin, S. J. (1972). Recognizing minimal cerebral dysfunction in the infant and toddler. *Clinical Pediatrics, 11,* 255–257.

Odom, S. L., & Fewell, R. R. (1983). Program evaluation in early childhood special education: A meta-evaluation. *Educational Evaluation and Policy Analysis, 5,* 445–460.

Oettinger, L. (1973). Discussion. *Annals of the New York Academy of Sciences, 205,* 345.

Ounsted, C. (1955). The hyperkinetic syndrome in epileptic children. *Lancet, 2,* 303–311.

Physicians' Desk Reference (39th ed.). (1985). Oradell, NJ: Medical Economics.

Renshaw, D. C. (1974). *The hyperactive child.* Chicago: Nelson-Hall.

Rivera-Calimlin, L., Nasrallah, H., Strauss, J., & Lasagna, L. (1976). Clinical response and plasma levels: Effective dose, dosage schedules, and drug interactions on plasma chlorpromazine levels. *American Journal of Psychiatry, 133,* 646–652.

Ross, D. M., & Ross, S. A. (1982). *Hyperactivity: Research, theory, and action* (2nd ed.). New York: Wiley.

Safer, D. J., & Allen, R. P. (1973). Single daily dose methylphenidate in hyperactive children. *Diseases of the Nervous System, 34,* 325–328.

Safer, D. J., & Allen, R. P. (1976). *Hyperactive children: Diagnosis and management.* Baltimore: University Park Press.

Schain, R. J., & Reynard, C. L. (1975). Observations on effects of central stimulant drug (methylphenidate) in children with hyperactive behavior. *Pediatrics, 55*, 709–716.

Schleifer, M., Weiss, G., Cohen, N., Elman, M., Cvejic, H., & Kruger, E. (1975). Hyperactivity in preschoolers and the effect of methylphenidate. *American Journal of Orthopsychiatry, 45*, 38–50.

Shirkey, H. C. (1971). The package insert dilemma. *Journal of Pediatrics, 79*, 691–693.

Shirkey, H. C. (1972). Clinical pharmacology in pediatrics. *Clinical Pharmacology and Therapeutics, 13*, 827–830.

Sleator, E. K., & von Neumann, A. W. (1974). Methylphenidate in the treatment of hyperkinetic children. *Clinical Pediatrics, 13*, 19–24.

Sleator, E. K., Ullmann, R. K., & von Neumann, A. (1982). How do hyperactive children feel about taking stimulants and will they tell the doctor? *Clinical Pediatrics, 21*, 474–479.

Sprague, R. L., Christensen, D. E., & Werry, J. S. (1974). Experimental psychology and stimulant drugs. In C. K. Conners (Ed.), *Clinical use of stimulant drugs in children* (pp. 141–164). Amsterdam: Excerpta Medica.

Sprague, R. L., & Gadow, K. D. (1976). The role of the teacher in drug treatment. *School Review, 85*, 109–140.

Stewart, M. A., Thach, B. T., & Freiden, M. R. (1970). Accidental poisoning and the hyperactive child syndrome. *Diseases of the Nervous System, 31*, 403–407.

U.S. Department of Education. (1985). *Seventh annual report to Congress on the implementation of P.L. 94-142: The Education for All Handicapped Children Act*. Washington, DC: Author.

Weinberg, W. A., & Brumback, R. A. (1976). Mania in childhood. Case studies and literature review. *American Journal of Diseases of Children, 130*, 380–385.

Weiss, G. (1975). The natural history of hyperactivity in childhood and treatment with stimulant medication at different ages: A summary of research findings.

Werry, J. S., Weiss, G., & Douglas, V. (1964). Studies on the hyperactive child. I: Some preliminary findings. *Canadian Psychiatric Association Journal, 9*, 120–130.

Zara, M. M. (1973). Effects of medication on learning in hyperactive four-year-old children. *Dissertation Abstracts International, 34*, 2407A. (University Microfilms No. 73-27, 620)

Zimmerman, F. T., & Burgemeister, B. B. (1958a). Action of methylphenidylacetate (Ritalin) and reserpine in behavior disorders in children and adults. *American Journal of Psychiatry, 115*, 323–328.

Zimmerman, F. T., & Burgemeister, B. B. (1958b). A new drug for petit mal epilepsy. *Neurology, 8*, 769–775.

APPENDIX A

Classification of Selected Psychotropic Drugs

Generic Name	Trade Name*
1. Stimulants	
Amphetamine	Benzedrine
Deanol	Deaner
Dextroamphetamine	Dexedrine
Methamphetamine	Desoxyn
Methylphenidate	Ritalin
Pemoline	Cylert
2. Antidepressants	
Tricyclics	
Amitriptyline	Elavil, Endep
Desipramine	Norpramin, Pertofrane
Doxepin	Adapin, Sinequan
Imipramine	Janimine, SK-Pramine, Tofranil
Nortriptyline	Aventyl, Pamelor
Protriptyline	Vivactil
Trimipramine	Surmontil
Monoamine Oxidase Inhibitors	
Isocarboxazid	Marplan
Phenelzine	Nardil
Tranylcypromine	Parnate

Appendix A (Continued)

Generic Name	Trade Name*
3. Antianxiety Agents (Minor Tranquilizers)	
Propanediols	
Meprobamate	Equanil, Miltown
Diphenylmethane	
Hydroxyzine	Atarax, Durrax, Vistaril
Benzodiazepines	
Alprazolam	Xanax
Chlordiazepoxide	Librium
Clonazepam	Clonopin
Clorazepate	Tranxene
Diazepam	Valium
Flurazepam	Dalmane
Halazepam	Paxipam
Lorazepam	Ativan
Oxazepam	Serax
Prazepam	Centrax
Temazepam	Restoril
Triazolam	Halcion
4. Neuroleptics (Antipsychotics, Major Tranquilizers)	
Phenothiazines	
	a. Aliphatic
Chlorpromazine	Thorazine
Promazine	Sparine
Triflupromazine	Vesprin
	b. Piperdine
Piperacetazine	Quide
Mesoridazine	Serentil
Thioridazine	Mellaril
	c. Piperazine
Acetophenazine	Tindal
Fluphenazine	Prolixin, Permitil
Perphenazine	Trilafon
Prochlorperazine	Compazine
Trifluoperazine	Stelazine
Thioxanthenes	
Chlorprothixene	Taractan
Thiothixene	Navane
Butyrophenone	
Haloperidol	Haldol

Appendix A (Continued)

Generic Name	Trade Name*
Dihydroindolone	
Molindone	Moban
Dibenzoxazepine	
Amoxapine	Asendin
Loxapine	Loxitane
Diphenylbutylpiperidine	
Pimozide	Orap
5. Sedative—Hypnotics	
Barbiturates	
Amobarbital	Amytal
Aprobarbital	Alurate
Butabarbital	Butisol
Mephobarbital	Mebaral
Pentobarbital	Nembutal
Phenobarbital	Luminal
Secobarbital	Seconal
Nonbarbiturates	
Chloral hydrate	Noctec
Ethchlorvynol	Placidyl
Ethinamate	Valmid
Glutethimide	Doriden
Methaqualone	Quaalude, Sopor
Methyprylon	Noludar
6. Anticholinergic Drugs	
Benztropine	Cogentin
Biperiden	Akineton
Ethopropazine	Parsidol
Trihexyphenidyl	Artane
Procyclidine	Kemadrin
7. Other Therapeutic Agents	
Lithium carbonate	Eskalith, Lithane Lithonate

*Only trade name products marketed in the United States are listed. In the case of drugs no longer protected by patent laws, the inclusion of trade names other than the original was arbitrary.

APPENDIX B

Conners' Abbreviated Teacher Rating Scale

Child's Name ______________________________

Completed on ______________________ by ______________________________________
(date) (teacher's name)

INSTRUCTIONS:
Please consider the last ______(day, week, month) only in filling out the checklist. Check the appropriate box for each item, *Not at all, Just a little, Pretty much,* or *Very much*, which best describes your assessment of the child. Please complete all ten items.

Observation	Degree of Activity			
	Not at all 0	Just a little 1	Pretty much 2	Very much 3
1. Restless (overactive)				
2. Excitable, impulsive				
3. Disturbs other children				
4. Fails to finish things he/she starts (short attention span)				
5. Fidgeting				
6. Inattentive, distractable				
7. Demands must be met immediately; gets frustrated				
8. Cries				
9. Mood changes quickly				
10. Temper outbursts (explosive and unpredictable behavior)				

OTHER OBSERVATIONS OF TEACHERS—Use Reverse Side.

APPENDIX C

Alphabetical List of Selected Psychotropic and Antiepileptic Drugs by Generic Name With Corresponding Trade Name (United States) and Drug Classification

Generic Name	Trade Name*	Classification
Acetazolamide	Diamox	Antiepileptic, Diuretic
Acetophenazine	Tindal	Antipsychotic
Alprazolam	Xanax	Antianxiety
Amantadine	Symmetrel	Antiparkinsonism
Amitriptyline	Elavil, Endep	Antidepressant
Amobarbital	Amytal	Sedative, Hypnotic
Amoxapine	Asendin	Antidepressant
Amphetamine	Benzedrine	Stimulant
Aprobarbital	Alurate	Sedative, Hypnotic
Benztropine	Cogentin	Anticholinergic, Antiparkinsonism
Biperiden	Akineton	Anticholinergic, Antiparkinsonism
Butabarbital	Butisol	Sedative, Hypnotic
Carbamazepine	Tegretol	Antiepileptic
Chloral hydrate	Noctec	Sedative, Hypnotic
Chlordiazepoxide	Librium	Antianxiety
Chlormezanone	Trancopal	Antianxiety
Chlorpromazine	Thorazine	Antipsychotic
Chlorprothixene	Taractan	Antipsychotic
Clomipramine	Not Approved	Antidepressant
Clonazepam	Clonopin	Antiepileptic
Clonidine	Catapres	Antihypertensive
Clorazepate	Tranxene	Antianxiety
Cyproheptadine	Periactin	Antiasthmatic
Dantrolene sodium	Dantrium	Skeletal muscle relaxant
Deanol	Deaner	Stimulant
Desipramine	Norpramin, Pertofrane	Antidepressant
Desmethylimipramine	Not Approved	Antidepressant
Dextroamphetamine sulfate	Dexedrine	Stimulant
Diazepam	Valium	Antiepileptic, Skeletal muscle relaxant, Antianxiety

Appendix C—Continued

Generic Name	Trade Name*	Classification
Diphenhydramine	Benadryl	Sedative, Hypnotic, Antihistamine
Diphenylhydantoin sodium	Dilantin	Antiepileptic
Doxepin	Adapin, Sinequan	Antidepressant
Ethchlorvynol	Placidyl	Sedative, Hypnotic
Ethinamate	Valmid	Sedative, Hypnotic
Ethopropazine	Parsidol	Anticholinergic, Antiparkinsonism
Ethosuximide	Zarontin	Antiepileptic
Ethotoin	Peganone	Antiepileptic
Fenfluramine	Pondimin	Anorectic
Fluphenazine	Prolixin, Permitil	Antipsychotic
Flurazepam	Dalmane	Sedative, Hypnotic
Glutethimide	Doriden	Sedative, Hypnotic
Halazepam	Paxipam	Antianxiety
Haloperidol	Haldol	Antipsychotic
Hydroxyzine	Atarax, Vistaril, Durrax	Sedative, Hypnotic, antianxiety
Imipramine	Janimine, SK-Pramine, Tofranil	Antidepressant
Isocarboxazid	Marplan	Antidepressant
Levoamphetamine	Not Approved	Stimulant
Lithium carbonate	Eskalith, Lithane, Lithonate	Antipsychotic
Lorazepam	Ativan	Antianxiety
Loxapine	Loxitane	Antipsychotic
Mephenytoin	Mesantoin	Antiepileptic
Mephobarbital	Mebaral	Antiepileptic
Meprobamate	Miltown, Equanil	Antianxiety
Mesoridazine	Serentil	Antipsychotic
Methamphetamine	Desoxyn	Stimulant
Methaqualone	Quaalude, Sopor	Sedative, Hypnotic
Metharbital	Gemonil	Antiepileptic
Methotrimeprazine	Levoprome	Antipsychotic
Methsuximide	Celontin	Antiepileptic
Methylphenidate	Ritalin	Stimulant
Methyprylon	Noludar	Sedative, Hypnotic
Molindone	Moban	Antipsychotic
Nortriptyline	Aventyl, Pamelor	Antidepressant
Oxazepam	Serax	Antianxiety
Paramethadione	Paradione	Antiepileptic
Pemoline	Cylert	Stimulant
Penfluridol	Not Approved	Antipsychotic

Appendix C—Continued

Generic Name	Trade Name*	Classification
Pentobarbital	Nembutal	Sedative, Hypnotic
Perphenazine	Trilafon	Antipsychotic
Phenacemide	Phenurone	Antiepileptic
Phenelzine	Nardil	Antidepressant
Phenobarbital	Luminal	Antiepileptic, Sedative, Hypnotic
Phensuximide	Milontin	Antiepileptic
Phenytoin	Dilantin	Antiepileptic
Pimozide	Orap	Antipsychotic
Piperacetazine	Quide	Antipsychotic
Piracetam	Not Approved	Nootropic
Parzepam	Centrax, Verstron	Antianxiety
Primidone	Mysoline	Antiepileptic
Prochlorperazine	Compazine	Antipsychotic
Procyclidine	Kemadrin	Anticholinergic, Antiparkinsonism
Promazine	Sparine	Antipsychotic
Promethazine	Phenergan	Sedative, Hypnotic
Propranolol	Inderal	Beta-Adrenergic Blocker
Protriptyline	Vivactil	Antidepressant
Reserpine	Serpasil	Antipsychotic
Secobarbital	Seconal	Sedative, Hypnotic
Temazepam	Restoril	Sedative, Hypnotic
Thioridazine	Mellaril	Antipsychotic
Thiothixene	Navane	Antipsychotic
Tranylcypromine	Parnate	Antidepressant
Trazodone	Desyrel	Antidepressant
Triazolam	Halcion	Sedative, Hypnotic
Thiethylperazine	Torecan	Antipsychotic
Trifluoperazine	Stelazine	Antipsychotic
Triflupromazine	Vesprin	Antipsychotic
Trihexyphenidyl	Artane	Anticholinergic, Antiparkinsonism
Trimethadione	Tridione	Antiepileptic
Trimipramine	Surmontil	Antidepressant
Valproic acid	Depakene	Antiepileptic

*In the case of drugs no longer protected by patent laws, the inclusion of trade names other than the original was arbitrary. Not apoproved = drugs not approved for general use by the Food and Drug Administration (FDA) as of 1984.

APPENDIX D

Alphabetical List of Selected Psychotropic and Antiepileptic Drugs by Trade Name (United States) With Corresponding Generic Name

Trade Name	Generic Name
Adapin	Doxepin
Akineton	Biperiden
Alurate	Aprobarbital
Artane	Trihexylphenidyl
Asendin	Amoxapine
Atabrine	Quinacrine
Atarax	Hydroxyzine
Ativan	Lorazepam
Aventyl	Nortriptyline
Benadryl	Diphenhydramine
Benzedrine	Amphetamine
Butisol	Butabarbital
Catapres	Clonidine
Celontin	Methsuximide
Centrax	Prazepam
Clonopin	Clonazepam
Cogentin	Benztropine
Compazine	Prochlorperazine
Cylert	Pemoline
Dalmane	Flurazepam
Dantrium	Dantrolene sodium
Deaner	Deanol
Depakene	Valproic acid
Desoxyn	Methamphetamine
Desyrel	Trazodone
Dexedrine	Dextroamphetamine
Diamox	Acetazolamide
Dilantin	Phenytoin
Doriden	Glutethimide
Durrax	Hydroxyzine
Elavil	Amitriptyline
Endep	Amitriptyline
Equanil	Meprobamate
Eskalith	Lithium carbonate
Gemonil	Metharbital
Halcion	Triazolam
Haldol	Haloperidol
Inderal	Propranolol
Janimine	Imipramine
Kemadrin	Procyclidine
Levoprome	Methotrimeprazine
Librium	Chlordiazepoxide
Lithane	Lithium carbonate
Lithonate	Lithium carbonate
Loxitane	Loxapine
Luminal	Phenobarbital
Marplan	Isocarboxazid
Mebaral	Mephobarbital
Mellaril	Thioridazine
Meprospan	Meprobamate
Mesantoin	Mephenytoin
Milontin	Phensuximide
Miltown	Meprobamate
Moban	Molindone
Mysoline	Primidone

Appendix D—Continued

Trade Name	Generic Name*
Nardil	Phenelzine
Navane	Thiothixene
Nembutal	Pentobarbital
Noctec	Chloral hydrate
Noludar	Methyprylon
Norpramin	Desipramine
Orap	Pimozide
Pamelor	Nortriptyline
Paradione	Paramethadione
Parnate	Tranylcypromine
Parsidol	Ethopropazine
Paxipam	Halazepam
Peganone	Ethotoin
Periactin	Cyproheptadine
Permitil	Fluphenazine
Pertofrane	Desipramine
Phenergan	Promethazine
Phenurone	Phenacemide
Placidyl	Ethchlorvynol
Pondimin	Fenfluramine
Prolixin	Fluphenazine
Quaalude	Methaqualone
Quide	Piperacetazine
Restoril	Temazepam
Ritalin	Methylphenidate

Trade Name	Generic Name
Seconal	Secobarbital
Serax	Oxazepam
Serentil	Mesoridazine
Serpasil	Reserpine
Sinequan	Doxepin
SK-Pramine	Impramine
Sopor	Methaqualone
Sparine	Promazine
Stelazine	Trifluoperazine
Surmontil	Trimipramine
Symmetrel	Amantadine
Taractan	Chlorprothixene
Tegretol	Carbamazepine
Thorazine	Chlorpromazine
Tindal	Acetophenazine
Tofranil	Imipramine
Torecan	Thiethylperazine
Trancopal	Chlormezanone
Tranxene	Clorazepate
Tridione	Trimethadione
Trilafon	Perphenazine
Valium	Diazepam
Valmid	Ethinamate
Vesprin	Triflupromazine
Vistaril	Hydroxyzine pamoate
Vivactil	Protriptyline
Xanax	Alprazolam
Zarontin	Ethosuximide

APPENDIX E

Dyskinesia Identification System—Coldwater (DIS-Co)

NAME: ______________________________

HOSPITAL NUMBER: ____________________

HOUSEHOLD: __________________________

DATE: ______________________________

TIME: ______________________ AM PM RATER: __________

I. FACIAL:

1. Tics	0	1	2	3	4	NA
2. Grimaces	0	1	2	3	4	NA
a. Other	0	1	2	3	4	NA

II. OCULAR:

3. Biopharospasm	0	1	2	3	4	NA
4. Blinking	0	1	2	3	4	NA
b. Other	0	1	2	3	4	NA

III. ORAL:

5. Lip Smacking	0	1	2	3	4	NA
6. Pursing/Puckering	0	1	2	3	4	NA
7. Sucking	0	1	2	3	4	NA
8. Upper Lip Tremor	0	1	2	3	4	NA
9. Thrusting Lower Lip	0	1	2	3	4	NA
10. Cheek Puffing	0	1	2	3	4	NA
11. Chewing	0	1	2	3	4	NA
12. Lateral Jaw	0	1	2	3	4	NA
c. Other	0	1	2	3	4	NA

IV. LINGUAL:

13. Clonic Tongue	0	1	2	3	4	NA
14. Tonic Tongue	0	1	2	3	4	NA
15. Tongue Thrusts	0	1	2	3	4	NA
16. Tongue in Cheek	0	1	2	3	4	NA
17. Tongue Tremors	0	1	2	3	4	NA

18. Lateral Tongue	0	1	2	3	4	NA
19. Myokymic Tongue	0	1	2	3	4	NA
20. Athetoid Tongue	0	1	2	3	4	NA
d. Other	0	1	2	3	4	NA
V. HEAD/NECK:						
21. Retrocollis	0	1	2	3	4	NA
22. Torticollis	0	1	2	3	4	NA
e. Other	0	1	2	3	4	NA
VI. TRUNK:						
23. Axial Hyperkinesia	0	1	2	3	4	NA
24. Shoulder/Hip Torsion	0	1	2	3	4	NA
f. Other	0	1	2	3	4	NA
VII. UPPER LIMB:						
25. Myokymic Finger/Wrist/Arm	0	1	2	3	4	NA
26. Athetoid Finger/Wrist/Arm	0	1	2	3	4	NA
27. Pill Rolling	0	1	2	3	4	NA
28. Finger Counting	0	1	2	3	4	NA
g. Other	0	1	2	3	4	NA
VIII. LOWER LIMB:						
29. Walking in Place	0	1	2	3	4	NA
30. Foot Tapping	0	1	2	3	4	NA
31. Ankle Flexion	0	1	2	3	4	NA
32. Toe Movement	0	1	2	3	4	NA
h. Other	0	1	2	3	4	NA
IX. GROSS BODY:						
33. Holokinetic	0	1	2	3	4	NA
i. Other	0	1	2	3	4	NA
X. AMBULATORY:						
34. Gait	0	1	2	3	4	NA
j. Other	0	1	2	3	4	NA

0—NOT PRESENT	Abnormal movements are *not observed.* Some movements may be observed but are not considered abnormal.
1—MINIMAL	Abnormal movements occur *infrequently and/or* are *difficult to detect.*
2—MILD	Abnormal movements occur *infrequently and* are *easy to detect.*
3—MODERATE	Abnormal movements occur *frequently and* are *easy to detect.*
4—SEVERE	Abnormal movements occur *almost continuously and/or are of extreme intensity.*
NA—NOT ASSESSED	The rater is not able to make an assessment.

Note. "From The Dyskinesia Identification System—Coldwater (DIS-Co): A Tardive Dyskinesia Rating Scale for the Developmentally Disabled." By R. L. Sprague et al., 1984, *Psychopharmacology Bulletin, 20,* p. 329. Reprinted by permission.

APPENDIX F

DIS-Co Item Identification

	I. Facial Movements
1. Tics	Brief, muscular contractions of small sections of the face.
2. Grimaces	Brief, muscular contractions of large sections of the face.
a. Other	
	II. Ocular Movements
3. Blepharospasm	Fine tremors of the eyelid(s)
3. Blinking	Rapid opening and closing of the eyelids.
	III. Oral Movements
5. Lip Smacking	Quick parting of the lips, which may produce a smacking sound.
6. Pursing	Puckering of the lips.
7. Sucking	Drawing in of lips, cheeks, air, etc., caused by lip-tongue action.
8. Upper Lip Tremor	Quivering of the upper lip (Rabbit syndrome).
9. Thrusting of the Lower Lip	Extending the lower lip similar to a child's pout.
10. Cheek Puffing	Forcing air into the cheeks producing a noticeable bulge.
11. Chewing	Circular or up and down jaw movements (similar to movements that occur during eating).
12. Lateral Jaw Movement	Side-to-side movement of the jaw.
	IV. Lingual Movements
13. Clonic Tongue	Rhythmic movement of the tongue in and out of the mouth
14. Tonic Tongue Protrusion	Extending the tongue and holding beyond the lips.
15. Tongue Thrusts	Abruptly moving the tongue in and out of the mouth.
16. Tongue in Cheek	Tongue pressed against the inside of the cheeks or lips, producing a noticeable bulge.

17. Tongue Tremors	Quivering of the tongue, observed with the mouth open and tongue resting inside or outside the mouth.
18. Lateral Tongue	Side-to-side movements of the tongue inside the mouth.
19. Myokymic Tongue Movements	Twitching movements of sections of the tongue, observed with the mouth open and tongue resting inside the mouth.
20. Athetoid Tongue Movements	Worm-like rolling and twisting movements.
V. Head/Neck Movements	
21. Retrocollis	Contractions of the muscles in the back of the neck which results in the head being tilted back.
22. Torticollis	Contractions of the neck muscles twisting the head to one side (similar to a stiff neck).
VI. Trunk Movements	
23. Axial Hyperkinesia	Front to back or circular movements of the pelvis.
24. Shoulder/Hip Torsion	Twisting, rolling movements of the shoulders and/or hips, involving large sections of the body.
VII. Upper Limb Movements	
25. Myokymic Finger/Wrist/Arm	Twitching movements observed of the fingers, wrists, and/or arms.
26. Athetoid Finger/Wrist/Arm	Worm-like rolling and twisting movements observed in the fingers, wrists, and/or arms.
27. Pill Rolling	Circular movements of the thumb against the fingers of the same hand.
28. Finger Counting	Tapping of the thumb against the fingers of the same hand.
VIII. Lower Limb Movements	
29. Walking in Place	Alternating from one foot to the other while standing.
30. Foot Tapping	An alternating heel-toe tapping or striking of the floor with the entire foot, heel, and/or toe.
31. Ankle Flexion	Circular, up and down and/or back and forth bending movements of the ankle.
32. Toe Movement	Movements or bending of the toe(s).
IX. Gross Body Movements	
33. Holokinetic	Sudden, unexpected, clumsy movements of large sections of the body.
X. Ambulatory Movements	
34. Gait	Shuffling of the feet while walking may be accompanied by arm extension and/or bent knees.

Note. "From The Dyskinesia Identification System-Coldwater (DIS-Co): A Tardive Dyskinesia Rating Scale for the Developmentally Disabled," by R. L. Sprague et al., 1984, *Psychopharmacology Bulletin, 20,* p. 329. Reprinted by permission.

APPENDIX G

Dyskinesia Identification System: Condensed User Scale (DISCUS)

NAME: ____________________

ID #: ____________________

UNIT: ____________________

DATE: ____________________

TIME: START ____ **STOP** ____ **AM/PM**

RATER: ____________________

COOPERATION LEVEL (circle one):

1 : NO CO-OP (passive or active resistance; few, if any, examamination steps done)

2 : PARTIAL CO-OP (at least one activation task done; some but not all examination steps)

3 : FULL CO-OP (most or all examination steps)

FACIAL:

1. Tics . . . . 0 1 2 3 4 NA
2. Grimaces . . . . 0 1 2 3 4 NA

OCULAR:

3. Blinking . . . . 0 1 2 3 4 NA

ORAL:

4. Chewing/Lip Smacking . . . . 0 1 2 3 4 NA
5. Puckering/Sucking/ Thrusting Lower Lip . . . . 0 1 2 3 4 NA

LINGUAL:

6. Tongue Thrusts/ Tongue in Cheek . . . . . 0 1 2 3 4 NA

OTHERS:

____________________ 0 1 2 3 4 NA

____________________ 0 1 2 3 4 NA

____________________ 0 1 2 3 4 NA

____________________ 0 1 2 3 4 NA

____________________ 0 1 2 3 4 NA

____________________ 0 1 2 3 4 NA

COMMENTS:

____

____

____

____

____

7. Tonic Tongue . . . . .0 1 2 3 4 NA
8. Tongue Tremor. . . . . . .0 1 2 3 4 NA
9. Athetoid/Myokymic/
   Lateral Tongue . . . . . . .0 1 2 3 4 NA

HEAD/NECK/TRUNK:

10. Retrocollis/
    Torticollis . . . . .0 1 2 3 4 NA
11. Shoulder/Hip
    Torsion . . . . .0 1 2 3 4 NA

UPPER LIMB:

12. Athetoid/Myokymic
    Finger-Wrist-Arm
    (*not* tremor) . . . . .0 1 2 3 4 NA
13. Pill Rolling . . . . .0 1 2 3 4 NA

LOWER LIMB:

14. Ankle Flexion/
    Foot Tapping. . . . . .0 1 2 3 4 NA
15. Toe Movement . . . . . . .0 1 2 3 4 NA

SCORING

0—NOT PRESENT (movements not observed *or* some movements observed but not considered abnormal)

1—MINIMAL (abnormal movements are difficult to detect *or* movements are easy to detect but occur only once or twice in a short nonrepetitive manner)

2—MILD (abnormal movements occur infrequently *and* are easy to detect)

3—MODERATE (abnormal movements occur frequently *and* are easy to detect)

4—SEVERE (abnormal movements occur almost continuously *and* are easy to detect)

NA—NOT ASSESSED (an assessment for an item is not able to be made)

Note: From "Dyskinesia Identification System: Condensed User Scale (DISCUS)" by R. L. Sprague, J.E. Kalachnik, and D. M. White, 1985, Champaign, IL: Institute for Child Behavior and Development, University of Illinois at Champaign-Urbana. Reprinted by permission.

APPENDIX H

Model of a Letter to Parents Regarding Side Effects

Dear ____ :

Attached is a list of possible side effects specific to the medication your child is or will be receiving. Please read this carefully. If the medication is classified as a "neuroleptic," please pay particular attention to the possibility of tardive dyskinesia. It is provided so that:

1. You are aware of possible side effects.
2. You can more accurately inform us if you observe any unusual events when you see your child.
3. You can call us if you have any questions or reservations regarding the medication.

All of the residents are assessed on a regular basis for side effects so that we can take appropriate action with the physician should they occur. If a new medication is prescribed, assessments are taken shortly thereafter. If no dosage changes occur, assessments are made every six months. If the medication is discontinued, assessments are also made. We are making all attempts to use the medication in the lowest possible dosages so as to further decrease the likelihood of side effects.

Thank you, and please call ______________________________ at phone number ______________________________________ if you have any questions or concerns.

Sincerely,

General List of Possible Side-Effects

Drug Class: Neuroleptics
Subclass: Butyrophenone
Specific Drug: haloperidol (Haldol)

Frequent: parkinsonism (tremor, drooling, shuffling, pill rolling, cogwheel rigidity, lack of movement)
akathisia (restlessness, inability to sit still, verbal comments such as "I feel like jumping out of my skin")
dystonia (rigidity, neck or back arching, eyes rolled up)

Occasional: sedation, fainting upon standing up, menstrual changes, secretions from the breast, blood dyscrasias (signs: pale, fever, bruising, sore throat)

Rare: cholestatic jaundice (signs: yellow skin), sunburn, rashes, weight gain, convulsions, impotence

****NOTE: ALL NEUROLEPTICS HAVE BEEN ASSOCIATED WITH TARDIVE DYSKINESIA, A POTENTIALLY IRREVERSIBLE SYNDROME OF INVOLUNTARY MUSCLE MOVEMENTS CONSISTING OF SUCH MOVEMENTS AS GRIMACING, TICS, BLINKING, LIP SMACKING, SUCKING, CHEWING, TONGUE THRUSTING, ARM WRITHING OR JERKING, AND/OR LEG WRITHING OR JERKING. THIS MAY DEVELOP AFTER ONE TO TWO YEARS OR MORE OF DRUG USE, ALTHOUGH A FEW CASES HAVE BEEN REPORTED BEFORE THIS. THE CONDITION IS PERSISTANT IN APPROXIMATELY 20% OF PATIENTS WHO RECEIVE NEUROLEPTICS. WHILE SUCH MOVEMENTS ARE GENERALLY MILD, THEY MAY BE COSMETICALLY OR FUNCTIONALLY DISABLING.

APPENDIX I

Alphabetical List of Selected United Kingdom Trade Names*

Trade Name	Generic Name	Trade Name	Generic Name
Allegron	nortriptyline	Liskonum	lithium carbonate
Almazine	lorazepam	Modecate	fluphenazine
Anafranil	clomipramine	Moditen	fluphenazine
Apsolol	propranolol	Nozinan	methotrimeprazine
		Phasal	lithium carbonate
Berkoldol	propranolol	Ponderax	fenfluramine
		Priadel	lithium carbonate
Camcolit	lithium carbonate	Rivotril	clonazepam
		Ronyl	pemoline
Domical	amitriptyline		
		Serenace	haloperidol
		Serenid-D	oxazepam
Emeside	ethosuximide	Serenid Forte	oxazepam
Epanutin	phenytoin	Soneryl	butabarbitone
Epilim	sodium valporate	Stemetil	prochlorperazine
Fentazin	perphenazine		
Fortunan	haloperidol		
		Tryptizol	amitriptyline
		Veractil	methotrimeprazine
Largactil	chlorpromazine	Vertigon	prochlorperazine
Lentizol	amitriptyline	Volital	pemoline

*Only trade names that are *not* used in the United States are listed.

Glossary

Abbreviated Teacher Rating Scale: a shortened, 10 item version of Conners' 39 Item Teacher Rating Scale (see Appendix B).

abdominal epilepsy: same as autonomic epilepsy.

aberrant: behavior that deviates markedly from what is considered normal.

absence seizure: same as petit mal seizure.

absorption: the process whereby a substance is taken into or across tissues, e.g., intestine; the movement of a drug into the bloodstream.

ACTH: adrenocorticotropic hormone.

acute: having a sudden onset and short duration.

acute dystonic reaction: characterized by uncontrolled muscle activity with stiffness or twisting of body parts; possible reactions include facial grimacing; torticollis, which may be associated with oculogyric crisis; and opisthotonos. A side effect of antipsychotic drugs occasionally seen with the initiation of treatment.

adaptive: having a capacity for modification to fit the demands of the environment.

adrenocorticotropic hormone: a hormone secreted by the anterior lobe of the pituitary gland which controls the secretion of adrenocortical hormones by the adrenal cortices; corticotropin; ACTH.

adverse reaction: same as side effect.

affective: pertaining to feelings or emotions.

affective disorders: characterized by changes in mood as the primary symptoms, e.g., mania, depression.

agitated: motor restlessness and increased activity level in association with anxiety and tension.

agitation: motor restlessness associated with mental distress.

akathisia: characterized by motor restlessness arising from a compulsion to move about; an extrapyramidal syndrome produced by antipsychotic drugs.

akinetic: cessation of movement.

akinetic seizure: a term used inconsistently in the literature to refer to the seizures associated with the Lennox-Gastaut syndrome; head nodding spells. The seizures are brief and typically consist of a sudden, violent jerk, either forward or backward. If standing the associated fall may cause severe, repeated head injury. Defined by The International League Against Epilepsy as "loss of movement without atonia" (Gastaut, 1970).

ambulatory: able to walk.

anemia: below normal number of red blood cells, amount of hemoglobin, or total drug volume.

anorexia: a lack or loss of appetite for food.

anoxia: absence or loss of oxygen.

antianxiety drug: same as minor tranquilizer.

anticholinergic: an agent that alters the effect of acetylcholine in cholinergic synapses; anticholinergic drugs are used in the management of some extrapyramidal syndromes produced by antipsychotic drugs.

anticonvulsant: an agent that reduces the frequency, magnitude, or duration of convulsions or seizures; antiepileptic.

antidepressant: an agent that prevents or suppresses the symptoms of depression; mood elevating.

antiepileptic: an agent that reduces the frequency, magnitude, or duration of convulsions or seizures; anticonvulsant.

antipsychotic: an agent that prevents or suppresses the symptoms of psychosis; major tranquilizer, neuroleptic.

anxiety: a feeling of uneasiness, apprehension, and fear over an anticipated experience.

ataxia: failure of voluntary muscle coordination; **gait ataxia:** a staggered walk with a wide base.

athetosis: characterized by slow, writhing movements of peripheral parts of the body.

atonic: loss of normal tone; **atonic seizure:** patient suddenly crumples and falls to the floor, muscles remain flaccid during the seizure.

ATRS: Abbreviated Teacher Rating Scale.

atypical febrile convulsion: epileptic convulsion in association with a fever illness.

aura: a warning that precedes an epileptic seizure often manifest as a sensation or motor movement.

autism: a subjective, self centered form of thinking that is not correctable with information from external reality.

automatisms: seemingly purposeful involuntary behavior that is out of context; a manifestation of psychomotor epilepsy; **simple automatisms:** repetitive smacking of lips, chewing, mumbling; **complex automatisms:** undressing, walking about.

autonomic nervous system: the part of the nervous system that regulates the muscles of the heart, smooth muscles, and glands.

autonomic epilepsy: an uncommon form of epilepsy in which seizures may be manifest as gastrointestinal disturbances (abdominal pain, vomiting, nausea, etc.), headache, or other symptoms of autonomic dysfunction; thalamic epilepsy, abdominal epilepsy, epileptic equivalent.

behavior modification: a treatment approach based on a model that views abnormal behavior as being acquired in response to environmental stress and learned and maintained in the same manner as normal behavior. The principles of experimental psychology are emphasized, particularly classical and operant conditioning. The importance of the cognitive mediation of behavior and vicarious and symbolic learning processes, e.g., modeling, is also recognized. Treatment conditions are explicitly stated and therapeutic outcomes are measured objectively.

behavior therapy: same as behavior modification.

benign: having a favorable outcome; not recurring.

benzodiazepines: a category of antianxiety agents (minor tranquilizers) which includes diazepam (Valium), chlordiazepoxide (Librium), and clonazepam (Clonopin).

bilateral: pertaining to both sides.

biotransformation: the chemical alteration of a compound within the body, e.g., the metabolism of a drug by liver microsomal enzymes.

blood brain barrier: refers not to an anatomical structure but to the fact that the capillaries of the brain prevent certain classes of compounds from entering and affecting brain neurons. A closeknit layer of glial cells surrounds the brain capillaries creating an additional barrier for compounds which are not lipid soluble.

brand name: same as trade name.

butyrophenones: a category of antipsychotic agents (major tranquilizers) which includes haloperidol (Haldol).

cardiovascular: pertaining to the heart and blood vessels.

central nervous system: consisting of the brain and spinal cord.

cerebral palsy: a variety of syndromes, characterized by a disorganization of motor control, that are the result of damage to the motor areas of the brain.

chorea: characterized by continuous, random, uncontrolled contractions of different muscle groups.

chronic: persisting over a long period of time.

clonic: pertaining to a series of alternate muscle contractions and relaxations.

coarse facies: marked by swelling of the lips, thickening of the subcutaneous tissue of the face and scalp, and broadening of the nose; adverse reaction associated with phenytoin (Dilantin) treatment.

cognitive performance: performance on a specified task generally regarded to measure perception, thinking, and remembering.

colic: acute abdominal pain.

combined drug regimen: the simultaneous treatment of two or more disorders with different drugs.

concomitant: accompanying; joined with another.

convulsion: a violent and involuntary contraction or series of contractions of the voluntary muscles.

convulsive disorder: recurrent seizures; epilepsy.

convulsive threshold: the point at which a stimulus, e.g., electrical discharge, produces a convulsion or seizure.

corticotropin: same as adrenocorticotropic hormone.

deinstitutionalization: the transfer of individuals (e.g., mentally retarded, mentally ill) from institutional or residential care to community placement (e.g., half way houses, group homes).

delusions: a false belief that cannot be changed by reason or evidence from the patient's own senses.

depression: a psychiatric disorder characterized by feelings of personal incompetence, listlessness, insomnia, loss of appetite, and psychomotor slowing.

dermatitis: inflammation of the skin.

diphenylmethanes: a category of antianxiety agents (minor tranquilizers) which includes hydroxyzine hydrochloride (Atarax) and hydroxyzine pamoate (Vistaril).

diplopia: double vision.

distribution: the movement of drug molecules in the bloodstream to the site of drug action; concentration of drug molecules in body compartments.

diuretic: an agent that promotes the secretion of urine.

dose: amount of medication administered.

double blind: characterizing a study of a particular treatment, e.g., drug, in which neither the person administering (evaluating) or receiving the agent is aware of whether the active or inactive (placebo) drug is being given.

drug: any substance other than food that has an effect on living tissue.

drug addiction: "A behavioral pattern of compulsive drug use, characterized by overwhelming involvement with the use of a drug, the securing of its supply, and a high tendency to relapse after withdrawal" (Jaffe, 1975, p. 285).

drug free period: a break in a chronic drug regimen for a period of time during which no medication is administered; drug holiday.

drug holiday: same as drug free period.

drug interaction: the modification of the effects of a drug by the prior or concurrent administration of another drug.

drug of (first) choice: the agent to be administered first in the treatment of a specific disorder, usually determined on the basis of safety and efficacy.

dysarthria: imperfect articulation of speech; slurred speech.

dyskinesia: fragmentary or incomplete movements that result from a diminished power to control voluntary movements.

dysphoria: disquiet; restlessness; malaise.

dystonia: disordered muscle tone.

early infantile autism: a rare disorder with onset during early infancy and characterized by autistic aloneness, absence of language or developmental language disorders, insistence on sameness, repetitive behaviors, and lack of demonstrable physical defect.

echolalia: the repetition of words spoken by other people as if echoing what is said.

edema: swelling resulting from an accumulation of fluid in subcutaneous tissues.

educable mentally retarded: an educational classification for children whose IQs range from 50 or 55 to 75 or 80.

EEG: electroencephalogram.

efficacy: effectiveness.

endocrine system: the glands and structures that produce hormones which are released into the blood.

endoplasmic reticulum: ultramicroscopic network of tubules and cavities within almost all cells; microenzymes in the endoplasmic reticulum of liver cells break drugs down into metabolites that are more easily removed from the body.

enteric-coated: a special coating applied to tablets and capsules that delays absorption until the drug reaches the intestine.

enuresis: involuntary discharge of urine.

enzyme: a protein that brings about or accelerates chemical reactions.

epidemiology: the study of the factors that influence the incidence, distribution, and control of disease.

epilepsy: recurrent seizures that are due to sudden electrical discharges in the brain.

epileptic equivalent: same as autonomic epilepsy.

epileptic seizure precipitated by fever: form of epilepsy characterized by seizures that are triggered by a fever illness.

equilibrium: a state of balance between two opposing forces.

etiology: the causes of a disease; the study of the factors that cause disease.

exacerbate: to make more severe or violent.

excretion: the elimination or discharge of substances, e.g., wastes, metabolites, from the cell, tissue, and blood; drugs are often excreted as water soluble metabolites by the kidney.

extensor: a muscle that extends a joint.

extracellular fluid: fluid outside the cell.

extrapyramidal syndromes: a group of disorders characterized by abnormal involuntary movements. Extrapyramidal syndromes produced by antipsychotic drugs include Parkinsonian syndrome, akathisia, acute dystonic reaction, and tardive dyskinesia.

extrapyramidal tract: not an anatomical structure, but a group of nuclei (a nucleus is a mass of nerve cells) and fibers that control and coordinate motor activities, especially gross intentional movements, patterns of movement, walking movements, and "background" muscle tone.

FDA: Food and Drug Administration.

febrile: relating to or characterized by fever.

Feingold diet: same as Kaiser-Permanente diet.

flexor: any muscle that bends a joint.

focal epilepsy: characterized by seizures associated with an abnormal electrical discharge originating in, or restricted to, a limited area of the brain.

folic acid: substance used by the bone marrow to form red blood cells.

gastrointestinal: pertaining to the stomach and intestines.

generalized seizures: seizures associated with abnormal electrical discharges that affect the entire brain; they may be focal at the onset and spread to become generalized or be generalized from the beginning. Grand mal, petit mal, and myoclonic seizures are all generalized seizures.

generic name: a drug name, not protected by a patent, that identifies a specific chemical structure; official name, nonproprietary name.

Gilles de la Tourette's syndrome: a rare disorder with an onset in childhood characterized by tics, particularly of the facial muscles, and involuntary vocalizations.

gingival hyperplasia: an excessive growth of gum tissue with a mulberry shaped appearance. Irritants lodged in the tissue cause secondary inflammation resulting in a red or bluish-red discoloration. This is an adverse reaction commonly associated with phenytoin (Dilantin).

gonadotropic hormones: Three hormones secreted by the anterior pituitary that have an influence on the ovaries and testes.

grand mal epilepsy: characterized by periodic attacks of unconsciousness and generalized tonic and clonic movements frequently lasting from 3 to 5 minutes. Interseizure EEG findings may be normal and seizures can begin at any age. Generalized seizures fall into four categories: Tonic-clonic, clonic, tonic, and atonic.

growth rebound: an increase in growth rate following the cessation of stimulant drug treatment in hyperactive children.

hallucination: perception of an object in the absence of corresponding stimuli.
hallucinogens: a category of psychotropic drugs capable of inducing hallucinations.
hirsutism: abnormal hairiness; an adverse drug reaction associated with phenytoin (Dilantin) therapy.
hydantoinates: a category of antiepileptic drugs with potent anticonvulsant properties that includes phenytoin (Dilantin), mephentoin (Mesantoin), and ethotoin (Peganone).
hyperactivity: a long term, persistent behavior disorder characterized by excessive restlessness and inattentiveness originating during early to middle childhood (2 to 6 years of age).
hypertonicity: characterized by excessive skeletal muscle tone; the muscle is more resistant to passive stretching.
hypnotic: a category of psychotropic drugs that induce sleep.
hypoplasia: failure of an organ to develop and reach its adult size.
hypotension: abnormally low blood pressure.
hypothalamic epilepsy: same as autonomic epilepsy.
hypsarrythmia: an exceedingly abnormal electroencephalographic pattern between seizures characterized by random, high voltage slow waves and spikes that originate from multiple foci and spread to all cortical areas. This EEG pattern is associated with myoclonic epilepsy of young children (infantile spasms, salaam seizures, massive myoclonia). Severe mental retardation is common.

idiopathic: a disease of spontaneous origin or unknown cause.
incidence: the number of new cases, e.g., of a disease, during a certain period of time.
infantile spasms: same as myoclonic epilepsy of young children.
induce: to bring about by stimulation; cause something to occur.
insomnia: inability to sleep.
intracellular fluid: fluid within the cell.
intractable: resistant to control.
intramuscular: within the substance of the muscle.
intravenous: within a vein.
in utero: within the uterus.
Isle of Wight: island of the southern coast of England.

Jacksonian seizure: a focal seizure characterized by unilateral clonic movements that start in one group of muscles moving systematically to adjacent groups of muscles. The seizures are due to an abnormal electrical discharge that originates in, and spreads across, the motor cortex.
jaundice: a syndrome characterized by an excess of bile pigment in the blood and yellow appearance of the skin resulting from the deposition of bile pigments in the skin; icterus.

Kaiser-Permanente diet: a treatment regimen for childhood behavior disorders, especially hyperactivity, which involves the elimination of low molecular weight chemicals, e.g., salicylates and artificial colors and additives, from daily food intake; K-P diet, Feingold diet.
ketogenic diet: a dietary regimen in which the total daily consumption of fat (in grams) is at least four times greater than proteins and carbohydrates combined (in grams). This maintains the state of ketosis achieved by a marked reduction in food intake at the onset of treatment. The diet is effective in treating myoclonic epilepsy in young children.
kg: kilogram.
kilogram: a unit of weight in the metric system being 1000 grams; equivalent to approximately 2.2 pounds.
K-P diet: same as Kaiser-Permanente diet.

learning performance: performance on a specified task generally regarded to measure learning rather than a more pure measure of the neural events associated with learning.
least restrictive alternative: handicapped children, including children in public and private institutions, are educated as much as possible with children who are not handicapped. Separate schools, special classes, or other removal of any handicapped child from the regular program is appropriate only if the regular educational environment accompanied by supplementary aids and services is not

adequate to give the child what he or she needs.

Lennox-Gastaut syndrome: one type of myoclonic epilepsy characterized by several types of seizures including staring spells, myoclonic seizures (sudden violent jerks with an associated fall, sudden falls without jerks, head nodding seizures, and sagging attacks (atonic seizures), and generalized tonic-clonic seizures. Age of onset is usually between 3 to 5 years of age. Mental and motor retardation are common. Interseizure EEG findings often show modified hypsarrhythmia (2 per second spike and wave). Also called petit mal variant, myoclonic epilepsy of older children.

lipids: a group of substances, such as fatty acids, that cannot be dissolved in water. Lipids are stored in the body, are used as fuel, and are an important part of all living cells.

lipid soluble: capable of being dissolved in lipids.

mainstreaming: an approach to the delivery of special education services that emphasizes the integration of the handicapped child with nonhandicapped peers in regular classrooms as opposed to segregation in self contained special classes. The educational needs of the child are met through modifications in the regular school program.

major motor epilepsy: same as grand mal epilepsy.

major tranquilizer: a category of psychotropic drugs that includes the phenothiazines, thiozanthenes, and butyrophenones; antipsychotic agents, neuroleptics. These drugs are used primarily in the treatment of psychotic disorders.

maladaptive: not promoting or assisting adaptation.

malaise: an indefinite feeling of bodily discomfort or lack of health.

MAO inhibitor: same as monamine oxidase inhibitor.

massive myoclonic seizures: same as myoclonic epilepsy of young children.

mcg: microgram.

μcg: microgram.

mcg/ml: microgram per milliliter.

μcg/ml: microgram per milliliter.

MCT: medium chain triglycerides.

megavitamins: massive doses of vitamins. A treatment of questionable efficacy for learning disabilities, hyperactivity, adult psychosis, and convulsions consisting of large doses of niacin, niacinamide, ascorbic acid, pyridoxine, and calcium pantothenate or other vitamins either individually or in combination. Possibly effective in the treatment of childhood psychosis.

mental retardation: "Significantly subaverage general intellectual functioning existing concurrently with deficits in adaptive behavior, and manifested during the developmental period" (Grossman, 1973, p. 11). Classification according to the severity of symptoms (IQ score) is as follows: mild (55–69), moderate (40–54), severe (25–39), and profound (below 25). The terms *borderline, dull-normal* and *slow learning* are occasionally used to refer to children with IQ's from 70 to 89.

metabolism: the sum of the processes in the building up and maintenance of living substance and the production of energy for vital activities; the sum of the processes by which the body transforms a substance, e.g., drug.

metabolite: any substance produced by a metabolic process.

mg: milligram.

mg/kg: milligram per kilogram.

microgram: a unit of weight in the metric system being one one-millionth of a gram or one one-thousandth of a milligram.

microsomal enzymes: enzymes within the cells of the liver that participate in the metabolism of many drugs.

migraine: a condition marked by periodic attacks of severe headaches often associated with nausea and vomiting. The attacks are preceded by constriction of cranial arteries and begin with the dilation of the arteries.

milligram: a unit of weight in the metric system being one one-thousandth of a gram; equivalent to approximately one twenty-eight thousandth of an ounce.

milliliter: a metric unit of capacity being one one-thousandth of a liter.

minimal brain dysfunction: a syndrome found "in children of near average, average, or above average general intelligence" and characterized by "learning or behavioral disabilities ranging from mild to severe, which are associated with deviations of function of the central nervous system. These deviations may manifest themselves by various combinations of impairment in perception, conceptualization, language, memory, and control of attention, impulse, or motor function . . .'' (Clements, 1966, p. 9–10).

minor tranquilizer: a category of psychotropic drugs with sedative and antianxiety properties which includes the benzodiazepines, propanediol carbamates, and hydroxyzine.

mixed epilepsy: two or more different types of epilepsy manifest at the same time.

ml: milliliter.

monoamine oxidase inhibitor: a category of antidepressant drugs that includes tranylcypromine (Parnate) and phenelzine (Nardil).

motor cotrex: the area of the brain that controls discrete movements of the skeletal muscles.

muscle tone: a slight degree of muscle tension produced by continuous neural stimulation.

mutism: inability or refusal to speak.

myoclonic epilepsy: consists of several different types of epilepsy including myoclonic epilepsy of young children (infantile spasms, West syndrome) and myoclonic epilepsy of older children (Lennox-Gastaut syndrome, petit mal variant), both of which appear to be the same disorder but with different age at onset of seizures. Classification of the other types of myoclonic epilepsy is incomplete but includes children and adolescents with myoclonic seizures who do not manifest the symptoms associated with infantile spasms or the Lennox-Gastaut syndrome.

myoclonic epilepsy of older children: same as Lennox-Gastaut syndrome.

myoclonic epilepsy of young children: characterized by brief (several seconds) myoclonic seizures that usually occur in clusters lasting several minutes and abnormal interseizure EEG findings called hypsarhythmia. Onset of seizures is commonly between 3 and 9 months of age. Severe mental retardation is common. Also called infantile spasms, West syndrome.

myoclonic seizure: flexor spasm of the musculature; extensor spasms much less common.

narcolepsy: a condition characterized by an uncontrollable desire to sleep or periodic attacks of deep sleep.

neuroleptic: same as antipsychotic agent.

neuropharmacology: the branch of pharmacology that investigates the effects of drugs on the nervous system.

nocturnal: pertaining to night.

nonproprietary name: same as generic name.

nystagmus: a rapid involuntary movement of the eyeball either horizontally, vertically, or in a rotatory manner.

oculogyric crisis: fixed upward gaze; a symptom associated with acute dystonic reaction, an extrapyramidal syndrome produced by some antipsychotic drugs.

official name: same as generic name.

opiates: a group of drugs consisting of opium and its derivatives.

opisthotonos: a type of muscle spasm in which the back is arched, head and heels are bent backward, and the body bowed forward.

organic: pertaining to, or arising from, the organs; affecting the structure of an organism.

organic epilepsy: epilepsy that develops subsequent to permanent, nonprogressive damage to the brain, e.g., head trauma, brain infections.

orthopedic: pertainint to the correction of musculoskeletal deformities; marked by crippling.

orthostatic hypotension: weakness or fainting on rising to an erect position.

osteomalacia: a condition that results from vitamin D and calcium deficiency characterized by softening of the bones, pain, anorexia, and muscular weakness.

oxazolidinediones: a category of antiepileptic drugs that include trimethadione (Tridione) and paramethadione (Paradione).

panic anxiety: a psychiatric disorder characterized by recurrent and unexplained panic attacks with feelings of impending doom. The attacks may be associated with physical symptoms such as breathing difficulties or heart palpitations.

Parkinsonian syndrome: an extrapyramidal syndrome characterized by psychomotor slowing, masklike facial expression, shuffling gait without free swing of the arms, rigidity, and tremor. "Pill rolling" movements may also be present. An adverse reaction associated with antipsychotic drug therapy.

parenteral: administration by a route other than the digestive tract; any of several routes of injection including subcutaneous, intramuscular, and intravenous.

pathognomonic: characteristic of a disease; a sign or symptom that is used to make a diagnosis.

pathology: the study of the structural and functional changes in tissues and organs of the body that are caused by disease; deviations from the normal that characterize disease.

pediatric psychopharmacology: the branch of pharmacology that investigates the behavioral effects of drugs in children.

petit mal epilepsy: characterized by periodic attacks of altered consciousness usually lasting from 5 to 30 seconds. The seizure is manifest as a sudden cessation of movement and vacant staring into space. In some children the eyes roll back into the head. Seizures may be associated with brief clonic movements that usually recur at a frequency of 3 per second or automatisms. An EEG finding of 3 per second spike-wave forms is pathognomonic of petit mal epilepsy; absence epilepsy.

petit mal variant: same as Lennox-Gastaut syndrome.

pharmacology: the science that deals with the chemical properties, biochemical and physiological effects, absorption, distribution, biotransformation, excretion and therapeutic uses of drugs.

pharmacotherapy: the treatment of disease with medicines.

phenothiazines: a group of antipsychotic drugs which includes chlorpromazine (Thorazine) and thioridazine (Mellaril).

phobia: a persistent abnormal fear.

photophobia: abnormal intolerance to light.

photosensitivity: abnormal reaction of the skin to sunlight.

pigmentation: an abnormal increase of coloration by melanin.

pill rolling: as if rolling a pill between the fingers; a symptom of Parkinsonian syndrome.

placebo: an inactive medication administered to satisfy a patient's need for drug therapy; an inert substance used to control for expectancy effects in pharmacological research; a procedure with no intrinsic therapeutic value.

polypharmacy: the simultaneous administration of two or more drugs.

post seizure phenomena: disturbances following the active stages of a seizure including weakness, nausea, fatigue, muscle soreness, headache, irritability, confusion, and abnormal behavior.

post seizure sleep: period of deep sleep following a seizure.

prevalence: total number of cases in a specific area during a certain period of time.

prolonged seizure: an individual seizure lasting for an uncharacteristically long time.

propanediols: a group of antianxiety agents that includes meprobamate (Equanil, Miltown); propanediol carbamates.

prophylaxis: preventive treatment.

proteins: any one of a group of complex compounds consisting of a combination of amino acids; the principal constituents of all living cells.

psychic seizures: a type of psychomotor seizure manifest as changes in perception, thought, self awareness, mood, or affect.

psychomotor: relating to muscular actions resulting from conscious mental activity.

psychomotor epilepsy: characterized by periodic attacks of altered consciousness lasting from one to several minutes. Seizures may be manifest as a cessation of movement starting with or without automatisms or as changes in perception, thought, self awareness, mood, or affect. EEG findings usually show interseizure temporal lobe abnormalities. Also called temporal lobe epilepsy or complex partial seizure disorders.

psychomotor slowing: manifest as an inability to respond spontaneously at a normal speed, weak voice and labored speech, deliberate body movements, fixed facial expression, and a slowed, dragging walk.

psychopathology: mental disorders; the study of such dysfunctions.

psychopharmacology: the branch of pharmacology that investigates the effects of drugs on behavior.

psychosis: a general term for any severe mental disorder involving a loss of contact with reality and usually associated with delusions, hallucinations, or illusions.

psychotropic drug: any agent that has its principal effect on mood, thought processes, or behavior; behavior modifying drug.

rebound effect: reaction to the withdrawal of medication that may be manifested as an aggravation of the symptoms of the disorder being treated.

refractory: unresponsive to treatment.

relapse: a return of a disease after it apparently ceased.

remission: the lessening or cessation of the symptoms of a disease.

rickets: a condition that results from vitamin D deficiency characterized by bending or distortion of the bones.

salicylates: a group of drugs with analgesic, fever reducing, and anti-inflammatory properties, e.g., aspirin.

schizophrenia: a psychotic disorder characterized by emotional distortion, ambivalence, disturbances of thought, retreat from reality, delusions, hallucinations, and withdrawn or bizarre behavior.

secondary epilepsy: same as organic epilepsy.

sedative: a category of psychotropic drugs that reduce excitement and having a calming effect.

seizure: a sudden attack; fit. **Epileptic seizure:** a loss or alteration of consciousness associated with involuntary muscle movement (or cessation of movement) and abnormal electrical discharges in the brain; convulsion, spell, fit.

self limiting: limited by its own nature and not by outside influences. Self limiting side effects run a limited course and terminate on their own.

separation anxiety: apprehension resulting from loss of contact with significant persons or familiar surroundings; common in infants 6 to 10 months old.

serial grand mal (major motor) seizures: characterized by recurrent grand mal seizures during which the person regains consciousness between attacks; frequently associated with the abrupt withdrawal of antiepileptic medication.

side effect: a consequence other than that for which an agent or treatment is being used; adverse reaction, toxic effects, untoward reaction.

simple febrile seizure: a benign, nonepileptic disorder characterized by brief generalized seizures that occur usually 2 to 6 hours after the onset of a fever. The disorder rarely lasts beyond 6 years of age.

spasm: a sudden and involuntary muscle contraction.

spasticity: increase over normal muscle tone; hypertonicity.

sphincter: a muscle that forms a ring around a body opening, e.g., urethra, and prevents passage via constriction.

spontaneous: occuring without external influence; voluntary.

status epilepticus: a series of seizures in succession during which the person does not regain consciousness between attacks; usually refers to grand mal status.

status seizure: a series of recurring seizures during which the patient does not regain consciousness between seizures.

stereotypic behavior: repetitive and often bizarre motor movements such as rhythmic rocking, head weaving, hand or arm flapping, and rubbing parts of the body; stereotypies.

stereotypies: same as stereotypic behavior.

stimulant: a category of psychotropic drugs that includes methylphenidate (Ritalin), dextroamphetamine (Dexedrine) and pemoline (Cylert).

subcutaneous: beneath the skin.

succinimides: a category of antiepileptic drugs particularly effective in the treatment of petit mal epilepsy that includes ethosuximide (Zarontin), methsuximide (Celontin), and phensuximide (Milontin).

symptomatic epilepsy: seizures are one of the symptoms of a specific disorder that involves the brain, e.g., cerebral degenerative disease.

syndrome: a set of symptoms that occur together and characterize a specific disorder.

tardive dyskinesia: a late appearing extrapyramidal syndrome characterized by involuntary, repetitive movements usually in the region of the mouth but may involve the limbs and trunk as well. Movements include tongue protrusion, licking or smacking of the lips, side to side movements of the chin, blowing of the cheeks, facial grimacing, and eye blinking. A side effect of long term antipsychotic drug treatment.

temporal lobe epilepsy: same as psychomotor epilepsy.

thiozanthenes: a category of antipsychotic agents that includes prothixene (Taractan) and thiothixene (Navane).

teratogen: a substance that causes physical defects in the developing embryo.

tic: spasmodic movement of a muscle; a twitching movement especially of a facial muscle.

titration: a method for determining the strength of a solution or the concentration of a substance in solution; used metaphorically to describe a procedure for adjusting the dose of a drug. The initial dose, usually too small to produce a therapeutic response, is gradually increased over time until the desired effect is achieved or unacceptable adverse reactions appear.

TMR: trainable mentally retarded.

tolerance: a lessened susceptibility to the effects of the same dose of a drug over repeated administrations.

tonic: characterized by continuous tension. The tonic phase of a grand mal seizure is marked by boardlike rigidity.

torticollis: characterized by contracted cervical muscles resulting in a twisting of the neck and unnatural positioning of the head. A symptom of an acute dystonic reaction, an extrapyramidal syndrome associated with antipsychotic drugs.

toxic: poisonous; causing disturbance of body function or structural damage to organs and tissues.

toxic reaction: same as side effect.

trade name: a brand name protected by trademark laws which restrict use to the original copyright holder indefinitely; proprietary name, unofficial name. The trade name of a drug refers to a particular formulation of a generic drug made by a specific manufacturer.

trainable mentally retarded: an educational classification for children whose IQ's range from 25 or 35 to 50 or 55.

trauma: a wound or injury.

tremor: an involuntary trembling or shaking.

tricyclics: a category of antidepressant drugs that includes imipramine (Tofranil), amitriptyline (Elavil), and nortriptyline (Aventyl).

unilateral: affecting but one side.

untoward reaction: same as side effect.

urticaria: a skin reaction marked by patches of skin either redder or paler than the surrounding skin, usually associated with severe itching, and often caused by emotional stress or certain foods, drugs, or infections; hives.

vitamin D: a substance that greatly accelerates the absorption of calcium from the gut.

water soluble: capable of being dissolved in water.

withdrawal syndrome: characteristic symptoms associated with the withdrawal of a specific drug.

REFERENCES

Dorland's Illustrated Medical Dictionary (25th ed.). Philadelphia: Saunders, 1974.

Author Index

C

G

H

T

Subject Index

U

V

W